Praise for *Yoga for Transformation*

"In *Yoga for Transformation,* Gary Kraftsow writes elegantly about Yoga, a subject he knows well and loves. He expands our awareness from the narrow view of Yoga as 'posture' to the broader and deeper understanding of Yoga as a whole system of health and self-awareness. I especially like the section on breathing."
—Judith Hanson Lasater, Ph.D, physical therapist, Yoga teacher, and author of *Living Your Yoga* and *Relax and Renew*

"Viniyoga is a hightly intelligent approach to Yoga, and Gary Kraftsow is a very skillful communicator of this integrated approach. *Yoga for Transformation* is superb."
—Georg Furstein, founder-president of Yoga Research and Education Center and author of *The Shambhala Encyclopedia of Yoga*

"Comtemporary yogis are really just beginning the task of translating and interpreting the treasure-trove of teachings that lie buried in the Yoga traditions. We should all be enormously grateful for Gary Kraftsow's clear-headed and practical approach to this task. *Yoga for Transformation* will certainly become an essential text for those of us willing to travel to the heart of this practical science of liberation."
—Stephen Cope, senior scholar in residence, Kripalu Center for Yoga and Health, author of *Yoga and the Quest for the True Self*

"Addressing the heart in its physical, emotional, and spiritual aspects, Gary provides a detailed and comprehensive approach to the practice of Yoga, giving practitioners a variety of tools to help reach their highest potential."
—Dean Ornish, M.D.

"As Yoga has become increasingly popular in America as a form of exercise and stress management, many Americans are now eager to explore its potential for spiritual growth and personal healing. Gary Kraftsow's *Yoga for Transformation* fulfills this need. Whether you are a beginner or a seasoned veteran of Yoga, this book will be a valuable aid in your practice."
—Larry Dossey, author of *Healing Beyond the Body* and *Healing Words*

Praise for *Yoga for Wellness*

"Gary Kraftsow . . . will inspire every Yoga enthusiast. I admire his ability to transmit ancient wisdom in the modern context."
—T. K. V. Desikacher

"Gary Kraftsow is one of America's leading sources on Yoga therapy. He represents the best of the generation of people who went to India in the seventies to learn Yoga. Because of his mature understanding and experience, *Yoga for Wellness* is a treasure. It should be included on every Yoga practitioner's bookshelf."
—Swami Chetanananda, Abbot, Nityananda Institute,
and author of *Choose to Be Happy*

"*Yoga for Wellness* is a timely, splendid, and indespensible contribution to sound Hatha Yoga practice and to the burgeoning field of Yoga therapy."
—Georg Furstein, Ph.D., President of The Yoga Research
and Education Center and author of *The Yoga Tradition*

"Gary has done a great service to the Yoga world by putting his understanding of Viniyoga on paper. There is so much valuable information within these pages. Read it and learn!"
—Erich Schiffmann,
author of *Yoga: The Spirit and Practice of Moving into Stillness*

"A profound and detailed guide to Yoga therapy and Yoga for healing. It contains one of the most sophisticated presentation of *āsana-s* in print, showing how to adapt the Yoga poses to special individual health and energy requirements."
—David Frawley,
author of *Yoga and Ayurveda* and *Ayurveda and the Mind*

"I highly recommend this fascinating, practical guide to the ancient art of Yoga."
—Mitchell L. Gaynor, M.D., Director of the Strang
Cancer Prevention Center and author of *Sounds of Healing*

ABOUT THE AUTHOR

GARY KRAFTSOW'S interest in the spiritual dimension of life was awakened at a very young age. His connection to Yoga and the spiritual traditions of India was strengthened through his studies at Colgate University, where he graduated with honors. At the age of nineteen, he traveled to Madras to meet T. K. V. Desikachar and T. Krishnamacharya, initiating a link to Viniyoga that has become his lifelong dedication.

Gary has taught Yoga and has practiced Yoga therapy since 1976. In 1983 he completed a master's program in psychology and religion at the University of California, Santa Barbara, focusing his study on health as a paradigm for spiritual transformation. In 1988 Gary received the Viniyoga Special Diploma, recognizing his ability to train teachers and therapists in this lineage.

Gary's twenty-eight-year relationship with this teaching lineage, and his deep knowledge of and respect for its precious roots, are the foundation for his unique ability to translate and communicate Yoga in a modern Western context as an educator, consultant, and therapist. Gary founded the American Viniyoga Institute, through which he offers in-depth training programs for teachers and therapists, as well as retreats and seminars in all aspects of Yoga. His first book, *Yoga for Wellness: Healing with the Timeless Teachings of Viniyoga,* continues to be discovered and appreciated by Yoga students and teachers, health professionals, and researchers from around the world.

Yoga for Transformation

Ancient Teachings and Holistic Practices for Healing Body, Mind, and Heart

Gary Kraftsow

Penguin Compass
New York
2002

PENGUIN COMPASS
Published by the Penguin Group
Penguin Putnam Inc., 375 Hudson Street,
New York, New York 10014, U.S.A.
Penguin Books Ltd, 80 Strand,
London WC2R 0RL, England
Penguin Books Australia Ltd, 250 Camberwell Road, Camberwell,
Victoria 3124, Australia
Penguin Books Canada Ltd, 10 Alcorn Avenue,
Toronto, Ontario, Canada M4V 3B2
Penguin Books India (P) Ltd, 11 Community Centre, Panchsheel Park,
New Delhi – 110 017, India
Penguin Books (N.Z.) Ltd., Cnr Rosedale and Airborne Roads, Albany,
Auckland, New Zealand
Penguin Books (South Africa) (Pty) Ltd, 24 Sturdee Avenue,
Rosebank, Johannesburg 2196, South Africa

Penguin Books Ltd, Registered Offices:
Harmondsworth, Middlesex, England

First published in Penguin Compass 2002
1 3 5 7 9 10 8 6 4 2

A NOTE TO THE READER

The information in this book is not intended as a substitute for the advice of physicians or other qualified health professionals. It is not intended to be prescriptive with reference to any specific ailment or condition or to the general health of the reader, but, rather, descriptive of one approach to fostering health and wellness. The reader is advised to consult with his or her physician before undertaking any of the practices contained in this book. The reader should also continue to consult regularly with his or her physician in matters relating to his or her health, particularly in respect to any symptoms that may require diagnosis or medical treatment. Neither the author nor the publisher shall be liable or responsible for any loss, injury, or damage allegedly arising from the use of any information contained in this book.

LIBRARY OF CONGRESS CATALOGING IN PUBLICATION DATA

Kraftsow, Gary.
Yoga for transformation : ancient teaachings and practices
for healing body, mind, and heart / by Gary Kraftsow.
p. cm.
Includes index.
ISBN 0-14-019629-3 (pbk.)
1. Yoga, Haòha. 2. Yoga—Health aspects. I. Title

RA781.7 .K677 2002
613.7'046—dc21 2002016971

Printed in the United States of America
Set in A Garamond
Designed by M. Paul

A NOTE TO THE READER

The information in this book is not intended as a substitute for the advice of physicians or other qualified health professionals. It is not intended to be prescriptive with reference to any specific ailment or condition or to the general health of the reader, but, rather, descriptive of one approach to fostering health and wellness. The reader is advised to consult with his or her physician before undertaking any of the practices contained in this book. The reader should also continue to consult regularly with his or her physician in matters relating to his or her health, particularly in respect to any symptoms that may require diagnosis or medical treatment. Neither the author nor the publisher shall be liable or responsible for any loss, injury, or damage allegedly arising from the use of any information contained in this book.

For Mirka

In Memory of

the Venerable Lama Tenzin

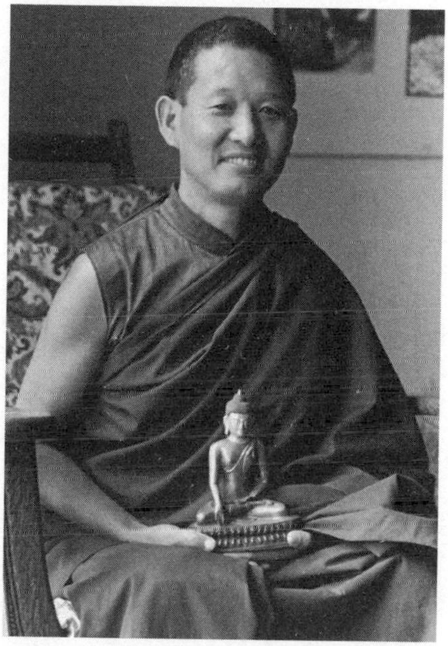

Our good and true personal and spiritual friend

"When I first met Gary in 1974 in Chennai, India, he was nineteen years old and a student at Colgate University. Gary took *āsana* lessons as part of the India study program at the University. Somehow, his relation with me clicked, and in spite of the many options he had—he was a very good student at Colgate—he chose to study Yoga and decided to become a Yoga teacher at a time when Yoga was hardly recognized in the West. We have met every year since then. He went through many obstacles, and the way he evolved step by step to become a good Yoga teacher is, for me, a testament to his conviction in the strength and value of Yoga. I am proud to be his friend."

—T. K. V. Desikachar

FOREWORD

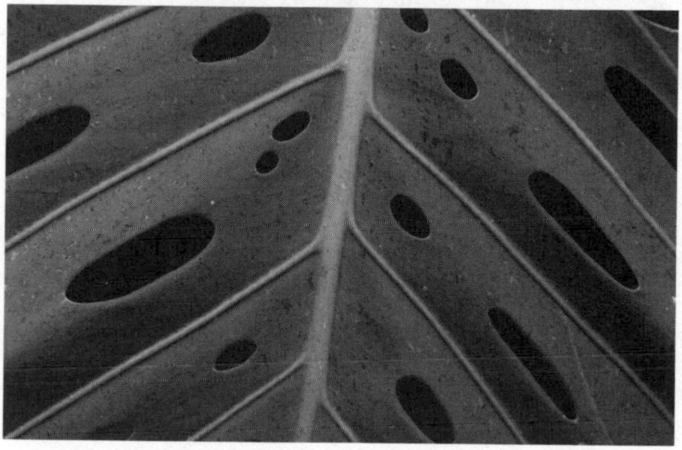

PERSONAL TRANSFORMATION has always been Yoga's prime directive. True to its etymological roots (the word *yoga* comes from a Sanskrit root meaning "to join"), Yoga seeks to join the several parts of an individual's life into a coherent whole. Whether we describe Yoga as "restraint of the fluctuations of the mind," as Patanjali did, or use Krishna's definition of "excellence in action," or take some other tack, any Yoga worthy of the name aims to optimize the relationship that people create with the world around them.

Thus far, Yoga has naturalized itself in the West chiefly as a system for arranging the body in particular poses, or *āsana-s*. While *āsana* practice is an important ingredient in many Yoga routines, particularly those that have emerged from the Yoga Sutra of Patanjali, too many Westerners are now convinced that Yoga consists of nothing but postures. Having peeled the fruit of Yoga, as it were, they have made a meal of its skin alone, unaware of the juicier flesh beneath it.

Until recently, the philosophical climate of the West found all of India's traditions substantially alien, but in the past few decades alternative perspectives have spread widely enough to permit Yoga and its sister sciences like *Ayurveda* (medicine) and *Jyotisha* (astrology) to transplant themselves into Western soil. The moment has now arrived for initial awareness of "Yoga as *āsana*" to burgeon into awareness of Yoga as a highly textured living tradition that has more to offer us than mere good posture.

Yoga however requires careful translation if its natal Indian idiom is to flower into a narrative that Westerners can clearly comprehend, for its theory can be abstruse, and its more refined practices mystifying. *Yoga for Transformation* is a fine example of how a work in English can coherently portray Yoga's breadth and depth, holding fast to the facts without sacrificing readability.

I have known Gary Kraftsow for some years now, and have found him a sincere and dedicated student of the totality of his Yoga tradition. In *Yoga for Transformation* he provides his readers the meat of Yoga's message in a form that any serious student should be able to digest. Beginning from the judicious premise that "the choice to orient one's practice in any direction is largely a function of one's own interests," he shows how the system of Yoga tailors itself to each individual who approaches it, according to age, ability, and aspiration. Know your goals in life, and you will find it easier to adapt your Yoga practice to fit them.

Far from limiting his canvas to the physical body (a failing of many popular books on Yoga), Gary clearly elucidates the significance of the Five *Koshas,* or Sheaths, that make up a human, in particular the Sheaths of Prāna and of Mind. The importance of *prāṇa* (the life force) to Yoga cannot be overstated, and Gary makes plain the nature of the relationships that link body, *prāṇa*, and mind.

Despite his commitment to portraying Yoga in the splendor of its wholeness, he in no way neglects *āsana*. Acclaimed as he is in Yoga circles for his ability to sequence *āsana-s,* he effectively directs his sequences to illustrate his assertions, cooking a Yoga repast that goes down easy, digests agreeably, and leaves its consumers well fed but hungry for more.

Yoga for Transformation is a book to assimilate and act upon. Sample its treats, and try out its principles in your own life. Adopt those practices that agree with your body and mind, and experience the results for yourself. Adapt your Yoga practice according to these guidelines, and some of that vigor and lightheartedness that you enjoyed as a child will begin again to flow into your life. Open yourself to transformation, and you will be transformed.

Robert E. Svoboda, Ayurvedacharya
TORONTO, OCTOBER 2001

PREFACE

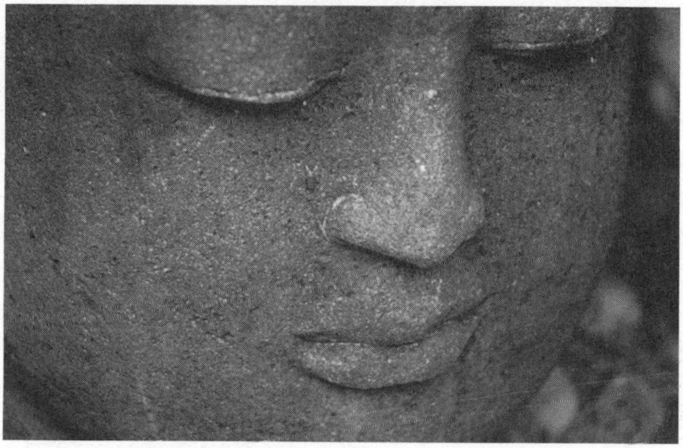

YOGA IS GOING MAINSTREAM. Yoga schools are appearing everywhere, and this is a good sign. But while a lot of new, modern Yoga styles are becoming popular, what is referred to as Yoga is often a synthesis of Western psychotherapy, various types of physiotherapy, and some *āsana* practice.

Perhaps integrating other modalities into Yoga is an important and useful development. The Yoga tradition is a living tradition, after all, and I applaud any and every attempt to help people improve the quality of their lives at any level. But, because most of these modern styles don't reflect the profound depth of that tradition, the deeper, inner teachings are not reaching a lot of Western students. The tradition is at risk of being lost with the rise of its popularity. The Yoga Sūtra of Patañjali, for example, which is perhaps the primary authoritative source of Yoga teachings, and which offers so much valuable insight and practical relevance for all of us in our day-to-day living, is known to the vast majority of Yoga teachers in the Western world only by name, if at all.

With this book, I would like to show the relevance of these ancient teachings to you, the modern student, while, at the same time, preserving the uniqueness of this beautiful tradition. To this end, I will try to lead you to an understanding not only of the development of the body but also of the mind, heart, and spirit.

Although people today turn to Yoga for different reasons, the underlying motivation for many is the hope that, through Yoga practice, they can transform recurring, troubling emotions and find greater meaning in life, even lasting peace. This is the promise of the Yoga tradition and, by following it, the potential to realize these goals is actually quite high.

Whether the journey is long or short will depend entirely on you, and on your own personal motivation. If you are mildly interested in this transformation, but, practically speaking, have too many other concerns to give it your full attention, the journey will indeed be long. If, on the other hand, you are ready to look deeply within and to abandon the many superficial distractions that usually occupy the mind, you can make great and rapid progress.

Finally, in presenting a deeper and broader view of what the Yoga tradition has to offer than is generally available, I am not interested in turning you into a Hindu or in teaching you how to imitate the ancient *yogī-s* in anything but what is most essential, which is that you become more deeply who *you* essentially are. For that is what it really means to study the ancient teachings, to take them to heart, and to make them part of your life.

ACKNOWLEDGMENTS

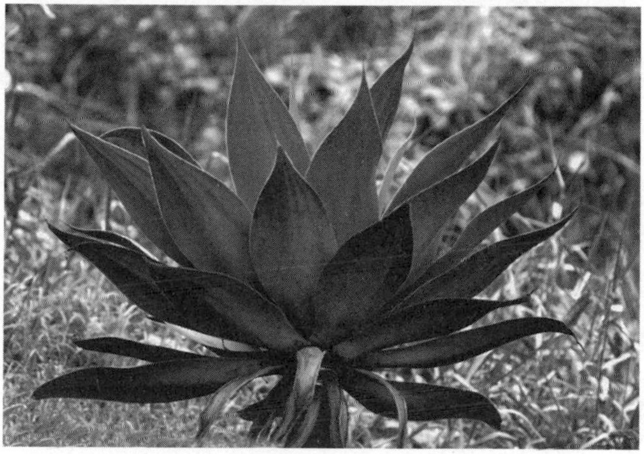

I WANT TO THANK MY YOGA TEACHER, SRI T. K. V. DESIKACHAR, and his teacher, Sri T. Krishnamacharya, for all that I have received, and continue to receive, from this lineage which has so fundamentally influenced my life.

I am grateful to my wife, Mirka, and our son, Matteo, for their love and support throughout the process of writing this book; and for the gift of family life that has furthered my understanding of the dynamics of relationship, and thus deepened my appreciation of these teachings.

I want to thank Barry Kaplan for his photography, Linda Getz for her illustrations, and Dr. Robert E. Svoboda for writing the Foreword to this book.

I also want to thank all of the models, most of whom are students and teachers of Viniyoga: Joshua Berman, Rachel Berman, Carlo Bressan, Laura Dotson, Gloria Kraftsow (my mother), Matteo Kraftsow, Mirka Kraftsow, Ted Kraftsow (my father), Sara Mata, Sasha Malek, and Juris Zinbergs.

I am grateful to my literary agent, Ling Lucas, for continuing to support me in my writing; to Mary Lou Mellinger, who continues to donate countless hours to help me with my work; to Pat Sheldon for her extensive editorial assistance on the first draft of the manuscript; to David Hurwitz for his comments in the early stages of writing this book; and to Steven Berger for generously sharing his insight into the Orthodox Christian tradition.

I also want to thank my editor at Penguin, Sarah Manges, for her detailed editorial assistance and her generous availability by phone during the completion of the final draft of the manuscript; Janet Goldstein for her support throughout the project; and the rest of the Penguin team, including Manuela Paul for the elegant design.

Finally, I want to thank Father Raimundo Panikkar, a great man with whom I had the good fortune to study, for his wisdom and inspiration.

About the Practices in This Book

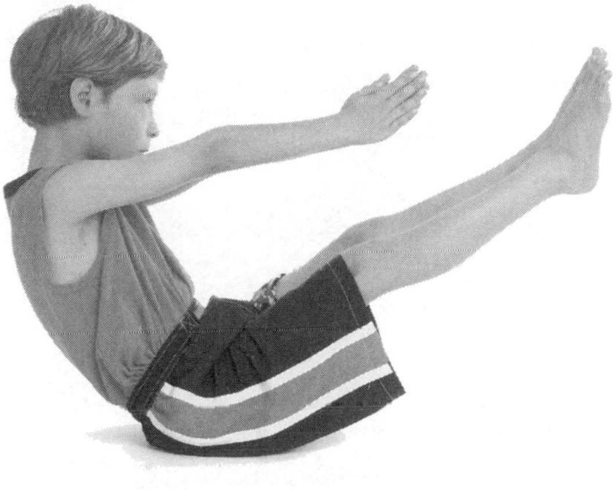

THIS BOOK IS INTENDED TO HELP you explore the full scope of Yoga practice including, but extending beyond, the practice of *āsana*. For this reason, I have intentionally selected certain key postures that appear repeatedly throughout the practices offered in this book. These postures represent a core of fundamental movements that will be relevant for almost every practitioner's daily practice. My intention is to show how the transformational potential of practice is furthered by progressively adding other elements—such as *prāṇāyāma,* chanting, meditation, prayer, and ritual—to the same or similar core postures, without having to master progressively more complex or difficult postures.

These practices are intended to be examples that demonstrate how Yoga can be adapted to refine and integrate the different dimensions of our system. They are not prescriptive for any individual, nor are they a substitute for a qualified teacher. Please read the information given in each chapter, and then feel free to experiment with these practices carefully, respecting any specific cautions given in the text. If at any time you feel excessive fatigue, strain, dizziness, or shortness of breath, please stop and rest in a comfortable position for some time before you go on. Remember that the purpose of these practices is to serve you in deepening your self-understanding, and to assist you in the process of self-transformation.

For a more extensive study of *āsana,* please see my previous book, *Yoga for Wellness,* published by Penguin in 1999.

Table of Contents

Foreword xv
Preface xvii
Acknowledgments xix
About the Practices in This Book xxi

Part I: The Ancient Foundation 1

Chapter 1: The Multidimensional Self 3
The Five Dimensions of the Human System 4
The First Dimension: The Physical Body 4
The Second Dimension: The Vital Body 5
The Third Dimension: The Intellectual Mind 6
The Fourth Dimension: The Personality 7
The Final Dimension: The Heart 9
The Ideal Condition of the Human System: An Integrated Whole 10
The Four Basic Aims in Life:
Dharma 11
Artha 12
Kāma 12
Mokṣa 12
The Integration Process: From *Rogī* to *Bhogī* to *Yogī* 13
The Imperfect Vessel 14
The Upside-Down Vessel 14
The Dirty Vessel 15
The Leaky Vessel 15
The Tilted Vessel 15

Chapter 2: *Kriyā Yoga*: Transformation Through Practice 17
Kriyā Yoga: A Threefold Approach to Practice 19
Tapas: The Purifying Heat 19
Svādhyāya: The Reflecting Mirror 22
Īśvara Praṇidhāna: The Refuge 27

Chapter 3: The *Viniyoga* of Yoga: The Art of Appropriate Application 31
Models and Related Approaches to Practice 32
The Age Model 32
The Orientation Model 36
The Developmental Approach to Practice 36
The Preventative Approach to Practice 38
The Therapeutic Approach to Practice 39
The Transcendental Approach to Practice 41

Part II: The Art of Personal Practice 43

Chapter 4: Nourishing the Physical (The *Annamaya* Level) 45
Becoming Aware of Our Bodies 45
Awareness of the Skeletal Structure 46
Awareness Exercises 47
Noticing the Alignment of Our Spine 54
Noticing the Condition of Our Joints 55
Awareness of the Muscular Structure 57
Awareness of Neuromuscular Patterning 58
Exploring *Āsana* in Personal Practice 59
Which *Āsana* to Pick 59
How to Do Postures 63
How to Adapt Postures 64
How to Breathe in Postures 66
How to Combine Postures 66
The Deeper Symbolism of *Āsana* 68
Annamaya Practice 69

Chapter 5: Energizing the Vital (The *Prāṇamaya* Level) 89
Prāṇāyamā and Personal Practice 89

The Five Aspects of the Vital Body:
Prāṇa, Apāna, Vyāna, Udāna, Samāna 90
Exploring the Breath 90
Exploring Your Inhale and Exhale 91
How to Inhale and Exhale 92
Five Types of Inhalation 92
Three Types of Exhalation 94
Prāṇamaya Practice 97
Exploring Ratio 113
Understanding Ratio 113
Developing Ratio 115
The Classic *Samavṛtti* Ratio 115
Viṣamavṛtti Ratios 116
Vinyāsa in *Prāṇāyāmā:*
Progressive Steps in Building a Ratio During Practice 117
Finding Our Threshold 118
Classic *Prāṇāyāma* Techniques 119
Ujjāyī 120
Anuloma Ujjāyī 121
Viloma Ujjāyī 121
Pratiloma Ujjāyī 121
Candrabhedana 122
Sūryabhedana 122
Nāḍī Śodhana 122
Śītalī 123
Sītkārī 124
Kapālabhāti 124
Bhastrikā 124
The Deeper Symbolism of *Prāṇāyamā* 125
Idā 125
Pingalā 125
Suṣumnā 126
The Classic *Bandha-s* 126
The Deeper Symbolism of *Bandha-s* 127

The *Bandha* Techniques 128
Jāladhara Bandha 128
Uddīyāna Bandha 128
Mūla Bandha 130
The Classical Theory of Practice 130
The Basic Paradigm 131
The Relationship Between Ratio and Technique 132
Application 132
Prāṇamaya Practice 134

Chapter 6: Educating the Intellect: The *Manomaya* Level 150
The Role of the Intellect 150
The Breakdown of Traditional Cultures 152
Training the Mind Through Chant 153
Learning to Listen 154
The Energetics of Sound 154
Transmitting Information Through Chant 155
The Symbolism of Sound 155
The *Cakra* Model 156
The Symbolism of Wheels and Lotuses 156
The Seven Major *Cakra-s* 157
Foundation: *Mūlādhāra* 158
Creation: *Svādhiṣṭhana* 158
Transformation: *Maṇipūraka* 159
Relation: *Ānāhata* 160
Communication: *Viśuddhi* 160
Evaluation: *Àjña* 161
Inspiration: *Sahasrāra* 162
Manomaya Practice 164

Chapter 7: Refining the Personality: The *Vijñānamaya* Level 184
The Nature of Personality 184
The Function of Meditation 185
One-Pointed and Self-Reflective Meditation 186
Initial Goals of Meditation Practice 187
Basic Steps in the Meditation Process 188
The First Step: *Dhāraṇā* 188

The Second Step: *Dhyānam* 188
The Third Step: *Samādhi* 189
Vijñānamaya Practice 191

Chapter 8: Fulfilling the Heart: The *Ānadamaya* Level 215
The Ultimate Goal of Our Practice 216
Developing *Ānanda* Through Relationship 216
Developing Relationship Through Ritual 217
Ritual and the Fulfillment of Our Highest Potential 217
The Ingredients of Personal Ritual 218
Taking Root in the Heart 218
The Natural Progression Toward Deeper Meaning 219
The Elements of Communal Worship 219
The First Step: Turning Within to the Source 219
The Second Step: Confessing Our Faith or Taking Refuge 220
The Third Step: Joyous Expression of Praise 221
The Fourth Step: Petitionary Prayer 221
The Fifth Step: Communion 222
The Sixth Step: Return to Ordinary Life and Thanksgiving 222
The Seventh Step: Expression of Commitment 222
The Eighth Step: Dedication of Merit 222
The Science of Personal Ritual 223
Preparation *(pūrvaṅga)* 223
Establishing Intention *(bhāvana)* 224
Using Symbol to Direct Our Attention 224
Using *Mantra* to Direct Our Attention 225
Meditative Absorption 226
Petition 226
Proclamation *(saṅkalpa)* 227
Gesture *(nyāsa)* 227
Dedication *(mangala)* 228
Ānandamaya Practice 231
Pronunciation Guide 247
Āsana and *Prāṇāyāma* Glossary 249
Index 251
Contact Information 259

PART I

The Ancient Foundation

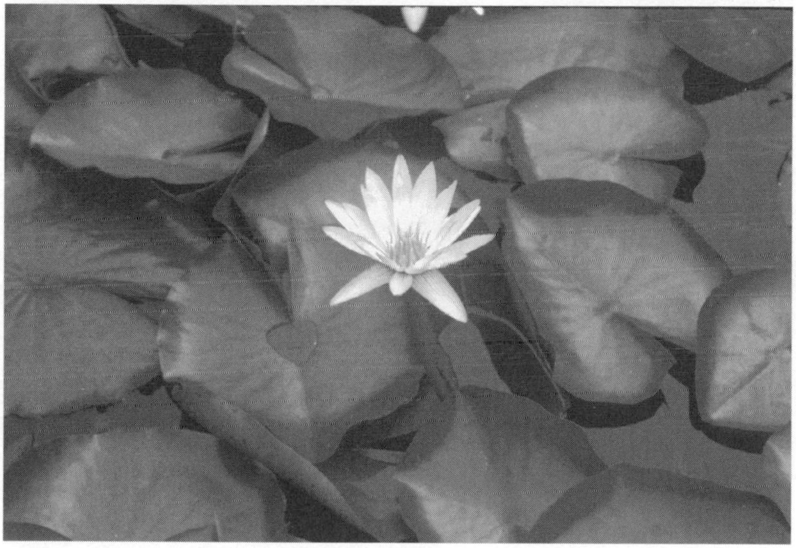

Chapter One

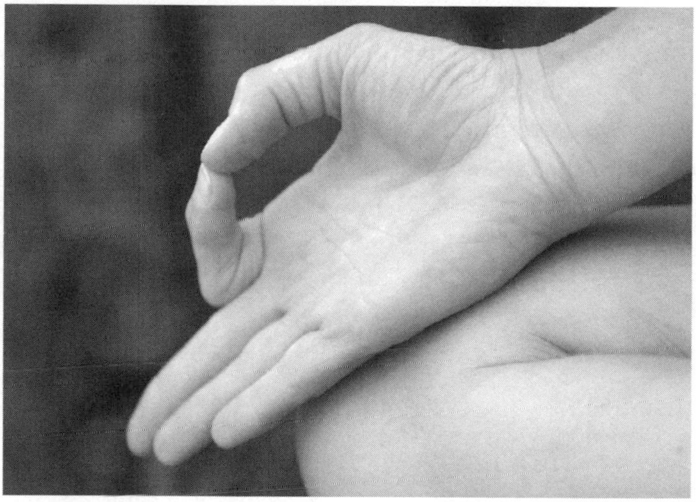

The Multidimensional Self

We are multidimensional beings. Therefore, holistic health practices, holistic therapies, and holistic *sādhana-s* or Yoga practices must also be multidimensional.

In the chapters that follow, we will explore multidimensional teachings about the human system based on an ancient model, found in the *Taittirīya Upaniṣad,* that have been transmitted by word of mouth from teacher to student over thousands of years.

Originally, these teachings came from the most authoritative scriptures of India, known as the *Veda-s.* Because the *Vedic* texts were considered to be revelatory, or *śruti,* they had to be passed on without any mistakes. They were first transmitted by great seers of the time, or *Ṛṣi-s,* who passed them on in the form of chants. The mode of transmission was through the oral instruction of the teachers, whose commentaries were added to the gradually expanding body of oral tradition. Both the original texts and these commentaries were passed on through students, who strove to realize their meaning and to actualize that meaning in their lives through the holistic art and science of personal practice, or *sādhana.* And thus these texts and commentaries have been preserved to our time through the reverence and devotion of countless people who have dedicated their lives to learning, understanding, and transmitting them.

The aim of this book is to explore the full extent to which the ideas and practices of the Yoga tradition can be applied and used as tools of integration and transformation in our own lives. In keeping with this aim, Part I, "The Ancient Foundation," will provide a brief explanation of certain basic philosophical tenets of the Yoga tradition, including the five recognized dimensions of the human system: the physical body, vitality, intellect, personality, and heart. Within the context of these five dimensions, Part II, "The Art of Personal Practice," will explore the practices through which each of these dimensions can be refined, applied, and integrated into the whole.

THE FIVE DIMENSIONS OF THE HUMAN SYSTEM

The First Dimension: The Physical Body

According to the ancients, the physical body consists of five aspects: the head, the torso, the two arms, and the two legs—and the related practice of *āsana*.

Our tendency today is to think of physical fitness and health in terms of measurements (the percentage of muscle to body fat or the target pulse rate, for example) and/or standards of performance (the ability to run a marathon or to bench-press our body weight). Bringing this mentality to *āsana* practice, many have the impression that it is about performance and that we can measure our progress by our ability to perfect the forms of the postures.

The ancients, however, based their concept of physical fitness and health on an entirely different set of criteria: a feeling of lightness in the body (*aṅgalaghavam*); an ability to withstand change (*dvaṅdvānabhighātaḥ*); and a stable body and focused mind, ready to sit for *prāṇāyāma* practice, in which the ancient science of the breath is applied.

They recognized that, from the moment of conception, all aspects of the physical body must be nourished. They understood that the needs of our bodies change from infancy through childhood, from adolescence into adulthood, and again from the child-bearing into the senior years. On the basis of this recognition and understanding, they developed the science of *āsana* practice (*āsanābhyāsaḥ*) as a way of promoting the balanced growth of the body and the maintenance of that balance into old age. And just as our bodies change through time, the ancients suggested that the purpose and methods of *āsana* practice must also change. In other words, traditionally, the practice of *āsana* was always considered as an integral part of a holistic practice, never as an isolated fitness system. And, in accordance with this understanding, one of the goals of this book will be to demonstrate how *āsana* practice can be adapted to serve the other dimensions of practice, such as *prāṇāyāma* and meditation.

The Second Dimension: The Vital Body

According to the ancients, the vital body consists of five identifiable aspects: *prāṇa*, *apāna*, *vyāna*, *ākāśa*, and *pṛthivī*.* All five of these aspects represent some manifestation of energy, and, although not equivalent, all may be understood in relation to the vital metabolic functions of the physical body.

Today we tend to think of health and vitality in terms of standards of measurement—the ratio of LDL to HDL in our blood serum cholesterol, the level of our PSA, the strength of our bones, for example. These measurements require professional medical tests. At best, most of us have a physical once a year, and many of us avoid doctors altogether.

According to the ancients, however, from the moment of our birth it is *prāṇa* that organizes, activates, and animates our physical bodies. By paying close attention to certain characteristics that reflect the balanced flow of *prāṇa* through our physical bodies, we can have a relatively accurate picture of our own health and vitality on a daily basis. These characteristics include how we fall asleep; the quality of our sleep, dreams, and morning energy; the nature of our digestion and bowel movements; and the regularity of our menstrual cycles, to name only a few examples. We can gain an even deeper understanding based on the quality of our respiratory rhythms, once we understand and can apply the science of the breath, called *prāṇāyāma*.

*I refer the reader to the *Taittirīya Upaniṣad,* Chapter II, section 2, verse 1.

As with *āsana* practice, the ancients also suggested that the purpose and methods of *prāṇāyāma* practice should complement each other and that they should change as we grow. Thus, another goal of this book is to show how, by becoming familiar with our threshold capacity for inhale and exhale, we can better assess our own physiological and emotional stress levels as a basis for improving the general quality of our lives.

The Third Dimension: The Intellectual Mind

The ancients recognized the inherent power of the mind and the tremendous influence that it has over the entire human system. They knew that it is through the mind that we are able to perceive, understand, and choose. They also knew that part of our problem in life is the fact that we do not perceive, understand, or choose correctly and that part of this is due to the nature of the mind itself. Thus they stressed the importance of educating and developing the mind in terms of its full capacity to learn, acquire knowledge, remember, and imagine.

As the basis for this education and development, the ancients identified the four great *Vedic* scriptures and the oral instruction of the teachers as the primary source and the teacher-student relationship as the primary mode. And, as pointed out above, both the texts of the scriptures and the commentaries of the teachers were traditionally transmitted through chanting. In other words, the method was to learn "by heart," that is, to memorize the texts and to be able to repeat them exactly.

In our modern secular world, certain subjects are a required part of all elementary and secondary education, and beyond that, education proceeds by choice and in accordance with our individual interests. In ancient times, while some *Vedic* teachings were given to all students, others were given according to family tradition, so that even the traditional models lack uniformity. Yet two things remained constant: in order to preserve these sacred texts without corruption through time, precise and detailed rules for chanting were always followed; and chanting itself was used as the primary tool for training and developing the mind. For example, the exacting process of repeating the chants without mistakes developed the students' ability to **listen**. Listening required and developed their ability to **direct and maintain attention**. And it also required the mind to remain **open to receive instruction**.

Of course, it is ever true that what we are able to receive is directly linked to what we are interested in. As humanity's interests have changed, so too have our methods of training and educating the intellect. And so as we proceed I will share not only the traditional methods of mind training and education but also others that can be adopted as part of a holistic practice for developing our intellects.

The Fourth Dimension: The Personality

The personality—the part of us that is deeper than the physical, the vital, or even the intellectual—has great potential for transformation through the combined practices of *āsana, prāṇāyāma,* chanting, and meditation.

According to the ancients, this personality dimension refers to the nature of our predispositions or conditioned responses, our drives, inclinations, motives, and basic beliefs. We may think of this part of ourselves as "who we really are" or our "true character" (*svabhāva*); not our essential nature, but our manifested nature based on conditioning. This dimension of ourselves determines the unique way in which we relate to our experience; how we take things; how we understand things in our own particular way. The ancients suggested that these aspects of ourselves are themselves influenced by an expression of things that have happened to us in our past, whether known or unknown. And they identified five aspects of this dimension of the personality: ***śraddhā, satya, ṛta, yoga,*** and ***mahat***.

In this context, *śraddhā* is our faith, confidence, and conviction in our choices. It is what leads us forward in action. *Ṛta* is our ability to recognize the underlying order and harmony of things. *Satya* is our ability to communicate this recognition with others. And Yoga is the state of mind—present, alert, and relaxed—from which we can understand the truth and, having understood, communicate that truth appropriately. In other words, when we are in the state of Yoga—understood as a state of clear, nonagitated mental awareness—we can know the truth of any situation and communicate that truth in a way that is beneficial, or at least not harmful, to others.

However, they also understood that, in actuality, we are not often in the stable frame of mind that enables us to perceive correctly and communicate appropriately. And they saw this as largely due to the fifth aspect of the personality—its conditioning, which they referred to collectively as *mahat*—and to the powerful effect of that conditioning on our attitudes, perceptions, and behavior.

According to this model, the nature of our personality is shaped by past conditioning. There are four levels of conditioning, which influence the structure of our personality. The first level is our genetic programming, because the personality develops in part as a tool for fulfilling the biological imperatives—survival and reproduction—that we share with other animals. The next level is our personal biography. Each of us has our personal stories, coming from early childhood into adulthood, that strongly shape what we become. All of us are also strongly influenced by the third level, society, in which we are raised and in relation to which we collectively share certain values and norms. And, finally, there is the fourth level, what might be called the transpersonal level of conditioning, which refers to the mysterious but observable truth that we seem to come into this life already carrying certain tendencies.

As we have said above, *mahat* refers collectively to all of these levels of conditioning, which actively influence our present attitudes, perceptions, and behavior. These conditioning influences manifest in our physical, emotional, and mental bodies. In other words, a basic tenet of Yoga philosophy is the idea that all patterns—from neuromuscular movement patterns, to strategies for manipulating our environment and relationships, to the defense mechanisms that we use to protect our own self-images—are based on some form of conditioning. What we call "personality" is, in fact, largely a collection of conditioned patterns. These influence its activities, which, in turn, reinforce our already acquired patterns—so that we find ourselves re-creating the same conditioning over and over again!

I remember when my wife first met my father. Her first comment to me after that meeting was, "I see." At that point she was just referring to the way I hold myself, and to the way I walk. She was able to recognize the same movement patterns in my father. As she got to know my parents better, she was also able to recognize the source of certain dynamics in my relationship to her, particularly the way I responded emotionally to stressful situations. And when our son was born, she was able to see parallels between the dynamics of my relationship to him and the dynamics of my father's relationship to me.

I was born with two wedged thoracic vertebra, giving me a naturally increased thoracic curve. My wife was born with a relatively flatten thoracic curve. When my son was born, I was happy to see that his upper back was more like my wife's than mine. And yet, though he has a relatively flat upper back, I notice that he sits more like me, rounding his upper back! It is mysterious, beautiful, and frightening! As the biblical scripture roughly says, ". . . the sins of the fathers are transmitted through seven generations."

The challenge, and the opportunity, that Yoga presents to us is the possibility of breaking the conditioning cycle. We do this by becoming aware of the depth and pervasiveness of our patterns and, at the same time, by working to change them. And true transformation begins at the moment that we become aware of our actual condition.

Proceeding from this awareness, the Yoga tradition uses this tendency to be conditioned itself as a means for transformation by working to displace dysfunctional patterns with beneficial ones. This is the key to any conscious orientation and sustained effort toward growth and development. And on this basis the ancients proposed the science of meditation to recognize, transform, evolve, and refine our personalities.

The Final Dimension: The Heart

The relational or heart level was considered to be the deepest dimension of them all, for two important reasons. Most basically, this was because the human system does not exist in isolation but in relationship—to a family, a society, and an external environment—and because these relationships are so instrumental in shaping our attitudes and behaviors they may even override our intelligence. But, above all, the ancients believed that the heart dimension is the deepest because the ultimate aim of our lives is to develop a conscious connection with our source and to realize the joy that results.

In light of this understanding, they identified five aspects of relationship—***priya, moda, pramoda, ānanda,*** and ***brahman***—which, taken together, lie at the basis of all relationships and enable us to evolve toward this ultimate goal. Within this context, *priya* is the feeling of strong, even passionate, attraction that arises when we think of, see, or hear about something that inspires us or awakens the feeling of joyfulness. *Moda* is the even deeper experience of joy that we have once we are able to connect to that which can arouse our passion. *Pramoda* is the desire that arises in us to experience this particular form of relatedness again and again. And *ānanda* is the unending joy that is possible when our passion for something, our experience of it, and our desire to continue in the experience are integrated and fulfilled.

The ancients taught that the only hope for eternal joy is to be linked to that from which we came, our source, because when we have a strong link to that source, nothing will disturb us. In this context, *brahman* refers to that eternal source from which we have come and to which we long to return.

We are constantly seeking joy and fulfillment through relationships, whether through a relationship with another person, teacher, family, or social group; through an intellectual or physical achievement; through new experience; or through material objects. With any of these or other relationships, there are inevitably ups and downs. The transient joy that comes from these objects is called *nanda* in Sanskrit. This constant seeking for joy and fulfillment, say the great mystics of the past and present, reflects the inner longing to return to our source. For, again, it is only in that relationship that we will find ultimate fulfillment. Thus the word *ānanda,* which implies an eternal joy.

We all have the potential for the limitless joy that is the promise of this ultimate relationship. It was to recognize, cultivate, refine, and ultimately celebrate it that the ancients evolved methods of purification and transformation, developed teachings on self-realization and illumination, composed hymns of praise and petition, and designed rituals of prayer and communion. And these gifts have been preserved through time in the various religious and spiritual traditions of the world.

THE IDEAL CONDITION OF THE HUMAN SYSTEM: AN INTEGRATED WHOLE

More and more of us long to discover and cultivate this spiritual dimension in our lives and, by so doing, to link with that which will enrich us, support us as we face the challenges of living, and inspire us to reach for our highest potential. Today, however, fewer and fewer of us remain connected to the spiritual heritage of our ancestors; and, despite a growing interest in the various spiritual, mystic, and shamanistic paths, most of us have difficulty forming an authentic relationship to a path whose origins are far from home.

Another way of saying this is that few of us are whole. According to the ancients, every human being has the inherent potential to function as an integrated whole—a unified expression of structural integrity at the level of the physical body, of balanced energy at the level of the vital body, of well-developed learning skills at the level of the mind, of clarity and a sense of purpose at the level of the personality, and of loving compassion at the level of the emotions and the heart.

As a means of developing and eventually actualizing this inherent potential for wholeness, the ancients taught four basic aims in life—***dharma, artha, kāma,*** and ***mokṣa***—and demonstrated how, in one way or another and in spite of our past conditioning, everything that we do relates to these aims.

The Four Basic Aims in Life

DHARMA

We all have certain fundamental responsibilities and obligations to fulfill in life. As parents, we have a responsibility to our children. As adult children, we have a responsibility to our elderly parents. As husbands and wives, we have a responsibility to our mates. As social beings, we have responsibilities to our employers, employees, society, and government. As students, we have responsibilities to our teachers. And, as teachers, we have responsibilities to our students.

These responsibilities must be fulfilled—they constitute a **personal *dharma*** from which there is no honorable escape. They are the basic requirements that give our lives the order and cohesion that hold us together and that support us on our journey through time. To see the truth in this we need only observe how rapidly our lives begin to fall apart once we become unable, or unwilling, to fulfill our basic personal responsibilities.

Beyond these personal responsibilities, there is also an **ultimate *dharma***—a responsibility to that which we all share in common, to a univesal common good. This is described variously according to different traditions, the common thread being the fulfillment of our highest potential as human beings. The ancients suggested that the first step toward fulfilling this ultimate aim lies in the fulfillment of our personal responsibilities. All too often we use our ideas of the spiritual realm as an escape from the real situations of our lives that face us day to day. And thus they taught *"dharma rakṣati rakṣata,"* which loosely translated means "as we take care of our responsibilities, wc will be taken care of."

Artha

In carrying out these obligations—this *dharma*—we also have certain fundamental material needs. At the most basic level, we all need food, clothing, and shelter to survive. In today's world, most of us also need such things as a means of transportation and a means of communication. And it is these necessary adjuncts to the fulfillment of *dharma*—personal and universal—that were referred to as *artha* by the ancients.

Kāma

Also basic to the fulfillment of *dharma* is that sensual attraction force—known in the ancient world as *kāma*—which acts as the primary motivating force in the fulfillment of desire. At its most basic level, this sensual attractive force manifests as that attraction between the sexes, which assures the continuity of all species. But beyond that, it is also about seeking pleasure through the senses, and, as such, it is a major force in all our lives and one with which we must learn to deal responsibly.

Mokṣa

Finally, at a level much deeper than the purely sensual, lies an inherent desire for freedom from bondage and suffering. It is this wish to be free—at all levels—that the ancients referred to as *mokṣa* and that they classified in two categories: freedom that is temporary or relative, and freedom that is permanent or ultimate.

Most of us are familiar with the first type of freedom: the type that comes with an ability to avoid getting caught in the same old stifling situations over and over again. But not so many of us are familiar with the second type: the ultimate freedom that goes hand in hand with *ānanda,* the ultimate joy of returning to one's source.

In both cases, however, *mokṣa*—the desire for freedom—is where we must begin. And because this desire for freedom always arises in relation to an awareness of suffering, our first step toward permanent freedom is to become aware that we suffer and to begin to understand why this is so. For only on the basis of this understanding can we start to face each situation with integrity, to build a strong foundation upon which to understand ourselves and our relationship to others, and to carry on a conscious and intelligent quest toward liberation.

Recognizing this, the ancients made certain basic suggestions. For example, they said that in our quests for freedom neither our material needs (*artha*) nor our sensual attractions (*kāma*) should compromise either our sense of responsibility (*dharma*) or our desire for freedom (*mokṣa*), and that both should be fulfilled within the boundaries of *dharma* and *mokṣa*. For example, when we fulfill our obligation to our parents by having children, *kāma* serves *dharma.* But, when we fail to resist the temptations of our sensual attraction and thus destroy our marriage, *kāma* compromises *dharma.* Or, while we may need a certain amount of material prosperity to fulfill our responsibilities, if we become so focused on making money that we neglect our families, *artha* no longer serves but compromises *dharma.*

THE INTEGRATION PROCESS: FROM *ROGĪ* TO *BHOGĪ* TO *YOGĪ*

Although, as human beings, we all share these basic aims, the way in which each of us seeks to fulfill them differs according to our character. How we grow as individuals is shaped by the way we act, according to these four aims. What is already in us strongly influences the way we act as well. And we all have our own sets of often conflicting motivations.

The general stages of human motivation and development were identified by three categories—the ***rogī,*** the ***bhogī,*** and the ***yogī.*** Although people rarely fit absolutely into any single category, considered together and in progressive relationship to each other, these categories provide a clear idea of how the ancients viewed human development.

The first and least developed type is the *rogī*. At this stage, the primary motivation is for personal gain, even at the expense of others. In other words, this type is pushed by its desire for pleasure, both material and sensual (*artha* and *kāma*). It is motivated primarily by self-interest, and is usually adept at manipulating circumstances with little or no consideration for anyone or anything but itself.

The next type is the *bhogī*. It is motivated primarily by the desire for enjoyment or pleasurable experience. It looks for what will be most comfortable or beneficial for itself in any situation, yet respects the interests of others.

The last type is the *yogī*. The primary goals of the *yogī* are to uphold responsibility (*dharma*), to serve the highest good, and, ultimately, to attain freedom (*mokṣa*). These goals are expressed in a dedication to helping others, even at the expense of personal self-interest. And, therefore, the *yogī* is an actualized expression of wholeness: a living symbol of the most basic goals of Yoga.

THE IMPERFECT VESSEL

While the ancients taught that we all have an inherent potential for wholeness, they were also keenly aware of the obstacles that keep us from it. And, in relation to our ability to practice those integrative and transformational techniques that eventually lead to freedom and wholeness, they spoke of four basic types of imperfect vessels, which they portrayed symbolically and in their esoteric teaching and practices as follows.

The Upside-Down Vessel

The upside-down vessel symbolizes fundamental disorientation. It represents an individual with a closed mind and a closed heart. The view of the ancients was that the first steps in personal transformation are the recognition of the reality of suffering, knowledge of the causes of sufferings, and the wish to change our condition. Those people who are represented by the image of the upside-down vessel are either unaware of their suffering, unwilling to accept their own role in it, or unable to envision the possibility of change. And in these cases there is no role for personal practice.

The Dirty Vessel

The dirty vessel represents those people whose systems are toxic at some level. This includes not only physical toxicity, but also psychological or emotional toxicity. In all such cases, the first step in personal practice is necessarily purification.

The Leaky Vessel

The leaky vessel is unable to hold whatever is put into it. It symbolizes those who are unable to sustain practice and to build energy in their systems. This condition may be the result of an unstable mind, too many distractions, and/or an unhealthy lifestyle. And in all such cases, the first steps in personal practice are disciplines that may include renunciation of certain activities as well as practices designed to seal the leaks.

The Tilted Vessel

The tilted vessel is able to contain a certain amount of whatever is put into it, but it loses some. It symbolizes those who receive practices and teachings and make progress, but who are unable to maximize their full potential. There are a variety of possible reasons for this condition, including, for example, a distorted perspective on the methods and purposes of practice. And, in these cases, certain practices were designed to "right" the vessel.

The most fundamental goal of the Yoga tradition is a holistic one. It involves the development of each dimension of the human system so that it can play its own unique role in the integration and transformation of the personality and its relationship with its own highest potential. This can only be accomplished through personal dedication, focused intention, and practice.

From the standpoint of practice, *Viniyoga*—the particular lineage that serves as a basis for this book—is based on the principle that each of us is different and that practice must respect these differences. As a methodology, it suggests that the practices we adopt must be relevant to who we are in our current life situation. Later we will look at some of the fundamental principles of *Viniyoga* in relation to personal practice, but first we must examine the general principles of *Kriyā Yoga,* which serve as a basis not only for this particular approach but for the Yoga tradition in general.

C H A P T E R   T W O

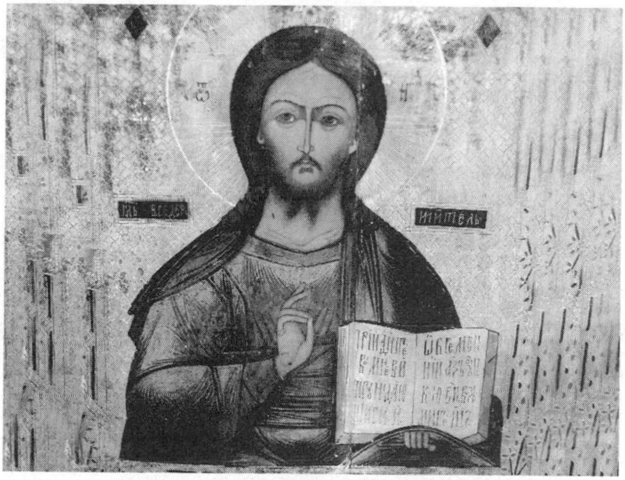

Kriyā Yoga: Transformation Through Practice

Tapaḥ svādhyāya Īśvara praṇidhānāni Kriyā Yogaḥ/
Samādhi bhāvanārthaḥ kleśa tanūkaranārthaś ca/

(Kriyā Yoga *is purification, self-reflection, and establishing a relationship to the highest for the purpose of reducing the seeds of suffering and actualizing the highest potentials of the mind)*

THE CLASSICAL YOGA TRADITION developed in the context of the spiritual traditions of India. It evolved as a means of recognizing and ultimately eliminating the root causes of suffering, which have plagued humanity since beginningless time.

According to this view, suffering is largely the result of a fundamental misapprehension, *avidyā,* lying at the root of our perception, about who we are and what is going on in this life. In short, we are confused at a very basic level about our own identity and, on the basis of this confusion, we develop all kinds of other misidentifications.

Perhaps the most telling of these misidentifications is the one we have in relation to our own self-image and, along with it, the pervasive sense of self-importance that allows us to remain unaware that this is a misidentification in the first place. In fact, the Yoga tradition maintains that this basic misapprehension and the subsequent identification with the "me" is the field in which the other seeds of suffering (*kleśa-s*) grow—the seeds of greed, anger, and fear, for example. So all the while, we not only remain confused about who we really are, we remain unaware of that confusion, therefore, helpless to deal effectively with the multitude of misidentifications that inevitably result.

A seed sprouts, shoots up, and becomes a plant or a tree. The ancients believed that our emotions—anger, frustration, sadness, jealousy, envy, fear, loneliness, anxiety, and depression, for example—exist within us as seeds waiting to sprout. We act continuously and our activity follows set patterns—patterns acquired in childhood and slavishly followed—so that every new opportunity serves mainly to reinforce old patterning. If we could see a video of ourselves—a digital recording of our walking sequence over time—we would recognize this unconscious patterning in the way we walk. And that is only an example of physical patterning—the outer expression of a condition that penetrates through all dimensions of our five-dimensional natures and impacts the way we breathe, communicate, and emote as well as the way we relate to food, sex, people, and the world around us.

The science of *Kriyā Yoga* developed primarily as an antidote to the basic problem of human misperception and the ignorance that results. It grew out of the realization that patterning is basic to everything we think and do. As human beings, we are constantly involved in activity that can affect our lives in two basic ways: it can either reinforce our conditioning or serve as the ground for positive change. These are the bases for Yoga practice. Thus, in his classical teachings, Patañjali poetically describes the purpose of *Kriyā Yoga* in terms of reducing the seeds of suffering and awakening the higher potentials of the mind. And this suggests that within each of us lies the potential to reduce and ultimately to eliminate undesirable characteristics, dysfunctional patterns, and impurities from our systems; to awaken our inherent potential, discriminative awareness, and the wisdom-mind; and to experience a still, quiet, untroubled, calm, joyous, and expanded consciousness.

KRIYĀ YOGA: A THREEFOLD APPROACH TO PRACTICE

The Yoga teachings are grounded in a recognition of the reality of suffering at any level. So, as long as we are aware of suffering in our own lives, this teaching has relevance for us. In fact, the ancients suggested that the first wisdom is the recognition of suffering. That it is from this recognition of suffering that the desire to end suffering arises. And that it is to accomplish the ending of suffering that the *Kriyā Yoga* teachings have been offered.

Within this context, *Kriyā Yoga* can be understood as a threefold practice (*sādhana*), or a threefold approach to practice, based on purification (***tapas***), self-reflection (***svādhyāya***), and recognition of and dedication to our source (***Īśvara praṇidhāna***).

Traditionally, *tapas, svādhyāya,* and *Īśvara praṇidhāna* referred to specific activities, but they may also be understood in the context of an overall relationship to action. In this chapter we will present these teachings as they apply to our day-to-day experience, giving examples to illustrate each point that we make along the way.

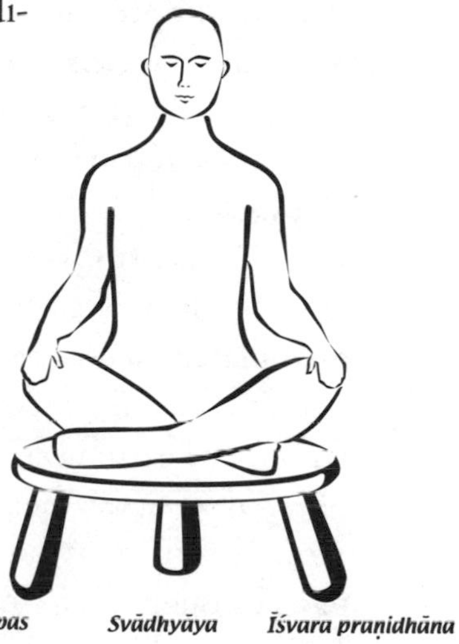

Tapas: The Purifying Heat

Kāya Indriya Siddhiḥ Aśuddhi Kṣayat Aśayāt Tapasoḥ
(The fire of disciplined practice destroys impurities
and leads to the mastery of the body and senses)

The purifying heat of *tapas* leads to the purification and mastery of the body and the senses; and, therefore, according to the ancients, there can be no Yoga without *tapas.*

The word itself comes from the Sanskrit root *tap,* which means to cook. And, in this sense, *tapas* is the means through which we purify and transform ourselves. Because it can also be translated as "austerities," the practice of *tapas* is also linked to renunciation and deprivation. In depriving ourselves of something to which we are habituated, we resist acting in our habitual patterns, and this resistance creates a kind of internal heat that purifies, strengthens, and transforms us.

Accordingly, we find in the religious traditions of the world a whole array of ascetic practices, ranging from fasting to self-flagellation—the former and most common form being widely practiced in association with holy days; the latter being reserved primarily for monks or ascetics.

The Christian Saint Francis of Assisi was one example of such extreme *tapas*. He renounced his wealth and, during most of his short life, went without shoes, dressed in rough clothes, and lived like a beggar. In medieval times, this extreme form of ascetic practice represented a widely held view that the soul was imprisoned in the body and that mortification of the flesh was the only way in which it could attain freedom. And yet, by the end of his life, Saint Francis rejected this idea. He confessed to his disciples that he had "abused this donkey," referring to his body, and exhorted them to avoid such extreme asceticism.

The life story of Buddha explains that he too practiced extreme asceticism until he discovered the Middle Way. It is said that he heard a simple fisherman playing a stringed instrument and realized that too loose a string would not sing and that too tight a string would break. And that at that point he renounced extreme asceticism.

Of course, the practices in this book are not about asceticism and certainly not about abuse. They are about purifying and strengthening our systems through disciplines designed to reduce physical, emotion, and mental impurities. In this context, *tapas* is primarily the process of getting rid of something undesirable in our system—from chronic subliminal muscular contraction, to toxicity in the colon, to deep-rooted emotions and behaviors. In order to do this we must break patterns. This requires energy. And thus the means and methods of personal practice that we suggest—postures (*āsana*), breathing exercises (*prāṇāyāma*), meditation, dietary restriction, fasting, refraining from idle gossip, and other forms of selective renunciation—are all designed to help us build sufficient energy to break free of our conditioned responses.

According to the ancients, the most important areas of *tapas* are restricting diet, limiting speech, and controlling breath. When we fast, we purify our bodies; we gain an appreciation of the nourishment that we usually take for granted; and we have an opportunity to recognize how much we rely on food for our sense of emotional well-being and even as a source of entertainment.

When we avoid idle gossip, we save energy and allow our minds to become more focused. And when we control our breathing we interrupt an automatic process that goes on at every moment of our lives, so that *prāṇāyāma* practice can function as a deep and profound method of *tapas* that is immediately accessible to any practitioner.

However, if we are to effectively apply *tapas,* we must be able to see beyond the specific actions of our lives to our entire relationship to activity. To this end, we might begin by observing the quality of attention that we bring to a given activity in a given moment. By practicing *tapas* in this way we might also begin to recognize how seldom it is that we are 100 percent focused on what we are doing. How often tensions and other preoccupations divide our attention. And thus we might come to appreciate why another basic requirement of *tapas* is to cut through distractions and to bring our full attention to the present moment.

In this way, we can bring a whole new level of discrimination to our practice. We can see clearly why a mechanical *āsana* practice does not function as *tapas*. We can see the value in modifying or giving up a certain *āsana* that we can apparently do well but that is causing harm to our structure, and we can see that to do so is *tapas,* even though the posture itself may no longer appear to be as picture-perfect as before. Carrying this idea of discrimination further, we might even come to see that if our *āsana* practice is strictly a mechanical one, it could be more *tapas* to discontinue that practice and go for a hike instead. And thus, on the basis of such discrimination, our own *āsana* practice can become a way of purifying and strengthening our systems so that they become a firmer foundation upon which to establish new and more useful patterns of movement.

As a result of this ability to discriminate, we can also recognize how we are slaves to our habits and addictions. We can take note of those things in our lives which, while generally attractive to us, are nonetheless harmful to some dimension of ourselves. (Consider New Year's resolutions, for example. Many of us are lucky if we survive the month of January before the strength of those habits take over and we find ourselves engaging in the same behavior that we intended to stop!) And thus, while we may enjoy a habit such as smoking cigarettes or drinking coffee, we can understand that they cause stress to our systems, that we could benefit from giving them up, and that to do so would be *tapas*.

On the basis of a yet more subtle level of discrimination, we may even learn to use *tapas* in the sense of renunciation. In other words, we may learn to give up certain things that we like and that are not at all harmful to us for the purpose of purification. This type of selective and disciplined renunciation is known as *tyāga*. And while the ancients advised that it be practiced carefully in order to avoid harm to body or mind, they also suggested that it could be a very effective way of accelerating our progress in personal practice.

At first, it may be difficult to understand that when *tapas* remains only at the level of the body, its beneficial effects will not be lasting; and that when it is done as a kind of penance without deep self-reflection, it may even be harmful. For example, one of my acquaintances, after making many mistakes in his relationship, decided to radically restrict his diet as a kind of penance. Though the diet was actually beneficial to his health, it became a mechanical process that didn't impact his behavior. Not long after, he repeated similar mistakes in his relationship and finally ended up divorced. I have also worked with many students who originally went to a gym or who had practiced extreme forms of *āsana* practice with the intention of improving their condition and who have ended up in surgery. In both of these cases, though effort was present, something was missing. In the first case, *tapas* without self-reflection was ineffective; in the second, it was harmful. So, taking a lesson from Saint Francis and the Buddha, we can say that our *tapas* should not be adverse to our physical health or to our mental composure (*citta prasādanam*).

Svādhyāya: The Reflecting Mirror

Svādhyāyāt Iṣṭa Devatā Saṁpra Yogaḥ
(Return to Oneself, dis-cover the Divine)

The second element of *Kriyā Yoga* is *svādhyāya*. It is a beautiful word. Its verbal root *i* (which becomes *aya*), means to go or to move. *Adhi* is a verbal prefix meaning "toward." *Adhyāya* is a verbal derivative meaning "to move toward." And *sva* is a reflexive pronoun meaning "self" or "one's own." Literally and etymologically then, *svādhyāya* means "to move toward one's self," "to return to oneself," "to come back (by some means) to who we are."

Tapas and *svādhyāya* exist in mutual relationship, *tapas* being the means whereby we purify and refine our systems, *svādhyāya* being the means of self-reflection through which we come to an increasingly deeper level of self-awareness and self-understanding. By cleaning the vessel, *tapas* makes us fit for *svādhyāya*; by examining the vessel, *svādhyāya* helps us to understand exactly where we should concentrate our practices of purification. And thus, in this relationship between purification and self-examination, we have a natural method for discovering who, in essence, we are.

When we use *svādhyāya* effectively, our actions become much more than a way to achieve something external; they become a mirror in which we can learn to see ourselves more deeply in terms of our true motivations. And, assuming a willingness to look at the behaviors, motivations, and strategies that we habitually use to maintain our own self-image, we can even use *svādhyāya* to pierce through the veil that it creates and into the nature of our own essential being.

Classically and in a technical sense, *adhyāyana* refers to the chanting of texts and *mantra-s* that pertain to freedom (*mokṣa*) and that were learned exactly from a teacher, and *svādhyāyana* refers specifically to chanting texts and *mantra-s* that were part of one's lineage and that were passed down by one's ancestors.

In a more general sense, however, *svādhyāya* suggests that any sacred or inspirational text that offers insight into the human condition can serve as a mirror, reflecting back to us our true nature. Classical texts of this sort might include the *Yoga Sūtra-s,* the *Bhagavad-Gītā,* the Bible, the Talmud, the *Tao Te Ching,* and the writings of the saints of any tradition. But the source might also be any spiritual or inspiring text that we use, not simply abstractly or academically, but as a means to deeper self-understanding.

IN SUMMARY, while there are various types of tapas, all have one thing in common: they are the means whereby we strengthen ourselves in order to break the cycle of habitual and addictive behavior that keeps us enslaved. And this they do by challenging us to wake up out of the momentum of our daily lives, to pay attention, and to look at life in a new way.

In fact, carrying the same logic a step further, *svādhyāya* can refer to any inspirational activity, from the simple act of chanting, using a *mantra,* or singing a hymn to receiving teachings from the guru or going to hear a sermon. Thus, even the rituals of the major religions can act as a type of *svādhyāya* process.

For example: The ritual of confession in the Roman Catholic faith is an example of a different kind of *svādhyāya* process. In confession, we reflect on our past actions and expose ourselves to ourselves before God. In this ritual, the priest serves primarily as a medium through which the confession is transmitted and the prescribed penance and absolution are received. In both the Jewish and Islamic faiths, to take a different example, repentance and forgiveness-seeking are integral parts of the process of purification and illumination. In yet another form of *svādhyāya,* the Tibetan Buddhist contemplates the "great thoughts that turn the mind to (ultimate) *dharma,*" thus turning the mind away from the worldly toward the spiritual life. Thus, in this context of *svādhyāya,* spiritually inspiring teachings are tools to help us understand ourselves, and, through that understanding, to change our attitudes and behavior.

This teaching is not meant only for those dedicated to matters of the spirit. It has great practical meaning for all of us who recognize that there is room for improvement in our lives. In this context, *svādhyāya* represents an ongoing process through which we can assess where we are in relation to many things at any given moment. It is like attuning our inner navigator and finding meaningful answers to questions such as: Am I at the right place at the right moment? Where am I now and also where am I going? What is my direction and what are my aspirations? What are my responsibilities? What are my priorities?

We often find ourselves on cruise control, acting habitually and being so swept up in the momentum of our daily lives that we don't take time to check where we are or where we are headed. And, since our lives are in motion, where we are today is probably different from where we will be tomorrow. The *mantra-s* and textual studies offered by the classical tradition function as references from which we can measure where we are. If we come back to the image of the inner navigator, then the *mantra-s* and texts can be seen as the polestar, which shows us true north.

One of the greatest opportunities we have to see ourselves is in the mirror of relationship. Therefore, another means of *svādhyāya* is the ability to look in the mirror of how people are responding to us and let that be an opportunity to understand something about the way we habitually operate. For example, it is difficult to hide aspects of our personality from our mates, our parents, or our children. Even with intimate friends, our pretenses are not likely to endure for long. And while we are quite able to play the games of avoidance and self-deception in our own company, in the mirror of our relationships it is not so easy to hide . . . that is, if we will look, avoid deflecting messages that we could benefit by hearing, and avoid playing victim or becoming self-righteous, of course.

In other words, *svādhyāya* suggests that we can use all of our activities—solitary and relational—as mirrors in which to discover something important about ourselves and to use what we discover as valuable information in the process of arriving at a deeper self-understanding.

Finally, the ultimate purpose of *svādhyāya* is to function as a mirror to remind us of our higher potential—in other words, as a way into the interior where our "true selves" reside. To this end, the classical means of *svādhyāya* include using a *mantra,* reading a text, or sitting with a spiritual master (guru).

In fact, the ancients used the word *darśana*—which means something like a mirror—to describe the teaching contained in a particular group of sacred texts; and they used the same word to describe what happens when we sit with a spiritual master. Because, in both cases, we can see our neuroses, our small-mindedness, and our pettiness mirrored completely. At the same time, we can also see beyond our current state to something like the divine potential. And that too is who we are.

Ultimately, *svādhyāya* is a means to reach that higher potential, a way to the interior where our "true selves" reside. Although the classical means of *svādhyāya* were *mantra-s*, texts, and masters, we can use our wives, husbands, lovers, friends, Yoga students, or Yoga teachers. Everybody. Everything. In fact, all of our activities can be an opportunity to see more deeply who we are and how we operate; and on that basis we can begin to refine ourselves and thus become clearer and more appropriate in our behavior. This is very important.

We cannot truly consider *tapas* (purification) apart from *svādhyāya*; and, therefore, an intelligent practice of *tapas* must of necessity include *svādhyāya*. For example, if we do an intensive *āsana* (posture) without being adequately self-reflective, we may end up destabilizing our hips, creating vulnerability in our lower back, and ruining our knees. If, however, we consider the *āsana* practice itself as a mirror, we are certainly more apt to avoid injury and may even come away with a better understanding of ourselves as well.

For many of us, who are drawn to styles of *āsana* practice that reinforce existing tendencies, this is a tricky point. For example, if we are the high-paced, hyperactive type, we might be drawn toward a very active practice—one that makes us sweat and that generates lots of heat—whereas what we may really need is a more soothing and calming practice. Or, if we are the slow-moving, sluggish type, we might be drawn to a very gentle and relaxing practice, whereas what we may really need is a more active and stimulating one. In either case, the result would be *tapas* without *svādhyāya*. And in both cases the result would most likely be a reinforcement of existing patterns or, even worse, a possible injury or illness.

When we practice, it is important to look carefully, both at who we are and what is actually happening to us in our practice. In our *tapas* there must be *svādhyāya* so that we have a constant feedback mechanism through which we accurately feel what is happening in our systems, and as a result of which we learn increasingly more about ourselves.

In short: *Tapas* accompanied by *svādhyāya* ensures that *tapas* is a transformational activity and not simply a mindless application of technology, or, worse yet, an abusive activity.

According to the ancients, *svādhyāya* develops *tapas*; *tapas* develops *svādhyāya*; and together they help us awaken to the spiritual dimension of life. Thus, as we go deeper and deeper into the process of self-investigation and self-discovery, we also go deeper and deeper into our Selves, until, eventually, we dis-cover or un-cover the Divine. One great teacher has described this process with the image of a drop of water dissolving into the ocean. At first we wonder

> IN SUMMARY, while the primary method of nourishing and cultivating the intellectual dimension is through learning, the use of chant as a primary tool of mind training and learning is not a part of our contemporary culture. Nevertheless, it remains a powerful tool for use in personal practice. So, recognizing this fact, we will now consider how to utilize chanting in the service of mind training, education, and for the purpose of deepening self-understanding in preparation for self-transformation.

whether we are the drop. But eventually we discover that we are not and have never been the drop, but only the water itself.

Īśvara praṇidhāna: The Refuge

Samādhi Siddhiḥ Īśvara Praṇidhānāt
(Open your heart, master your mind)

The third element of *Kriyā Yoga* is *Īśvara praṇidhāna.*

Although *Īśvara* is the Sanskrit equivalent of the word "God," it is not personalized. The ancient teachers of Yoga were not offering a theological testament on the Godhead, but rather a depth-psychological analysis of the tranformational potential inherent in opening the human heart and mind to the Divine.

In the *Yoga Sūtra* of Patañjali, *Īśvara* is described not as the Creator God of the traditional religious doctrines, but as a being without suffering or the seeds of suffering. In fact, it is for this reason that the traditional religious schools of Hinduism rejected Yoga philosophically, though they appropriated its practices.

In this context, *Īśvara* represents that living symbol of the Divine that is in our hearts. For the Christian, it could be Jesus; for the Muslim, Allah; for the Hindu, Krishna; for the Buddhist, Buddha; and for the atheist, it could represent whatever is of highest value.

Praṇidhāna is a technical term usually translated as "surrender." It consists of the root *dhā* (to sustain) plus two verbal prefixes: *pra* (in all directions) and *ni* (deeply or intensely). Implied in this word is the profound recognition of that which sustains us and gives meaning to every dimension of our lives—a kind of faith in the sense of a "place where we put or surrender our hearts." It also implies an element of self-sacrifice, for in this act of surrender we must give up our own self-importance.

In a traditional religious context, *Īśvara praṇidhāna* implies a recognition of God as the source of one's being. For the mystic, it means that God is present at every moment, in everyone, in everything, and in every situation—that all that is seen is God, and that God is all that is seen. For the devotee, it means standing in awe before the mystery of life, expressing gratitude for the gift of life, and dedicating that life to God. It is a recognition that is celebrated by the religious of all faiths through communal and personal songs of praise as well as through blessings, prayers, rituals, rites, and offerings.

Consider, for example, the ritual of Communion at the pinnacle of the Roman Catholic Mass. In this ritual, the individuals of the congregation are communing—indeed, merging—with the mystical body of Christ through the sacrament of bread and wine. Consider the completion stage practices at the pinnacle of the tantric Buddhists' deity Yoga. In this ritual, the individuals of the *saṅga* (congregation) merge and become one with the deity.

However, these rituals are for the faithful; and, in our contemporary and secular society, fewer and fewer of us are able to embrace the spiritual heritage of our ancestors with confidence. Unfortunately, for many of us the rituals through which our ancestors celebrated their faith have lost their meaning. At the same time, we are constantly being exposed to faiths and religions distinctly different from the ones of our childhood. Science and technology are rapidly and radically changing the way we live. Yet, many of us long to have this experience, this quality, in our lives. But we must ultimately be authentic and true to ourselves. We cannot fake at this level. It's as if we are entering a collective identity crisis. And, in the midst of this crisis, we are longing to find our way back to faith.*

And herein lies the greatness of *Kriyā Yoga,* which from ancient times has echoed a nonsectarian path along which we can travel beyond suffering toward realization. For example, stripped of all sectarian religious images, *tapas* can be understood as "being present" and *svādhyāya* as "being reflective." And, in this same context, *Īśvara praṇidhāna* can be understood in relation to attitudes of openness, availability, humility, and gratitude. It expresses implicit understanding that we are not in control of everything, that we cannot know what lies ahead, and that we can safely surrender control and stay open to receiving whatever life shows us. This attitude is the antithesis of, and antidotal to, the pervasive fixation around "me and mine" that dominates most all of us most of the time. It implies an open attitude toward our own mistakes and a sincerity in relation to repentance. Ultimately, it is a faith, deep in our hearts, that we have the potential to become free from suffering and to achieve our destiny as

*I refer the reader to *The Silence of God,* by Raimundo Panikkar. Orbis: 1989, Maryknoll, N.Y.

human beings. The ancients believed that when this quality is in our hearts all our action is done as an offering, without regard to personal gain.

I remember a woman asking me to help her with the idea of surrender. She told me that her husband was a marine and would never go for the idea of surrender. Of course she was referring to surrendering to the enemy, and not the necessary self-surrender implicit in being the member of a group. After considering the implications of what she was saying, I asked if he could relate to it better as "dedication to the mission."

Another woman came to see me who had been a Yoga teacher for five years. She was a professional psychotherapist and an avid trekker—very bright and very tough. She had also been doing mindfulness meditation, a popular form of Buddhist meditation, for ten years. However, at a certain point, in one of her private sessions with me, she realized that, in her own words, "something was missing." She was strong. She could sit straight. She could control her breath. Yet she realized that something was missing in her heart. It was the *Īśvara* element: the sweetness of devotion. I discovered that she used to go to church as a child so I taught her the following Italian chant, composed by Saint Francis of Assisi, which praises the beauty of nature and gratefully acknowledges it as a gift of God's immense love. An Italian chant, not a *Vedic* chant. And that filled her heart and made her practice more meaningful.

How sweet it is to feel how, in my heart
Now, humbly, love is being born
How sweet it is to know that I am no longer alone
But am part of an immense life
How generous the splendor that surrounds me
Gift of Him and His immense Love.

What we can learn from this is that *Īśvara praṇidhāna* is fundamentally about a relationship to something higher than or beyond ourselves. It may be a higher force, as in the context of religious traditions. Or it may be in relation to human values, such as kindness and compassion. In either case, it will manifest in our lives as the ability to let go of the tyranny of our own self-importance—whether that self-importance is manifesting as pride and arrogance or self-pity and low self-esteem. It will awaken in us attitudes such as gratitude and appreciation. As a result, we will be able to simply wake up in the morning and say, "Ah, I'm alive another day." We will feel grateful in our heart for the gift of this life. We will take the time to look and appreciate the beauty around us. In our relationships, we will become open to receiving each other with respect and appreciation. And if we make this the spirit and foundation of our practice then surely, as the Buddhists say, we will have attained the stream that will lead us to the river, that will return us to the ocean from whence we have come.

IN SUMMARY: *Svādhyāya* leads back into *tapas* on the one hand, and forward into *Īśvara praṇidhāna* on the other, for in a rightly oriented practice, each of these elements of *Kriyā Yoga*, while independent, is interdependent and mutually supportive.

CHAPTER THREE

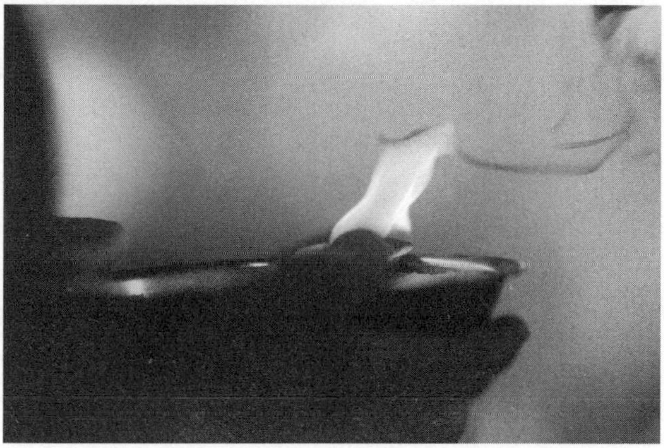

The *Viniyoga* of Yoga: The Art of Appropriate Application

IF *KRIYĀ YOGĀ* REPRESENTS a generalized description of the process of transformation, *Viniyoga* represents the way to actualize this process personally. The very essence of the *Viniyoga* of Yoga lies in the adaptation of the practice to the individual, not in the adaptation of the individual to the practice.

One of the key insights of *Viniyoga* is that in developing a personal Yoga practice, it is essential to respect our individual situations and requirements and to take into account constitution, place, gender, time, age, capacities, aspirations, and activities. In keeping with this insight, its practices are concerned with not only the development of our bodily structure, but of our breath, voice, memory, intellect, character, and heart as well. And its specific methodologies—which include physical postures (*āsana*), breathing exercises (*prāṇāyāma*), chanting, meditation, ritual, prayer, and study—are all designed to work deeply into the root of our being, to release our tensions, transform our conditioning, and unlock our highest human potential.

As we use its methods and apply its principles, we not only achieve greater harmony and balance within ourselves and in relation to our environment, we also begin to realize and actualize that higher potential. This deep, individualized application of the science of *Viniyoga* is "the art of personal practice."

MODELS AND RELATED APPROACHES TO PRACTICE

As a basis for developing this art, the principles of appropriate application developed in the *Viniyoga* teaching lineage can be represented by two models: **age** and **orientation**. These models represent different approaches to practice.

The Age Model

The movements of the sun throughout the day can represent the age model, in which sunrise represents childhood, midday represents midlife, and sunset represents old age.

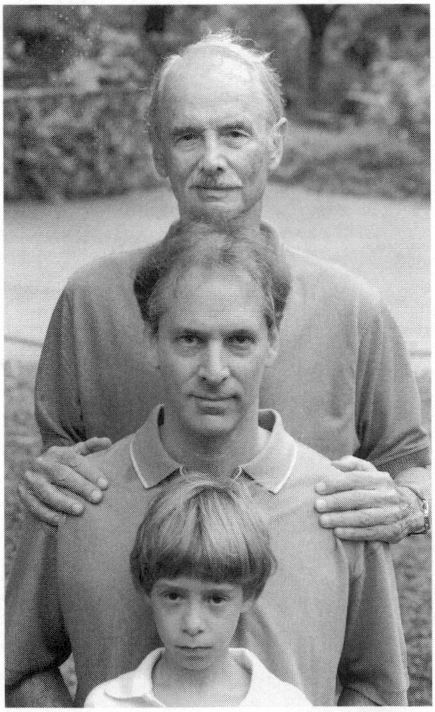

SUNRISE

This stage covers roughly the first twenty-five years of life.

Because in a very real sense the related methodology of practice is always adapted to map the natural development of the human system, during this first stage all the resources of the individual are utilized to promote growth and development. Practice is designed to promote the balanced growth and development of the body, including its structure and vital organs; the development of the mind, including the strengthening of memory and the development of its intellectual capacities; the control of the senses; the instilling of values; and the developing of character.

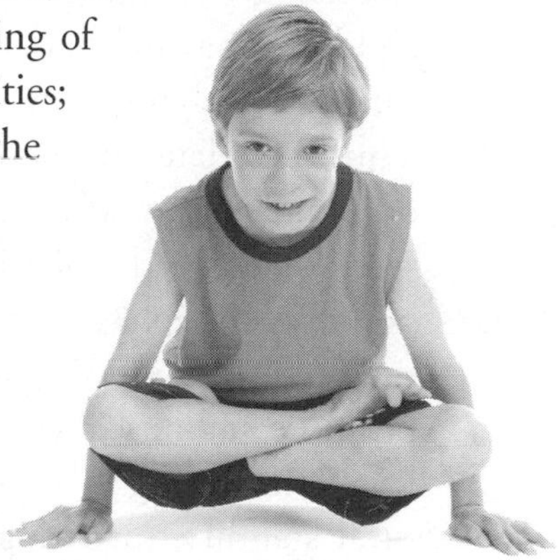

Lolāsana

While today we may extend the application of this strong emphasis on physical development—in some cases, until approximately forty years of age—classically it was known as *śṛṣṭikrama*: a methodology of personal practice considered most appropriate for the youth. In fact, in classical Hindu thought, this stage of life was referred to as the student or *brahmacarī* phase or primary development stage. In this sunrise stage, besides the strong emphasis on education, the most important emphasis in practice is considered to be *āsana,* which serves the growth and development of the body.

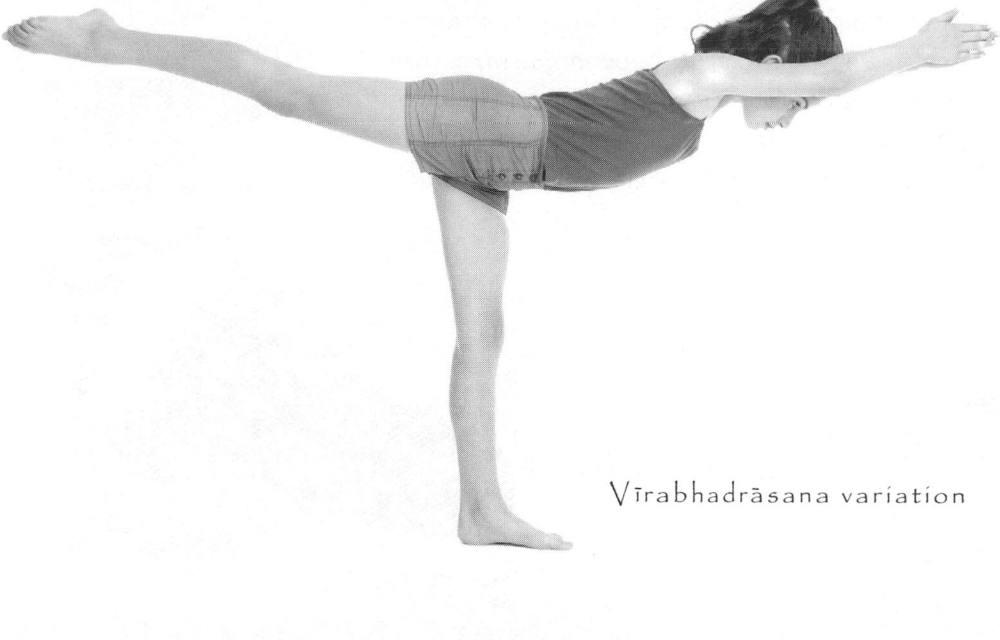

Vīrabhadrāsana variation

MIDDAY

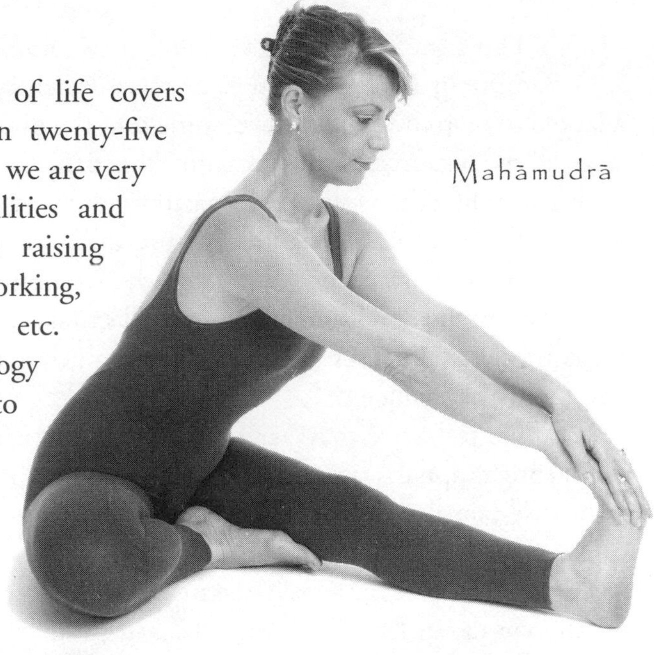

Mahāmudrā

The midday stage of life covers roughly the years between twenty-five and seventy, at which time we are very busy with the responsibilities and challenges of family life: raising children, paying bills, working, caring for aging parents, etc. Thus the related methodology of practice was adapted to serve the needs of this householder phase, and their orientation was to promote stability at every level—including structural stability, physiological immunity, emotional balance, and even financial stability—so that we are able to fulfill our responsibilities.

Known as *sthiti krama* (to stabilize), this methodology is most appropriate for the *gṛhasta* (householder), and the most important aspect of practice is considered to be *prāṇāyāma* (breath work). Of course, *āsana-s* are also important in this phase of life, but the intention shifts so that *āsana-s* become practices in the service of *prāṇāyāma.*

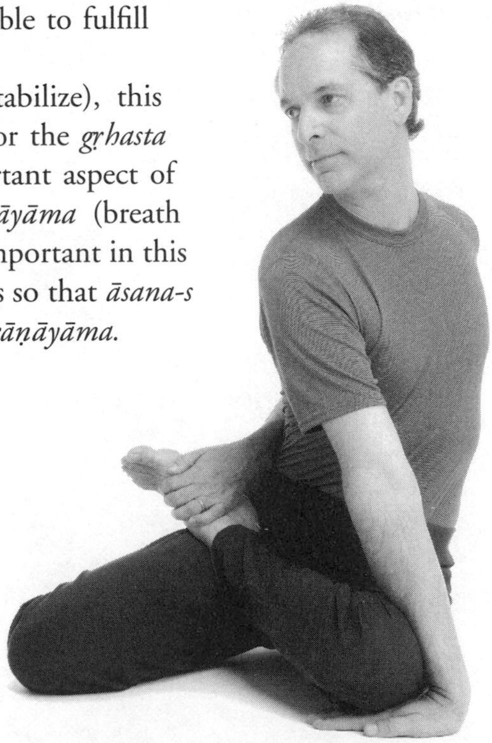

Bhāradvājāsana

SUNSET

The sunset phase of life covers the senior years, from roughly seventy until the end of life. It is known as *laya krama* (to merge). In classical Hindu thought, it was referred to as the *sannyāsin* (renunciate) phase. And because the methodology of practice was specifically adapted to serve the needs of the elderly, its orientation was designed to facilitate the progressive turning away from involvement in and attachment to the external material world, and toward the interiorization of the mind and heart in preparation for death and for merging back to one's source.

In the sunset phase of life, the most important aspect of practice is considered to be meditation and prayer. Of course, *āsana* and *prāṇāyāma* are important in this phase of life, but the intention shifts so that they are practiced in the service of meditation and prayer.

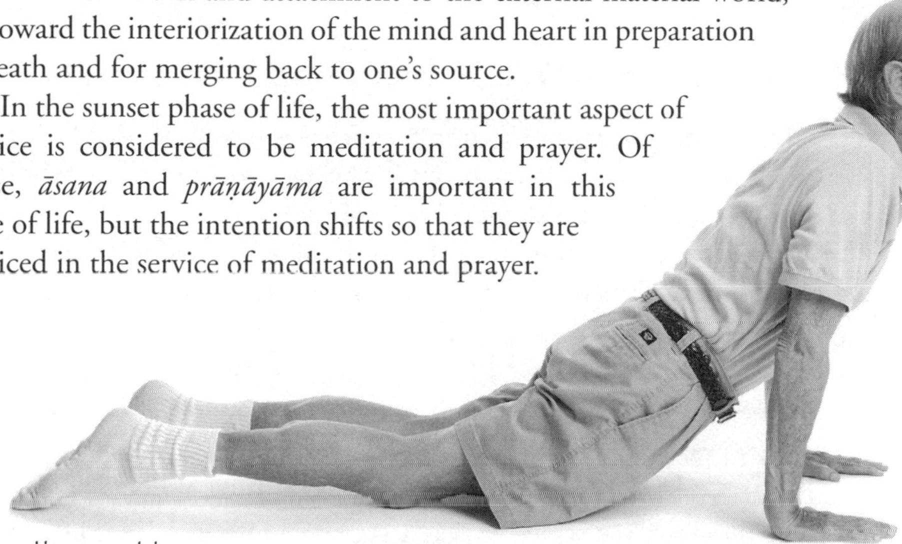

ūrdhva mukha śvānāsana variation

As we have seen, there are some generalizations regarding practice that can be made in relation to where an individual is in his or her life cycle. However, there are also generalizations that can be made on the basis of one's orientation, people differing in terms of aspiration and character as well as in terms of age. And it is this orientation that is the model for all of the following methods of approach to practice.

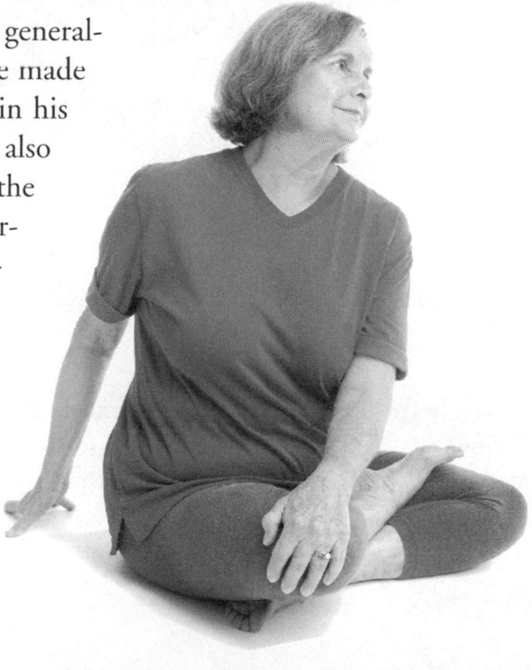

sukhāsana parivṛtti

The Orientation Model

The orientation model reflects the fact that we all have different interests, regardless of our age, and that practice can be adapted respecting those interests.

THE DEVELOPMENTAL APPROACH TO PRACTICE

Traditionally, this approach to practice was recommended for the sunrise stage of life. However, today people of all ages come to Yoga practice because they would like to develop themselves in some way.

Perhaps the most common goal is to develop our body through *āsana* practice. This development can range from simply refining our movement and postural skills to a complete mastery of the body, known as *śarīra saṃyama*. Refining our movement and postural skills can be accomplished through a careful selection and practice of *āsana-s* designed to stretch and strengthen key muscle groups that help maintain the integrity of the spine. Completely mastering the body, on the other hand, requires years of dedicated commitment to the practice of a full range of *āsana-s,* moving progressively from the simplest to the most complex, working to refine movement and postural skills. This process, know as *śikṣana krama,* requires strict and disciplined training in which all postures must be precisely executed without com-

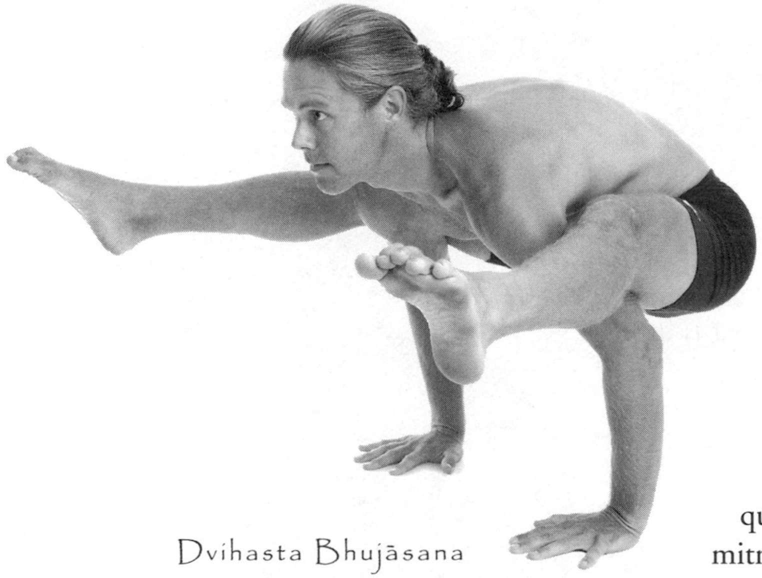

Dvihasta Bhujāsana

promise. Mastery of these postures reveals a tremendous degree of structural integration, strength, flexibility, and balance.

Another common developmental goal is to build our energy level. This can mean several things, including an increased ability to sustain physical or mental work without fatigue, an increased ability to withstand social and environmental changes, and a strengthening of the immune system and improved organ function. We can work toward the development of these goals through intensive *āsana* practice combined with *prāṇāyāma* practice and, specifically, with the select applications of controlled breathing and internal visceral locks know as *bandha-s*. In this approach to practice, we would emphasize increasing the sustainable length of inhalation, retention of the breath after inhalation, exhalation, and suspension of the breath after exhalation.

Another developmental goal is to improve memory, deepen concentration, develop the intellect, and expand knowledge. We can work toward these goals in personal practice through a variety of *prāṇāyāma,* chanting, and meditation techniques.

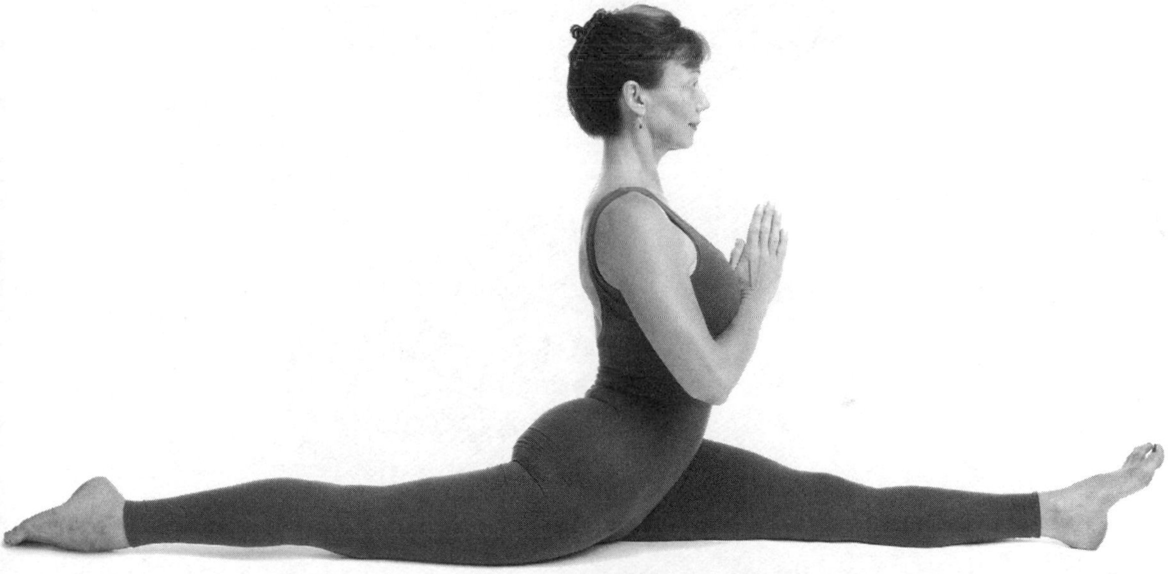

Hanumānāsana

The Preventative Approach to Practice

In the preventative approach to practice, known as *rakṣana krama,* we design our practices so as to protect and preserve what we have achieved. Traditionally, this approach to practice was recommended for the midday stage of life because once we have achieved something in ourselves, it is natural to want to avoid losing it. With this as our intention, for example, we may avoid practicing *āsana-s* that might threaten the stability of our joints by excessive stretching and contortion and emphasize *āsana-s* that will preserve and enhance structural stability (*sthiti krama*) by strengthening muscles that support the spine and the joints.

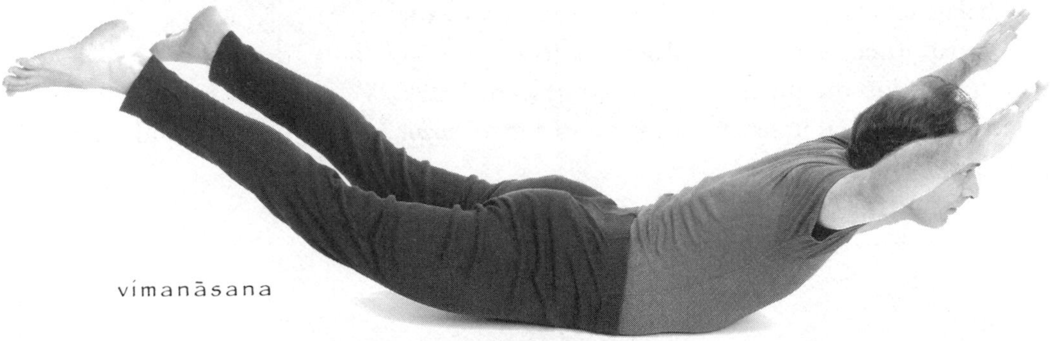

vimanāsana

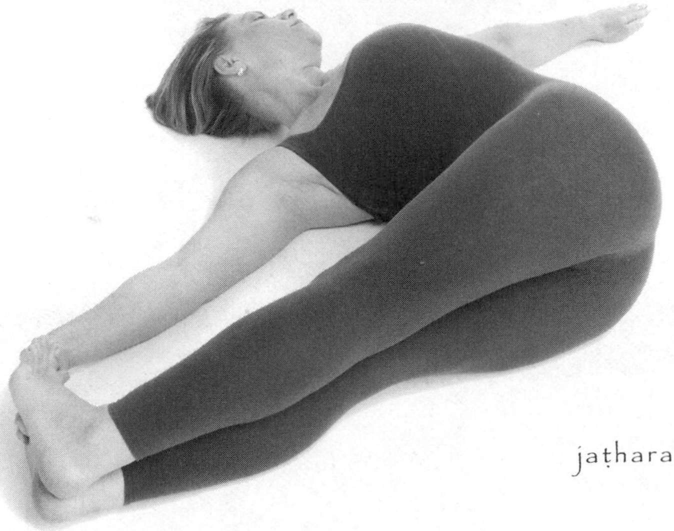

jaṭhara parivṛtti

This emphasis on prevention and protection will also involve the appropriate use of *prāṇāyāma,* adapted to help energize the system when it is fatigued and to calm the system when it is stressed.

Another important and often overlooked aspect of personal practice is lifestyle education and reeducation. In order to protect our condition, it is important to learn more about what can be harmful. Many people have come to Yoga classes with the intention of improving their health, for example, and ended up with mild to serious structural injuries. This may be the result of having inappropriate goals in *āsana,* or of practicing without adequate understanding of our own condition and the potentially harmful effects of certain practices. We can gain more education through contact with qualified teachers, studying available literature, and experimenting with lifestyle adjustments.

THE THERAPEUTIC APPROACH TO PRACTICE

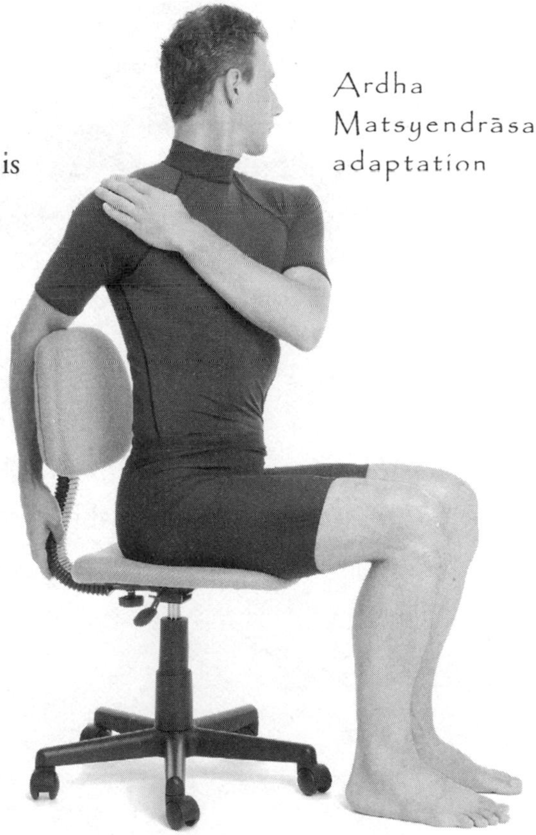
Ardha Matsyendrāsana adaptation

The therapeutic approach to practice is appropriate when we are suffering at some level and we want to use personal practice to help reduce the suffering. This approach to practice is relevant for any stage of life.

The main orientation in this approach is to alleviate suffering, support rehabilitation, and improve the quality of life. We should be clear that this approach is not a substitute for allopathic or other medical therapies, whether contemporary or traditional. It is first and foremost a complementary treatment, oriented toward helping the person who suffers from a condition, rather than an actual treatment for that condition.

In this approach to personal practice, we not only strive to alleviate suffering at the level of its manifest symptoms, such as back pain, but to reduce suffering at a deeper level—for example, fear of the future. This requires an ability to understand our condition, what has gone wrong, what the origins of the problem are, and what we can do to fix it. Using the body, breath, senses, and mind, we develop a personal practice that strives to stabilize our structure, enhance our physiological functioning, and balance our emotions.

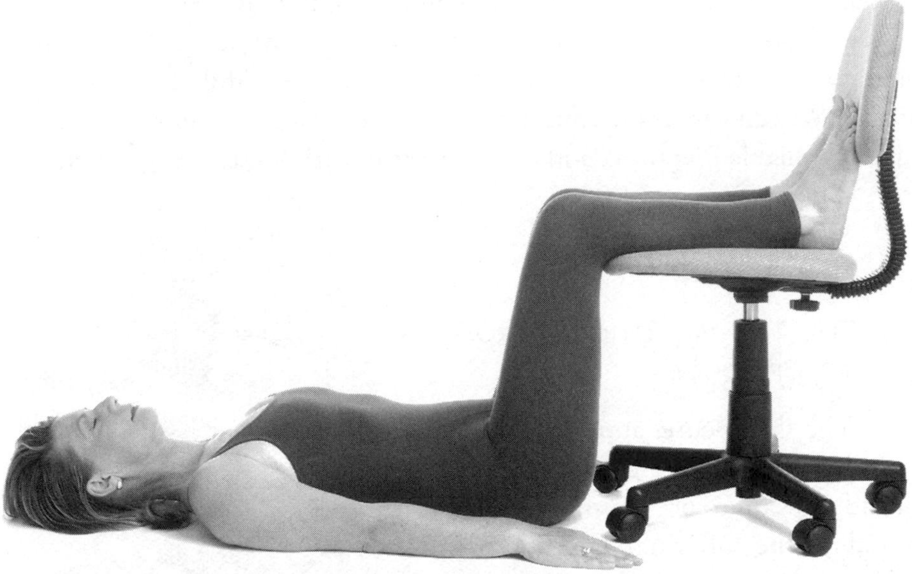

śavāsana variation

I refer readers to my first book, *Yoga for Wellness: Healing with the Timeless Teachings of Viniyoga,* which presents the teachings of this approach, known as Yoga *cikitsā* in detail.

THE TRANSCENDENTAL APPROACH TO PRACTICE

Traditionally this approach was recommended for the sunset stage of life.

Most of us go through a natural evolution in our lives. When we are young we are full of curiosity about life and the world around us. After puberty, we become interested in exploring ourselves as sexual beings. As young adults, we find ourselves faced with the responsibilities of supporting ourselves and possibly our new family. When we reach old age, however, a time comes when the outward and worldly orientation of our lives shifts and attention naturally turns inward and toward the end of life. It is at this time that the ancients recommended that the focus of practice be on meditation and prayer.

There are, of course, many examples throughout history of individuals who dedicated their lives to God or self-realization from a very young age. Monks, priests, nuns, and renunciates on different paths have chosen to give

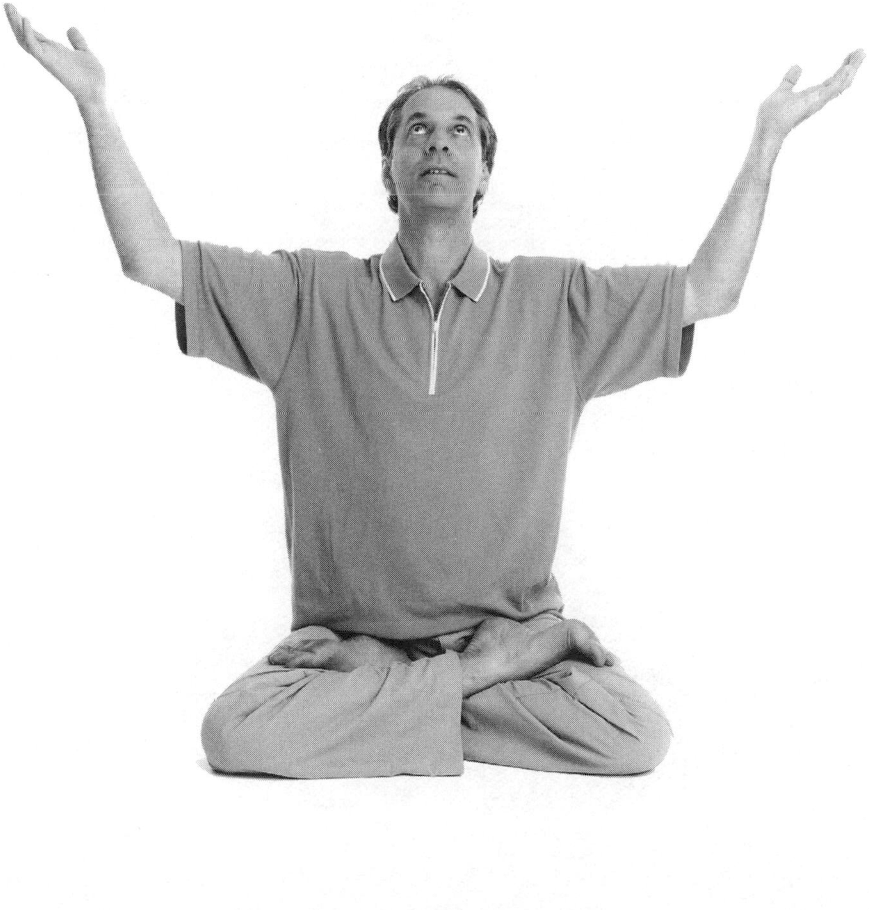

up worldly life at different times in their lives. And there are many secular people who have a deep interest in this approach to practice, balancing their worldly responsibilities with their deep faith in God or their deep interest in self-realization. The choice to orient one's practice in any direction is largely a function of one's own interests.

Known as *adhyātmika* (self-realization), this orientation to practice emphasizes meditation and prayer. There are those of us who have a passion to know, to find the deeper meaning in life. There are others who turn in this direction after an illness or a loss. In either case, there are practical means of developing oneself in this direction that have been developed, refined, and transmitted since ancient times. Examples of these means and methods will be examined further on in this book.

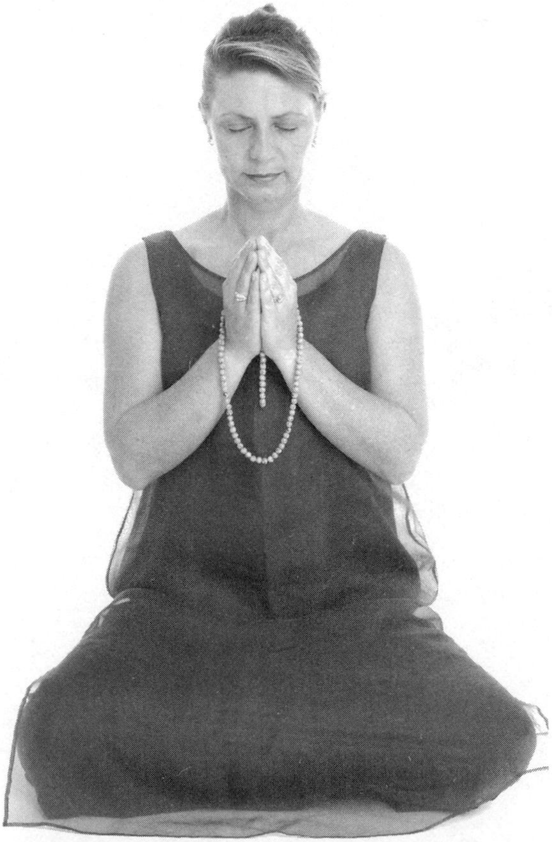

PART II

The Art of Personal Practice

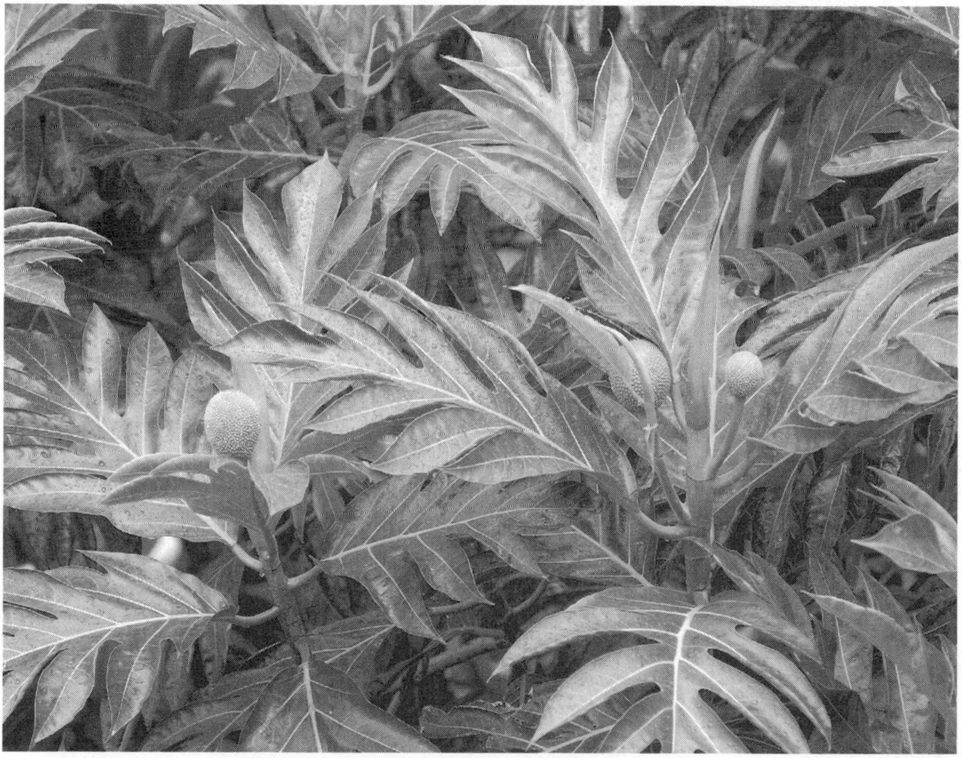

CHAPTER FOUR

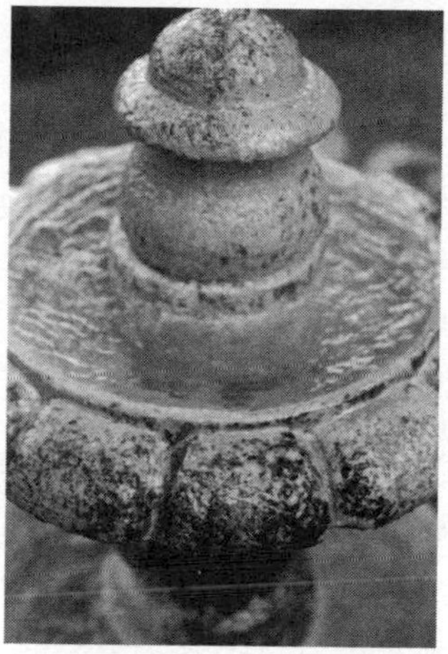

Nourishing the Physical

STABILITY, RELAXATION, AND EXPANSION:
WORKING THROUGH THE BODY
THE *ANNAMAYA* LEVEL

BECOMING AWARE OF OUR BODIES

THE *ANNAMAYA* REPRESENTS our physical body. In our ordinary day-to-day experience, we carry in our systems a level of subliminal stress that depletes our energy and leads to both restlessness and fatigue. The ancients conceived of the science of *āsana* as a tool to benefit this aspect of our human system. *Āsana* practice helps to release that tension and to bring us to a state that is both energized and relaxed. As we have seen, we can take a variety of approaches to the practice of *āsana,* depending on our needs and interests. No matter whether we are taking a developmental, preventative, therapeutic, or transcendental approach to our personal practice, it is important to remember that *āsana* practice is not fundamentally about the *āsana-s,* but about the practitioner. The more we become reflectively self-conscious of our actual condition, the more we will be able to adapt our practices to the needs of our system. Thus, the starting point in any process of self-improvement is increased self-awareness. And, therefore, the tools of personal practice must serve both as a means to increase our self-understanding as well as a means of self-transformation.

As a tool of personal transformation, *āsana* can function at many levels of our human system. At this point in our study, we will restrict our discussion to three aspects of our physical bodies: the skeletal structure, the muscular structure, and neuromuscular patterning.

Awareness of the Skeletal Structure

The skeletal structure consists of the vertical axis of the spine, known as the axial skeleton; and the attached pelvic girdle and legs and shoulder girdle and arms, known as the appendicular skeleton. It includes not only the bony structures but also the ligament tissues, intervertebral discs, and joint capsules.

As we begin our personal practice, a good starting point is to understand the unique condition of our skeletal structure. Because, as this is understood, we can adapt and apply *āsana* to effect desirable change. The following simple exercises will help you begin to see the functional relationship between the three spinal segments and the pelvis. As you become progressively more self-conscious of these relationships, you will be able to identify how and where your body compensates during *āsana* practice, avoiding useful work and reinforcing dysfunctional patterns.

Awareness Exercises

1.

Lie on your back. Take a moment to feel your body on the floor. Notice the points of contact that your body makes with the floor. Feel that:

- your heels touch the floor, your ankles do not
- your calves touch the floor, your knees do not
- your thighs, hips, and part of your sacrum touch the floor
- your lumbar spine rises off the floor
- part of your thoracic spine touches the floor
- your shoulders and arms touch the floor, your neck does not
- your head touches the floor

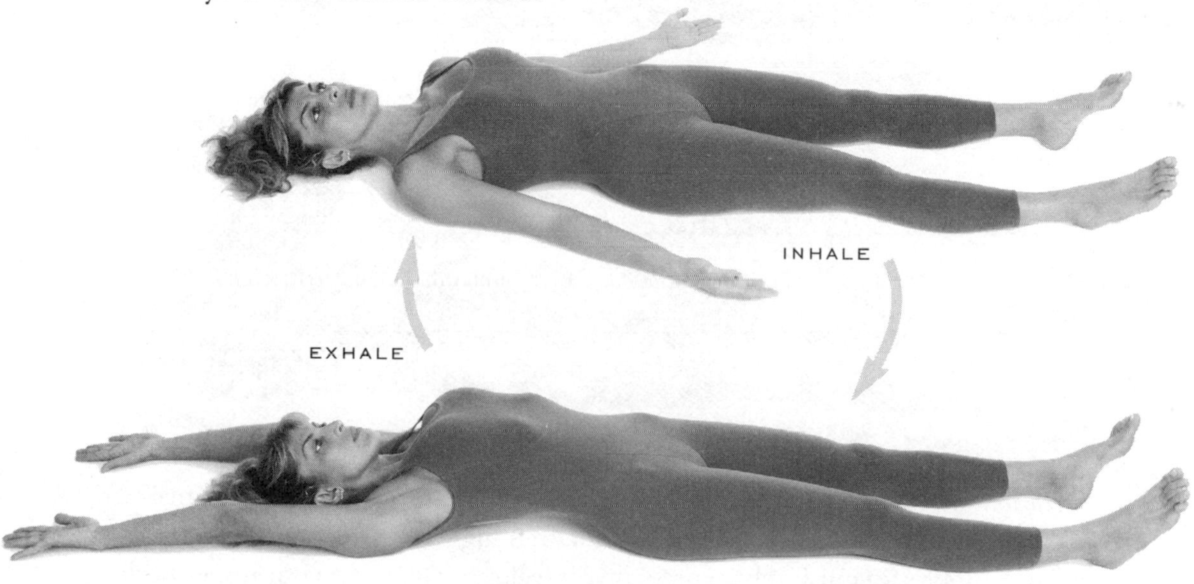

Notice in particular the relationship between your spinal curves and the floor.

On inhale: Raise your arms over your head to the floor behind you. Notice if your lumbar spine arches higher off the floor. Notice if your arms reach all the way to the floor. Notice if the position of your head changes.

On exhale: Return to the starting point. Notice how your spinal curves change their position relative to the floor.

Repeat several times.

2.

Bend your knees, bringing your thighs toward your chest and your feet off the floor. Notice that now your lumbar spine is flattened onto the floor. Notice if there is a change in the position of your head and neck with the knees bent.

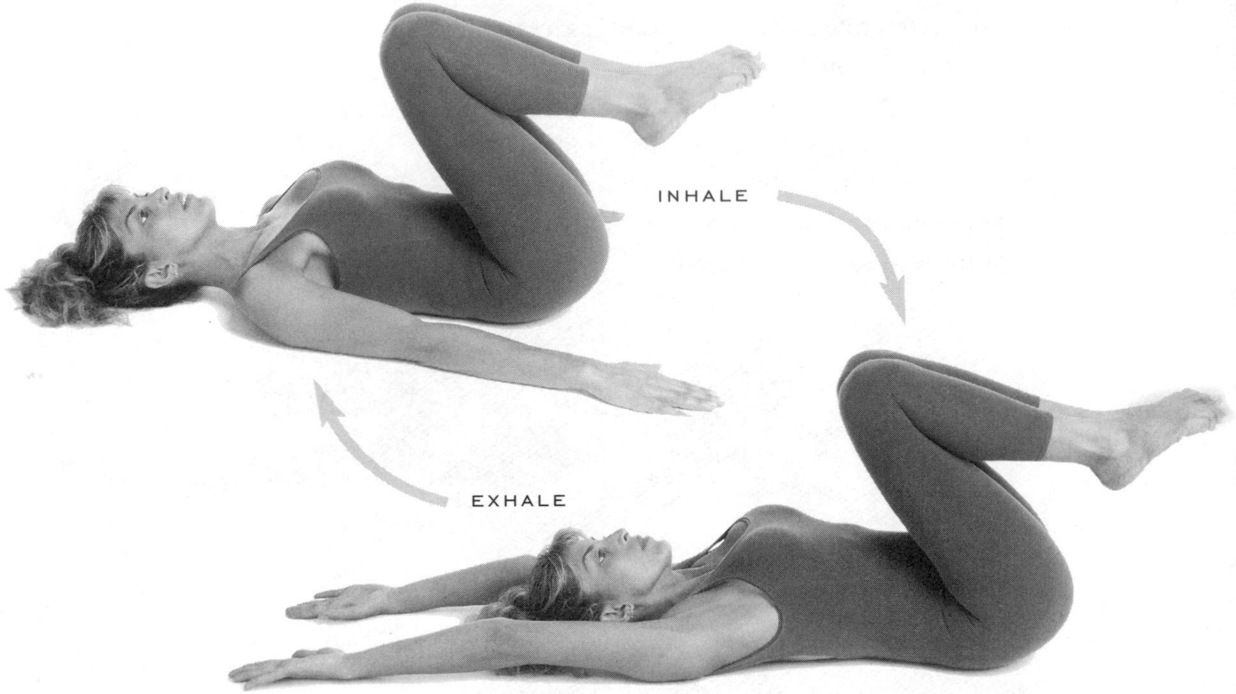

On inhale: Raise your arms over your head to the floor behind you. Notice that now your lumbar spine cannot arch higher off the floor. Notice, as you block your lumbar curve, if you feel more effect in your upper back. Notice if your arms are able to reach as far to the floor as they were when your legs were straight. Notice if the position of your head changes.

On exhale: Return to the starting point. Notice how your spinal curves change their position relative to the floor.

Repeat several times.

3.

Now sit on your heels with your spine straight. Notice how the position of your buttocks on your heels tends to encourage the forward rotation of your pelvis.

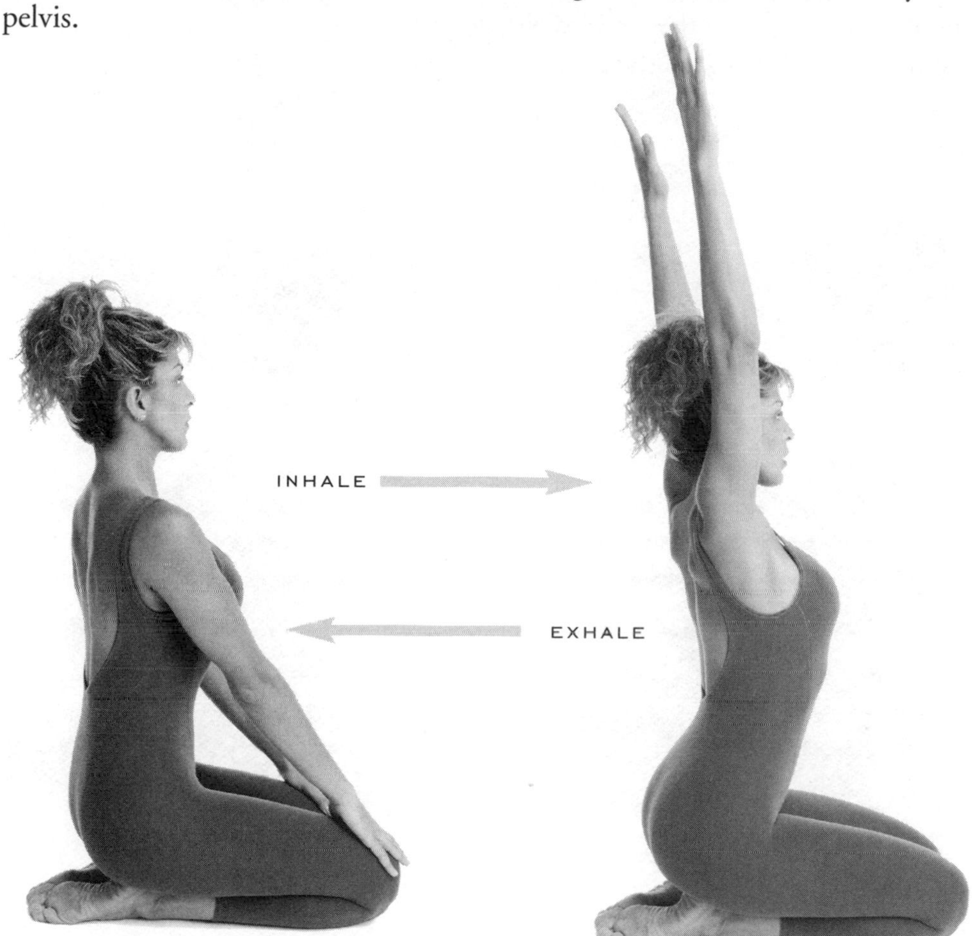

On inhale: Raise your arms over your head and slightly behind your ears as you arch your upper back. Notice as you arch your upper back that your pelvis rotates further forward and your lumbar curve increases.

On exhale: Lower your arms to your knees.

Repeat several times.

4.

Now sit cross-legged, with your spine straight. Notice how the position of your buttocks on the floor slightly inhibits the forward rotation of your pelvis compared to the previous exercise.

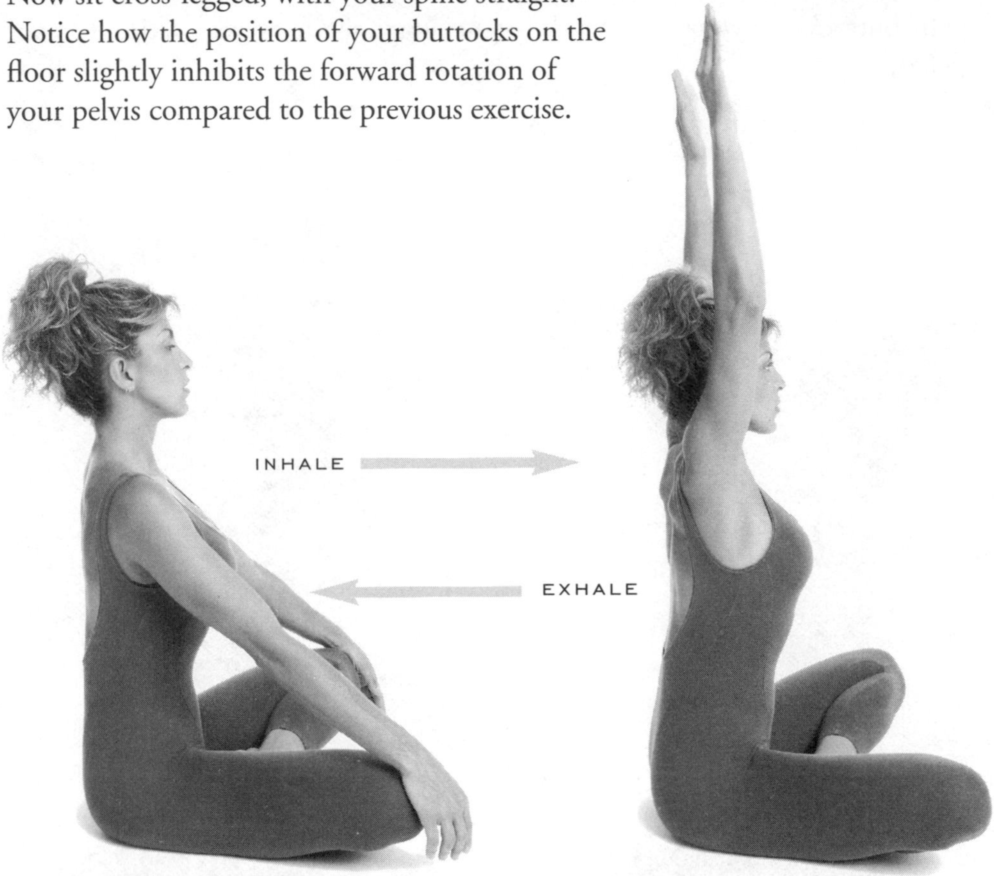

On inhale: Raise your arms over your head and slightly behind your ears as you arch your upper back. Notice, as you attempt to arch your upper back, that the forward rotation of your pelvis, and corresponding increase of the lumbar curve, is more inhibited here than in the previous position.

On exhale: Lower your arms to your knees.

Repeat several times.

5.

Now sit with your legs extended straight in front of you, with your spine straight. Notice that this position further inhibits the forward rotation of your pelvis, and that it is more difficult to keep your spine straight.

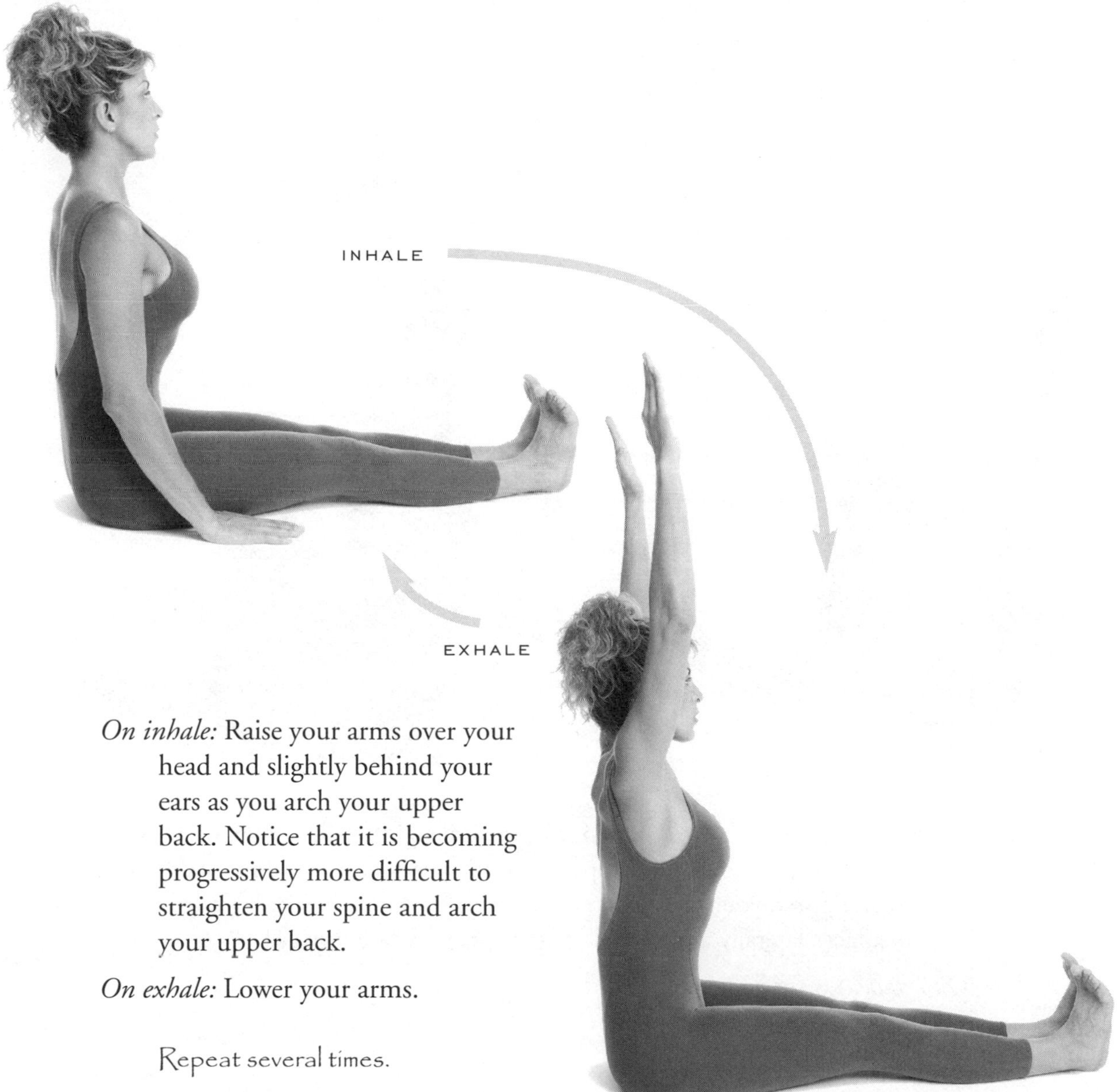

On inhale: Raise your arms over your head and slightly behind your ears as you arch your upper back. Notice that it is becoming progressively more difficult to straighten your spine and arch your upper back.

On exhale: Lower your arms.

Repeat several times.

6.

Now sit with one leg extended in front of you and the other knee bent and pointing straight up, with that heel close to its corresponding sitz bone. Notice that now the pelvis tends to rotate backward, and the chest tends to round forward.

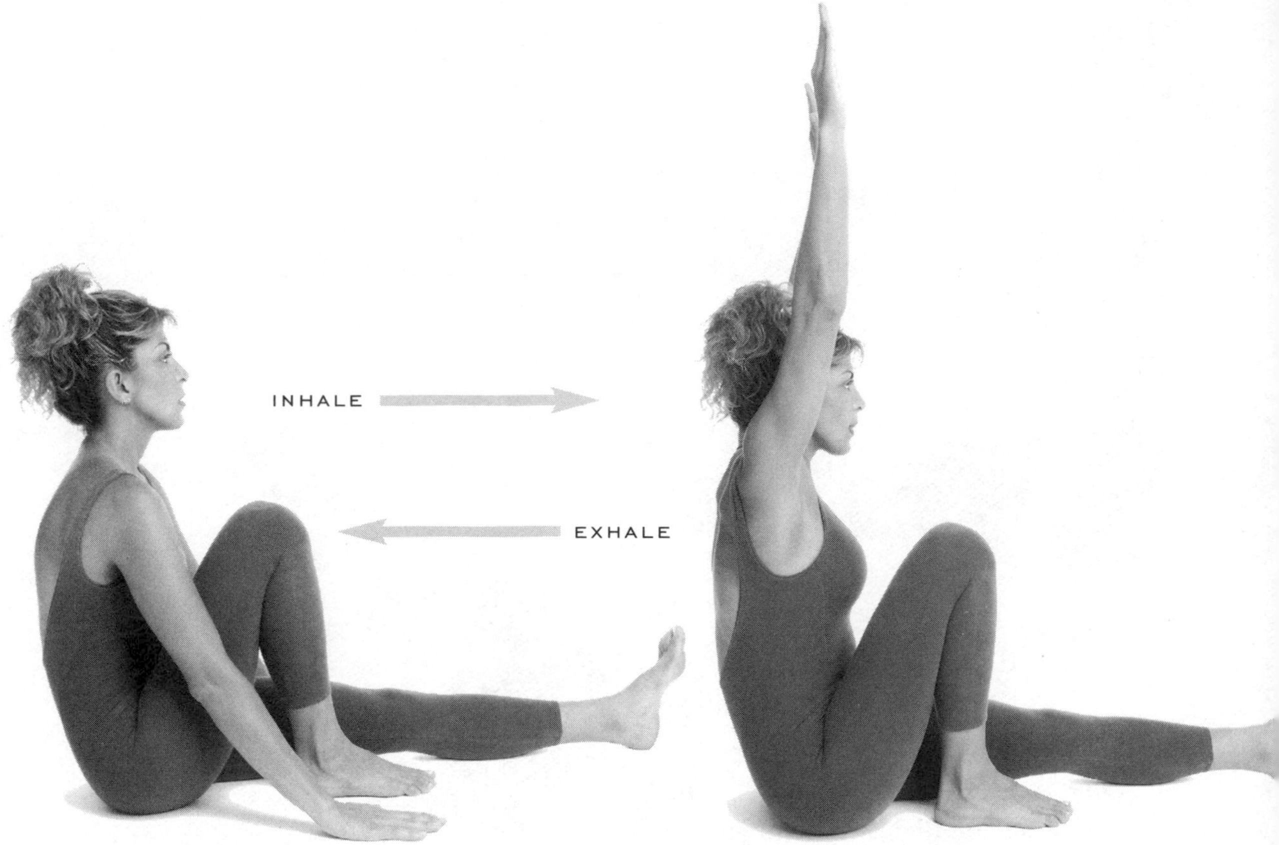

On inhale: Raise your arms over your head and slightly behind your ears as you attempt to arch your upper back. Notice that it is still more difficult to straighten your spine and arch your upper back. Notice if your knee displaces laterally as your pelvis attempts to rotate forward.

On exhale: Lower your arms.

Repeat several times.

7.

Now sit with both knees bent and together, and your heels by their respective sitz bones. Notice that it is practically impossible for you to sit straight. Notice that the tendency for your pelvis to rotate backward is more pronounced than in the previous position, and that it is even more difficult to straighten your spine.

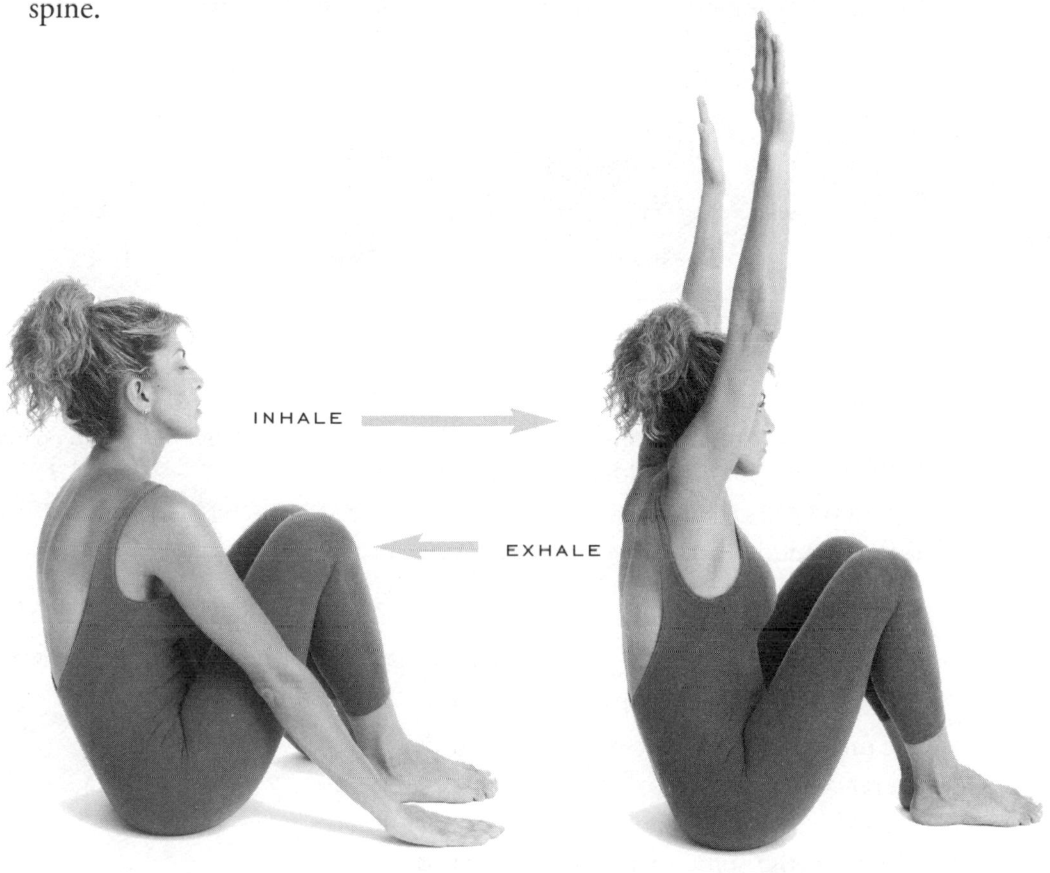

On inhale: Raise your arms over your head and slightly behind your ears as you attempt to arch your upper back. Notice that it is yet again more difficult to straighten your spine and arch your upper back. Notice if your knees widen as your pelvis attempts to rotate forward.

On exhale: Lower your arms.

Repeat several times.

Noticing the Alignment of Our Spine

Now let's consider the vertical axis of the spine in relation to the limbs (axial skeleton in relation to the appendicular skeleton) and, in particular, the relative alignment of the spine.

In the following positions, try to sense the degree of lateral displacement (see below).

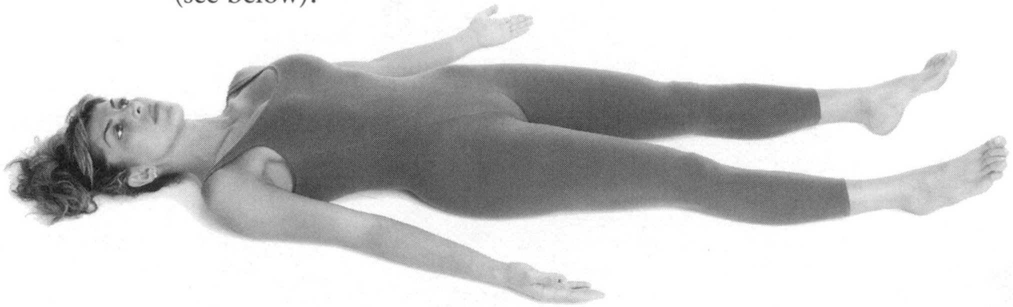

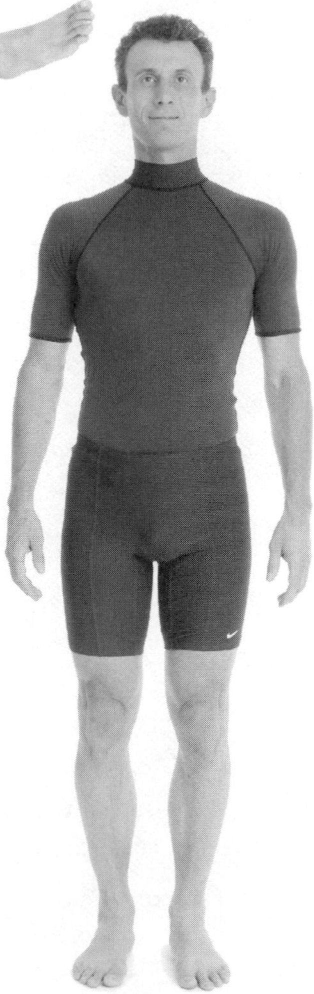

- While lying on your back, notice if one leg or arm seems longer than the other.
- Does one hip or shoulder seem higher than the other?
- Stand and look at yourself in a full-length mirror. Is there symmetry in your shoulders and hips?
- Look to see if any apparent asymmetry can be linked to the spine itself, or if it appears to come from the pelvic or shoulder girdles. Lateral displacement of the axial skeleton in known as scoliosis. This condition can originate in the spine or be causally linked to imbalances in the pelvic girdle and legs, or even in the shoulder girdle and arms. Try to notice if apparent imbalances in your hips are linked to apparent imbalances in your shoulders.

It is important to become progressively more self-conscious of your condition, so that the *āsana* practice you develop will serve you.

Noticing the Condition of Our Joints

Now let's look at the condition of your joints and, in particular, the condition of your ligaments. Range of motion at the joint is largely a function of the ligament, and the ligamentous condition is largely congenital. Some children, for example, tend to be very flexible while others tend to be stiff. The polarity is hypermobility and rigidity. The hypermobile joint can be stabilized to a certain extent, and the rigid joint can be mobilized to some extent. However, the possibilities for ligamentous change are limited, so it is important to understand your own condition.

Unfortunately, many people in the growing Yoga community consider increased flexibility to be the measure of progress in Yoga. However, at one extreme, there are those with congenitally shortened ligaments, who will never achieve certain postures, whose self-esteem has been negatively impacted by this idea. And, at the other extreme, there are those who are hypermobile, but who continue to do postures that, while satisfying their image of good *āsana* practice, reinforce this condition.

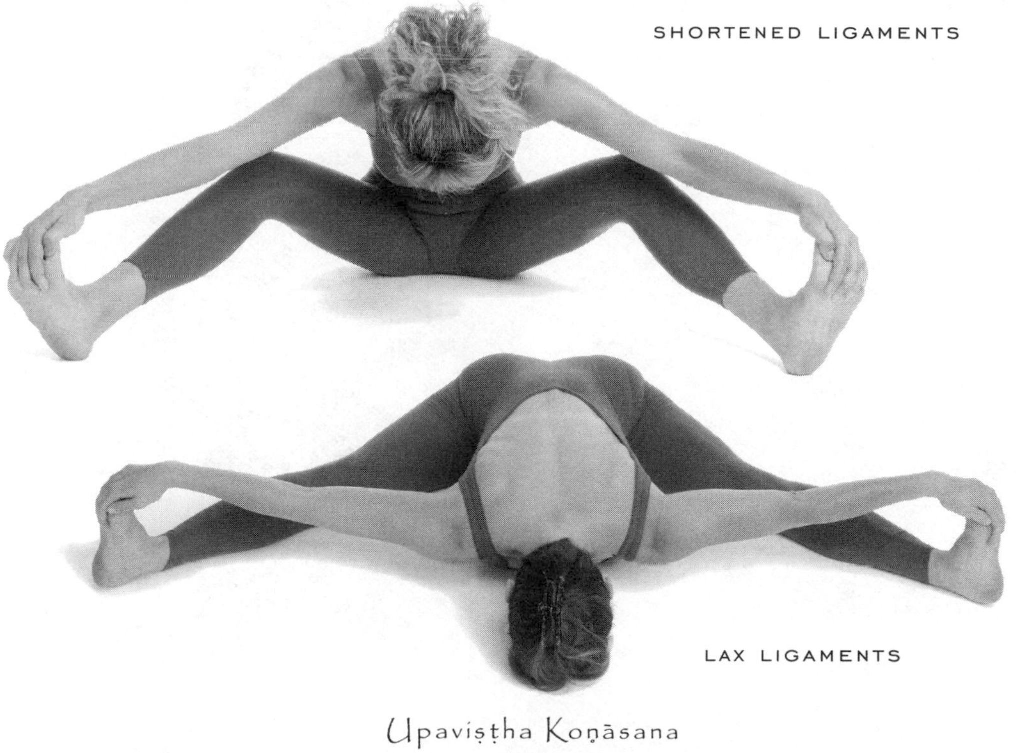

SHORTENED LIGAMENTS

LAX LIGAMENTS

Upaviṣṭha Koṇāsana

In addition, the condition of our ligaments may not be consistent throughout our body. We can have, for example, lax ligaments in our hips and relatively short spinal ligaments. Most people will find that they have certain kinds of postures that they can move into with relative ease and others that are extremely challenging. Again, it is important to understand where the limitation comes from.

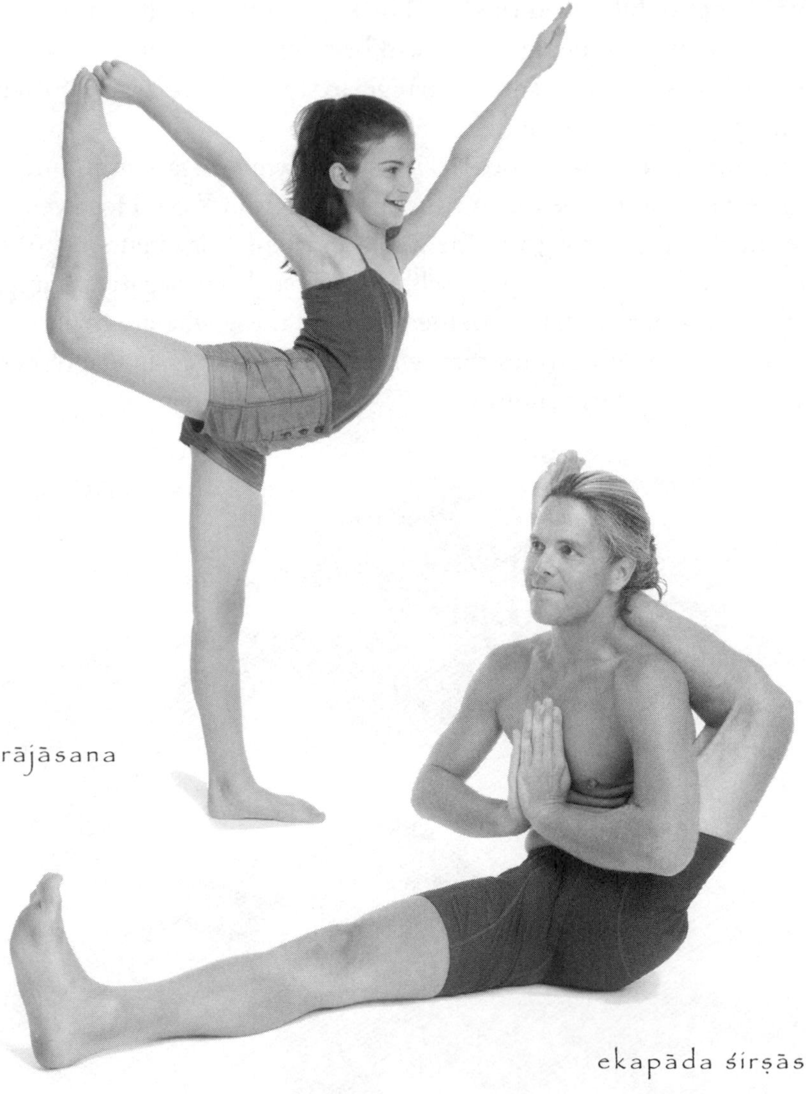

Naṭarājāsana

ekapāda śirṣāsana

Awareness of the Muscular Structure

The next area to consider is the musculature. The muscle is a relatively simple tissue. Basically, it is either in a state of contraction or in a state of relaxation. A muscle can contract in three ways: concentric, eccentric, and isometric. In addition, it can be passively stretched when it is antagonist to an opposing muscle in a state of contraction. In our practice we want to develop core muscles by utilizing all three methods of contraction as well as by stretching. As we will see later, this way of working the muscles is built into our methodology of practice. At this point it is important to consider the general and particular condition of our muscles. Are the muscles chronically tight and contracted, are they weak and lacking tone, or are they strong and yet relaxed when not at work? As with ligaments, the condition of the muscles will vary in different parts of the body. So it is important to recognize these differences.

It is also important to identify the primary muscles we wish to develop through our practice. In this approach to *āsana,* we will emphasize those fundamental muscles that help maintain the integrity of the spine. These include the erector spinae, the abdominal rectus, the iliopsoas group, and the rhomboids.

And, finally, it is important to examine the symmetric development of the muscle groups. If there is a degree of skeletal asymmetry, there is likely to be a corresponding asymmetry in the musculature.

FRONT

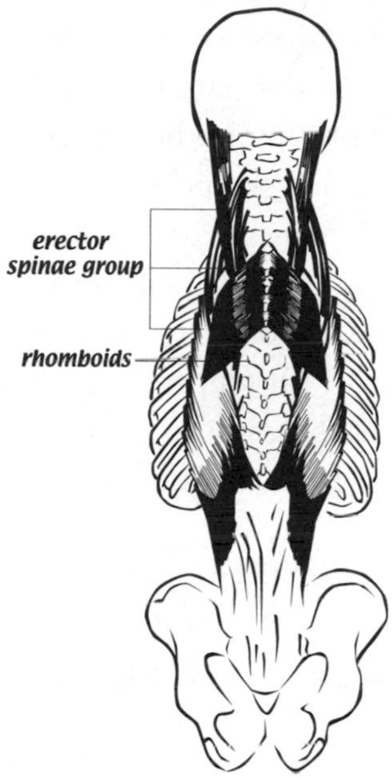

BACK

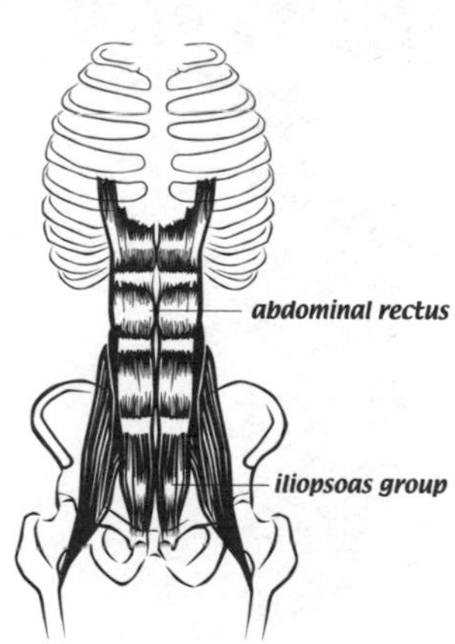

Awareness of Neuromuscular Patterning

The last aspect we will consider for now is the phenomenon of neuromuscular patterning. We want to become reflectively self-conscious of our movement patterns and how they may contribute to structural stress. Patterns can be seen in the way we hold our head, the way we use our arms, and the way in which the pelvis rotates around the transverse axis between our hips.

Movement patterns translate into release valves or avoidance mechanisms. When you bend forward, for example, what is the proportional relationship between forward hip rotation and the transformation of the lumbar curve? Of course, if your hips are very loose and your back stiff, there will be more hip rotation. This proportional relationship, however, may have more to do with a movement pattern than a structural condition. It is interesting to begin to identify these movement patterns and to see which derive from actual structural limitations and which result from habit or poor training. Common patterns to look for when forward bending include hip rotation, the use of the head, and the collapse of the chest over the belly.

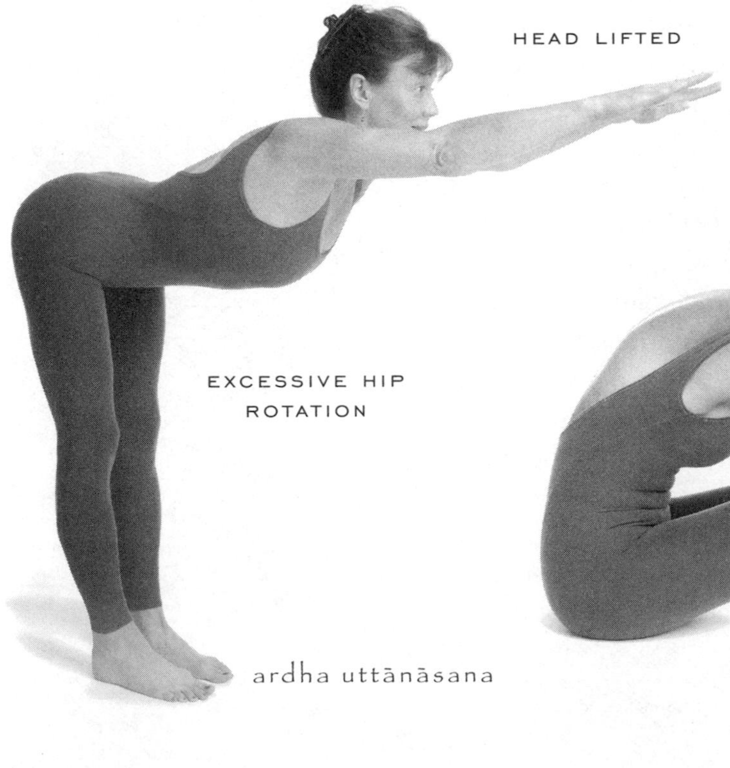

ardha uttānāsana

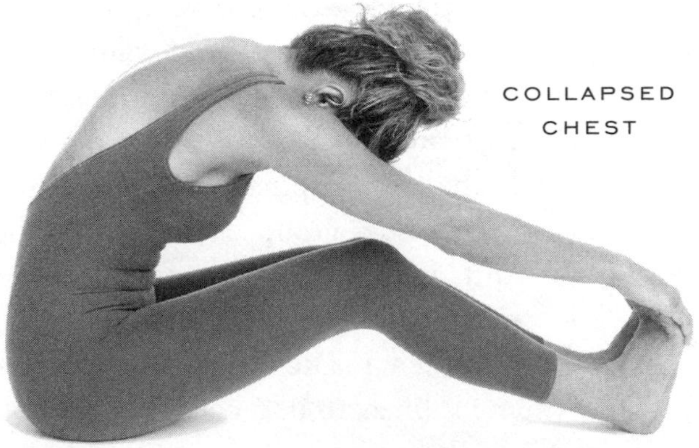

paścimatānāsana

EXPLORING *ĀSANA* IN PERSONAL PRACTICE

As we begin to understand more about our structure, we can begin to adapt *āsana* practice so that it serves our particular needs or interests. The first step is to determine what our particular goals in practice will be.

The orientation to and goals for our *āsana* practice will influence the way we practice. From a purely structural point of view, specific goals can include increasing our ability to practice difficult postures, perform preventative maintenance in order to protect our structure from injury, or provide relief for acute or chronic conditions. *Āsana* can also be used to prepare for *prāṇāyāma* (breathing exercises) and meditation. In each of these different scenarios, the nature of the *āsana* practice will differ. A traditional view is that *āsana* practice has a major role to play in maintaining balance (*samakāya*) in the body, and that it can and ultimately should relate to and engage every part of the body (*sarvāṅga sādhana*). I say "ultimately" here because it may not be necessary, or even possible, to relate to every part of the body every day. You may have enough time to do an extensive *āsana* practice each day. Many of us, however, are too busy to dedicate that much time to our practice. In that case, we might create a series of four or five shorter practices that can be rotated over a period of one or two weeks, thus ensuring that all parts of our bodies are engaged.

When ready to begin our practice, we ask ourselves:

- Which *āsana* to pick
- How to do postures
- How to adapt postures
- How to breathe in postures
- How to combine postures

Which *Āsana* to Pick

Out of the vast number of possible postures to practice, how do we determine which *āsana-s* are the ones for our practice? This is, of course, a large topic of study. The following list represents the traditional way in which *āsana-s* were categorized and chosen. If you want to explore all of the different types of *āsana* and their primary purpose in practice, I refer you to my first book, *Yoga for Wellness.*

PŪRVATĀNA

This category represents all back-bending *āsana-s*. These postures are particularly useful when there are conditions of increased thoracic curve, tightness in the front of the torso, and when there's a need to expand the chest—for example, to deepen the capacity for inhalation, and to energize the system.

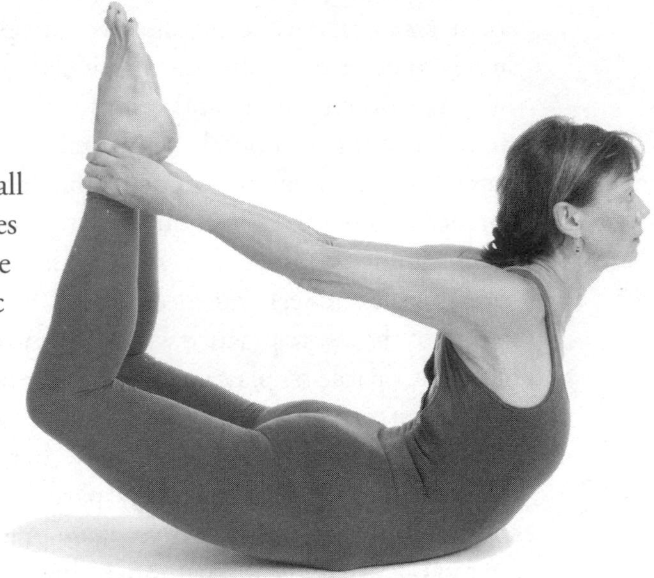

dhanurāsana

PAŚCIMATĀNA

This category represents all forward-bending *āsana-s*. These postures are particularly useful when there are conditions of increased lumbar curve or tightness in the back, when there's a need to compress the belly in order to enhance digestion and elimination, or when there is a need to calm the system.

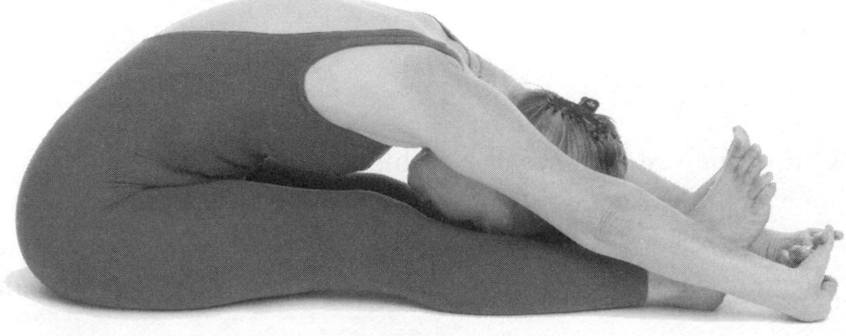

paścimatānāsana

PARIVṚTTI

This category represents all twisting postures. These postures are particularly useful when there are conditions of scoliosis, asymmetries in the body, tightness in the shoulder or pelvic girdles, and when digestion and absorption need to be stimulated.

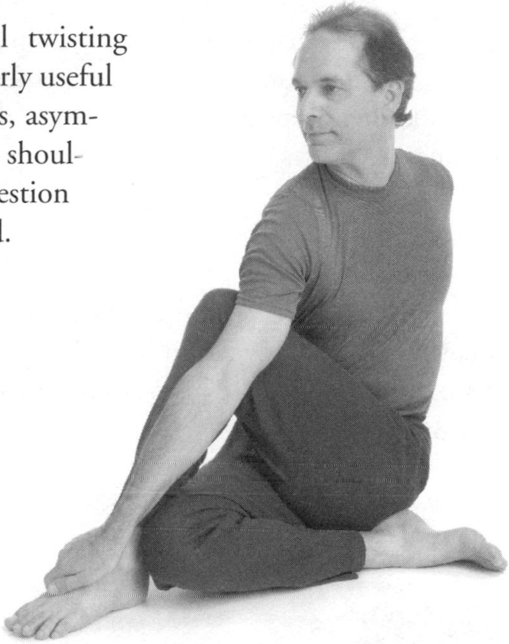

bhāradvājāsana

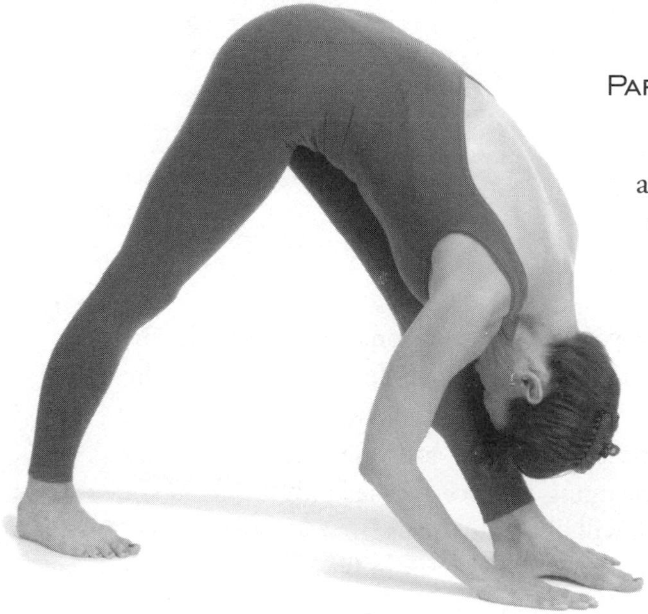

PARŚVA

This category represents all asymmetric and lateral bending postures. Like *parivṛtti* postures, these postures are also useful when there are conditions of scoliosis, asymmetries in the body, tightness in the shoulder or pelvic girdles, and when the metabolic function is in need of stimulation.

pārśvottānāsana

VIPARĪTA

This category represents all inverted postures. These postures are useful for strengthening the spinal musculature, deepening the respiratory rhythms, and reversing the effects of gravity on our systems.

VIŚEṢA

This category represents all unusual postures. They are particularly useful in building a sense of confidence, strengthening the body, and increasing concentration.

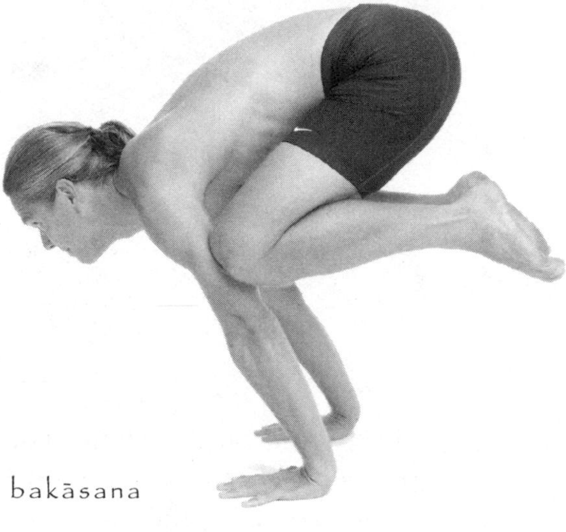

bakāsana

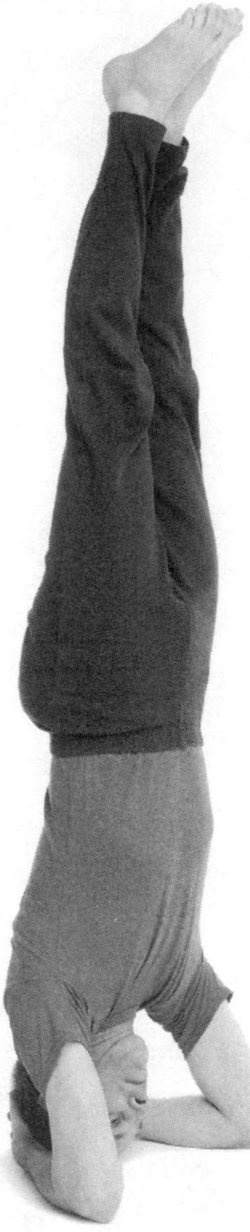

śirṣāsana

No matter the particularities of your goals in personal practice, it is important that, at the minimum, you select postures that help you to increase the strength and flexibility of your spine. The section at the end of this chapter is designed to give you an example of a practice that addresses the whole body (*sarvāṅga*) and is oriented toward bringing balance to the body (*samakāya*). Practices that appear later in the book will illustrate the use of *āsana* in the service of the other dimensions of practice and will therefore be more limited in scope.

How to Do Postures

There is a general notion that the way to do an *āsana* is to bring the body into the configuration of the posture and to stay there and work, through subtle muscular actions, to perfect the form of the postures. In our view, there are two fundamentally different ways we should work postures: through repetition and by holding.

Repetition involves actively moving the frame of the body into and out of postures from their neutral starting point. This action of repetition is considered to be the most effective way of effecting musculoskeletal transformation. Repetitive movement tends to increase circulation and to promote elimination. It is a means of facilitating neuromuscular reeducation. And this way of doing postures is also useful for overcoming heaviness of body and mind, known by the ancients as *tamasic* energy.

The second way to do postures is to achieve the form of the postures and then, while holding the external frame of the body still, to work the posture through the deep action of inhalation and exhalation. This way of doing postures is classically used to promote inner purification. These postures are also useful for overcoming the agitation of the mind and body, known by the ancients as *rajasic* energy.

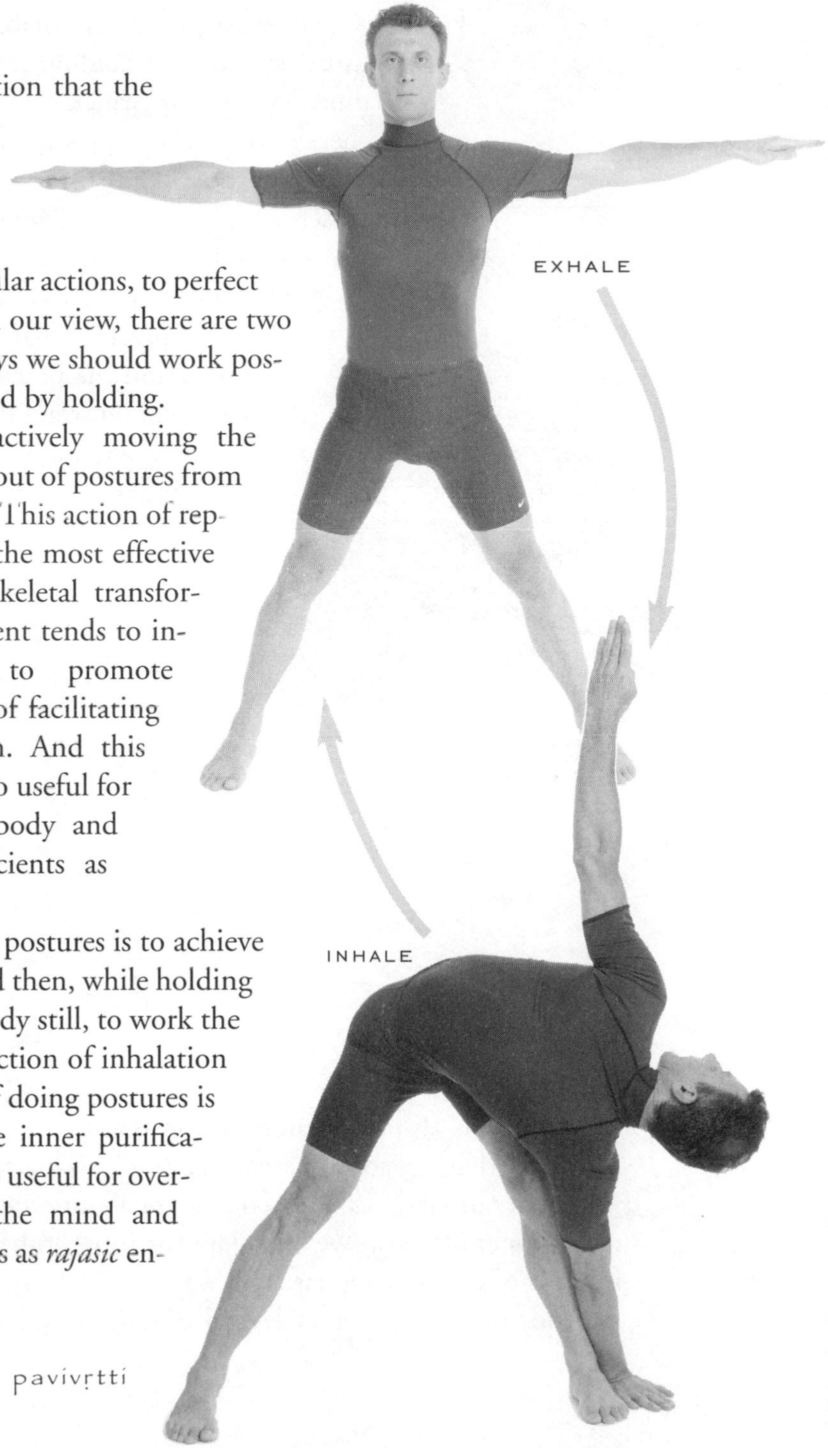

utthita trikoṇāsana pavivṛtti

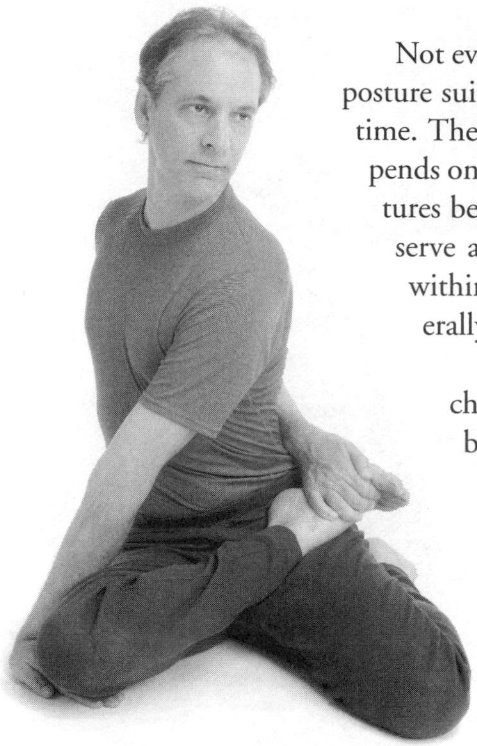

Bhāradvājāsana

Not every posture is suitable for repetition, nor is every posture suitable for holding statically for longer periods of time. The way in which you choose to do a posture depends on the role it plays within the sequence. Some postures become the main focus of a practice, while others serve a preparatory, compensatory, or traditional role within the practice. These secondary postures are generally done repetitively rather than statically.

The practice that follows at the end of this chapter, and the practices that appear later in the book, will illustrate the appropriate use of repetition into and out of postures as well as the static holding of postures.

How to Adapt Postures

There is also a common notion that each posture has a correct classical form and that the goal of *āsana* practice is to master the form of each posture. Again, in our view, *āsana* practice is not about *āsana,* but, rather, it is about the practitioner of *āsana*. We can adapt the form of the posture to suit the needs or interest of the practitioner. The way in which the posture should be adapted depends on the answer to several questions: What is the role of the posture

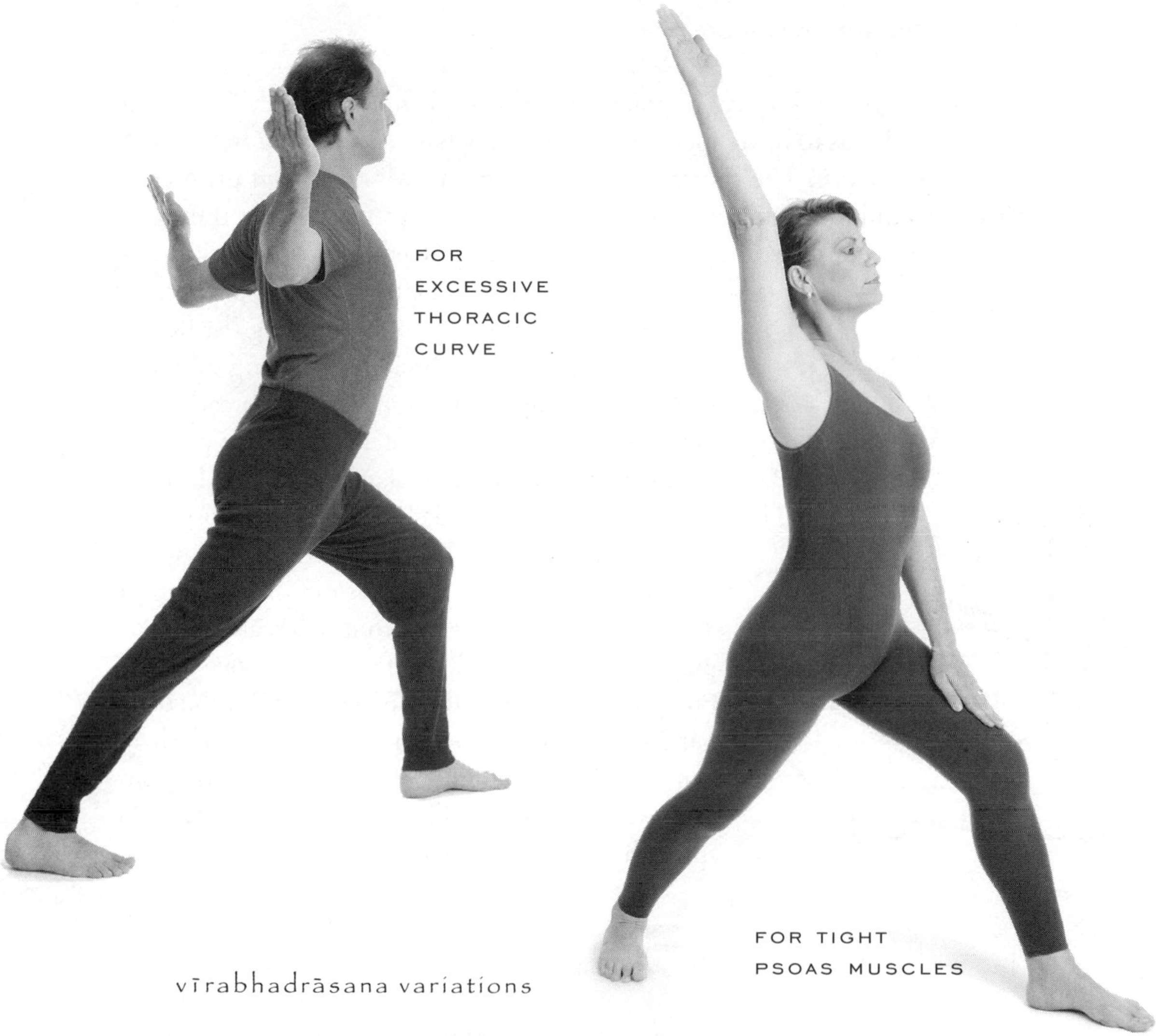

FOR EXCESSIVE THORACIC CURVE

FOR TIGHT PSOAS MUSCLES

vīrabhadrāsana variations

within the overall sequence? What is the overall purpose of the practice? Is it meant to prepare you for *prāṇāyāma* (breathing exercises), to help you with some structural problem, or is there some other intention? The same posture can be done in multiple ways, each producing a slightly different effect. The practice that follows, and the practices that appear later in the book, will illustrate the art of adaptation.

How to Breathe in Postures

In this approach to *āsana* practice, the breath is fundamental. The breath is what enables us to bring focused attention to what is happening in our bodies during practice. The breath has two important roles in *āsana* practice: it helps us to link our attention to the spine and it helps us to move the spine. The ancients considered the breath to be like a steed, which consciousness mounts and rides into the body during practice.

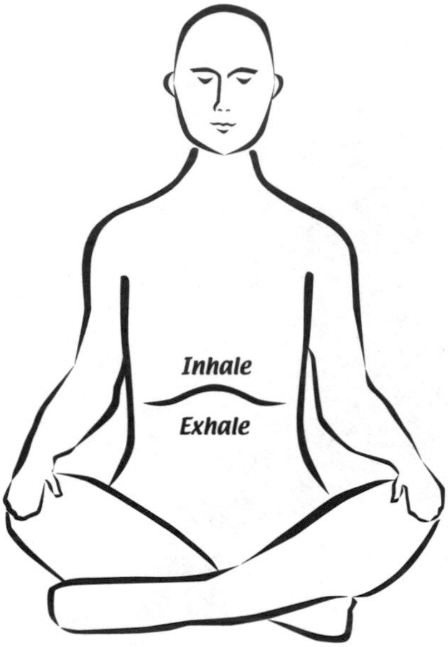

There are many ways of controlling the flow of inhale and exhale in conscious breathing exercises. A detailed analysis of these ways of breathing is presented in the next chapter. For *āsana* practice, according to our view, inhalation is adapted to emphasize the spine. The technique that is most effective in straightening the spine and improving the posture involves chest expansion on inhalation. Therefore, unless otherwise contraindicated, we emphasize expanding the area of the chest above the diaphragm during inhalation. Exhalation, on the other hand, is adapted to emphasize keeping the belly firm and the pelvic lumbar spine stable. And, therefore, we emphasize pulling the belly in toward the spine throughout exhalation.

How to Combine Postures

The key to setting up a personal practice is the ability to combine all the different elements of your practice into an integrated whole. The topic of combination, or sequencing, is about all of the elements of your personal practice, not simply the *āsana* aspect. The integration of *āsana* with the other dimensions of practice will be illustrated in the practices that appear later in this book. The discussion here will be restricted to the topic of *āsana* per se.

There are two general categories to consider in the selection of postures: the direction of movement with respect to the spine and the position in which these directions can be accomplished. In relation to the first category—the direction of movement with respect to the spine—there are five fundamental groupings of postures: forward-bending, backward-bending, twisting, lateral-bending, and axial extension postures. The second category—the position in which these directions can be accomplished—includes standing, kneeling, supine, inverted, prone, seated, and lying on the side.

Direction of Movement with Respect to the Spine:

In sequence-building, there are a few basic principles to follow. Regarding the directions of movement, consider the following drawing:

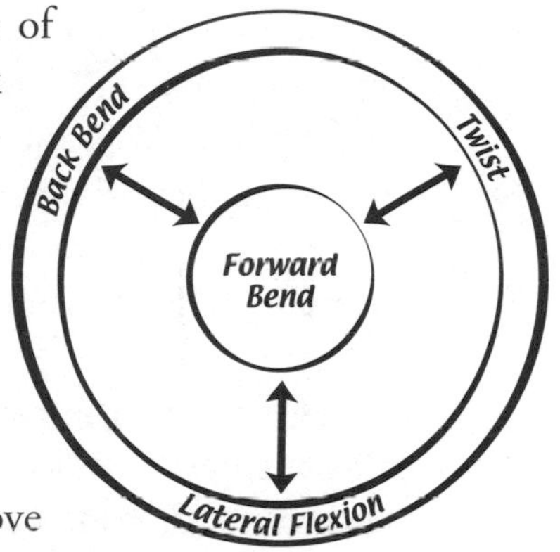

Forward-bending can be understood as the hub of the wheel, or, perhaps more practically, you can think of forward-bending as the neutral of an automobile's standard shift transmission. We must go through neutral when we want to transition from forward to reverse. In a similar way, we use forward-bending as neutral when we want to transition between, for example, backward-bending and twisting.

As we proceed into a practice sequence, we must respect the need to gradually prepare the body to move from ordinary to unusual positions in order to maximize our ability to achieve particular postures and to minimize risk to the body. This idea of preparation is know as *vinyāsa*. In addition, we must respect the need to compensate for any stress created by the postures we use in our practice. This idea of compensation is known as *pratikriyā*.

Using Various Positions in Sequencing:

The other aspect of sequence-building involves the use of the various positions, and movement from one position to another. For example, standing postures are generally most effective for warming up the body because they involve large movements and engage the large muscle groups in our bodies. Kneeling postures, on the other hand, are often used to transition from standing to either supine or prone postures. Supine postures generally require less effort and are more relaxing, though they can be adapted to do specific work on the legs and hips.

Inverted postures—although very much out of the ordinary and requiring a good deal of preparation and compensation—are considered to be an important part of *āsana* practice because of their ability to reverse some of the effects of gravity on our bodies. Prone postures involve backward-bending and are therefore strong and useful. And seated postures, where there is a certain amount of inevitable stress in the lower back, are usually done at the end of the practice to be sure we have adequate preparation. Seated postures also serve as preparation for seated breathing and meditation exercises. Finally, it is important to take adequate rest at the end of an *āsana* practice. And the best position for that is lying supine on the back.

Whatever the orientation to practice, we must integrate the above principles to develop our *āsana* practice. If the orientation is fundamentally developmental, we will work toward mastering a full range of *āsana-s,* moving progressively from the simple to the complex. Our emphasis will be to stretch and strengthen all the muscles of the body, to stabilize the joints, to increase the range of motion, to improve structural alignment, and to enhance structural integrity. If the orientation is preventative, however, certain postures may also be contraindicated.

Of course, the value of *āsana* practice exceeds its structural benefits. In the next chapter we will see how *āsana* practice can be adapted to serve our constitutional needs and to support the work done in *prāṇāyāma.*

THE DEEPER SYMBOLISM OF ĀSANA

Discussing *āsana* from a structural perspective might give the impression that *āsana* is fundamentally an ancient system of physical culture. It is important to emphasize that the ancients regarded *āsana* from a much deeper perspective, as an integral part of a complex and profound science of personal transformation.

In order to appreciate the depth of this system, let's consider some of its fundamental symbolism.

In their esoteric anatomy, the ancients conceived of a system of channels within the body, known as *nāḍī-s,* as well as a series of reference points, known as *cakra-s.*

We will consider the details of the *nāḍī* and *cakra* symbolism in Chapters 5 and 6, respectively. At this point, we will briefly consider the role of *āsana* relative to these symbols. According to this model, all *cakra-s* are located in the center of the main channel, known as the *suṣumnā,* which is located in the center of the body and supported by the spine. In an ideal situation, the flow of energy (*prāṇa*) through the channels (*nāḍī-s*) is balanced and unobstructed, and all of the *cakra-s* are placed exactly where they should be. In actuality, however, this is usually not the case. And when the flow of energy through the channels is out of balance or obstructed, and the *cakra-s* are displaced from their proper locations, our systems are out of balance and afflictions arise.

The ancients conceived of *āsana* as an aid to spinal alignment (*rekhā*)—a way of balancing and enhancing the flow of energy through the channels; of moving the *cakra-s,* at their gross level, into their proper place (*sthāna*); and of reestablishing their correct relationship to each other. They also saw it as a way to help maintain balance in some of the other systems of the body that will be discussed later in the book.

ANNAMAYA PRACTICE

The following sequence represents a practice that will meet both of the classic goals of *āsana* practice: to maintain the balance of the body (*samakāya*) and to engage all of its parts (*sarvāṅga sādhana*). The headstand posture that is present in this sequence is very challenging, and we recommend practicing it only after being initiated by a qualified teacher. Practitioners may delete the headstand, posture #8, and practice the rest of the sequence as shown below. Alternately, for a shorter course, practice postures #1–#5, skip postures #6–#9, and then practice postures #10–#16.

1.

POSTURE: *Tāḍāsana*

EMPHASIS:

To encourage balance.
To extend the spine.
To strengthen calves and feet.

TECHNIQUE: Stand with arms at side, feet parallel.

On inhale: Raise up on toes while simultaneously raising arms up over head, fingers interlocked, palms up.
Stay in position one breath longer with each successive repetition, from one to four breaths.

On exhale: Return to starting point.

Number: Four times.

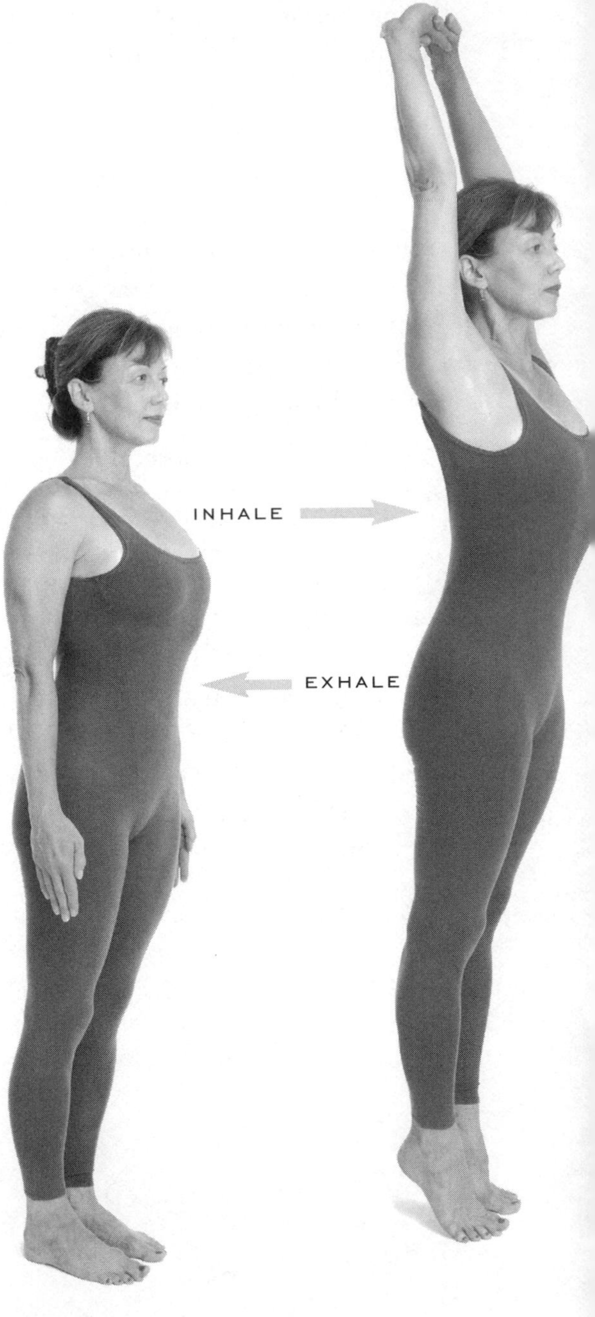

DETAILS:

On inhale: Slightly arch back and lift head.

On exhale: Slightly flatten lower back, chin down.

2.

POSTURE: *Parśvottanāsana*

EMPHASIS:

To stretch and strengthen muscles of back and legs.

TECHNIQUE: Stand with left foot forward, right foot turned slightly outward, feet as wide as hips, and arms over head.

On exhale: Bend forward, flexing left knee, bringing chest toward left thigh, and bringing hands to either side of left foot. *Stay in position one breath longer with each successive repetition, from one to four breaths.*

On inhale: Return to starting position.

Number: Four times each side.

DETAILS: Stay stable on back heel and keep shoulders level throughout movement.

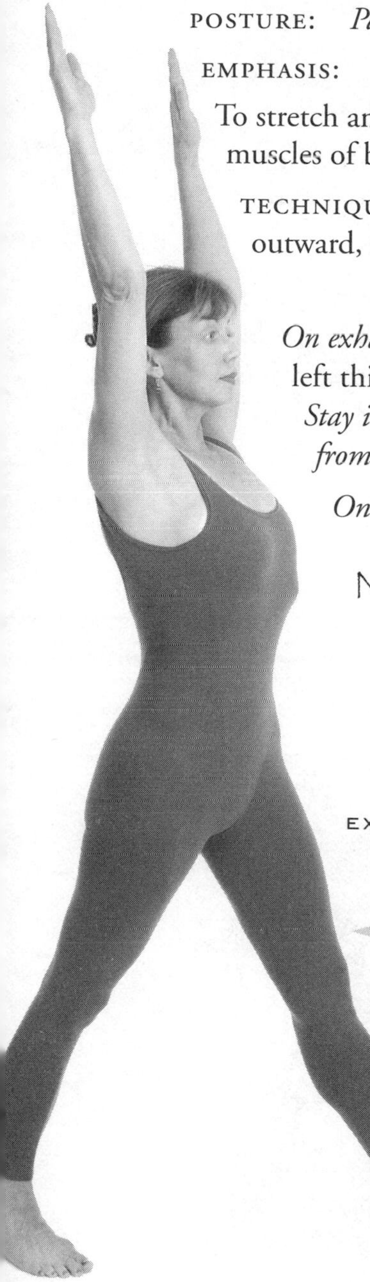

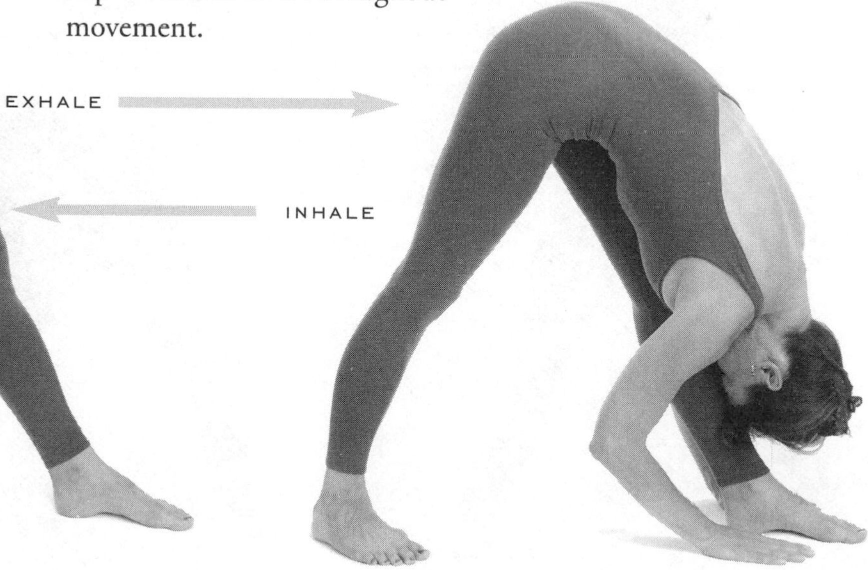

3.

POSTURE: *Utthita Trikoṇāsana*

EMPHASIS: To laterally stretch torso and rib cage.

TECHNIQUE:

A: Stand with feet spread wider than shoulders, left foot turned out at ninety-degree angle to left foot, left arm over head, and right arm straight down at waist, which is slightly rotated externally.

On exhale: Keeping shoulders in same plane as hips, bend laterally, lowering left shoulder and bringing left hand below left knee while turn ing head up toward right hand.

On inhale: Return to starting position.

Repeat.

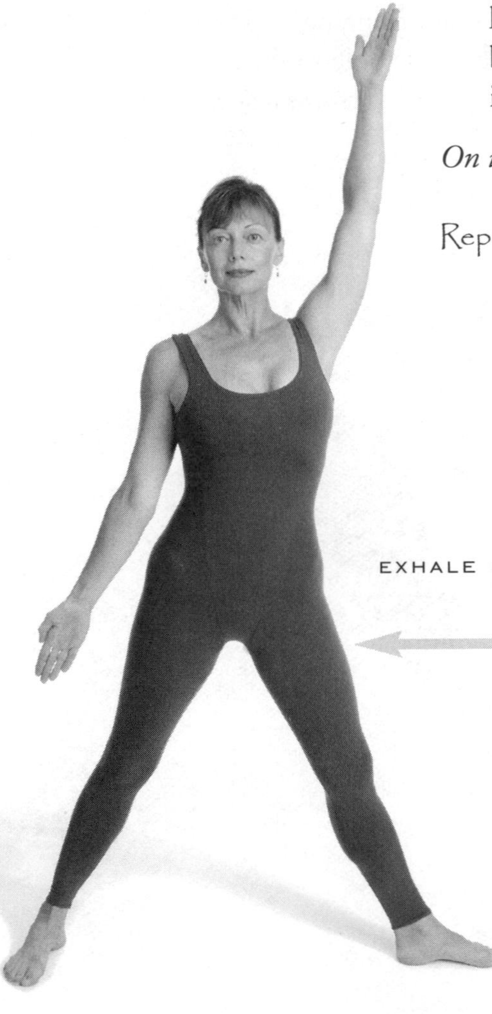

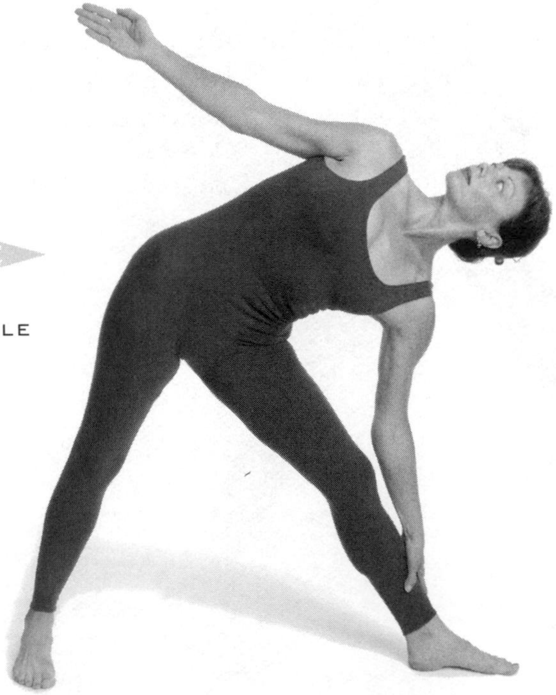

B: With left hand down along left leg:

On inhale: Bring right arm up and forward while turning head forward toward right hand.

On exhale: Return right hand to starting position while turning head up toward right hand.

Repeat.

Number: Repeat A and B four times each on each side, one side at a time.

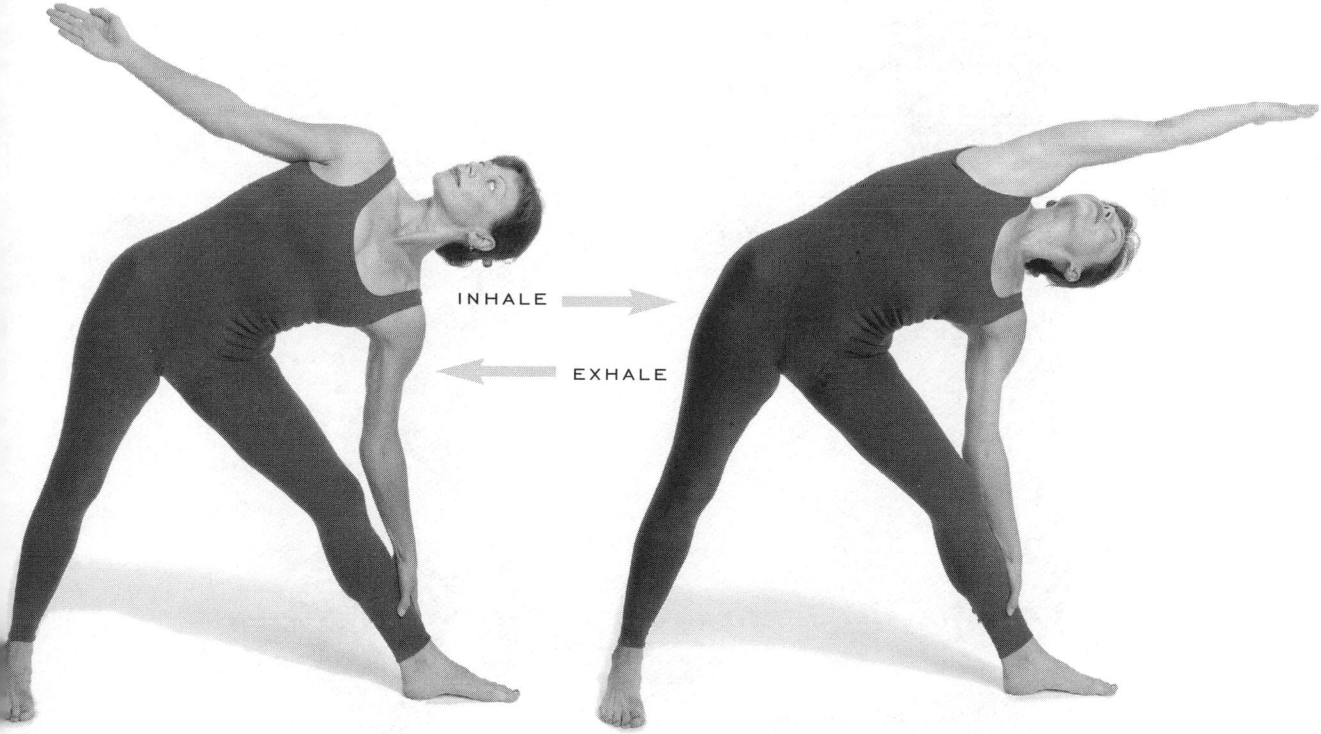

4.

POSTURE: *Uttānāsana/Pādahastāsana*

EMPHASIS: To stretch back symmetrically.

TECHNIQUE:

A: Stand with feet slightly apart, arms over head.

On exhale: Bend forward, bending knees slightly, bringing chest to thighs, and palms to sides of feet.

On inhale: Return to starting position.

Repeat

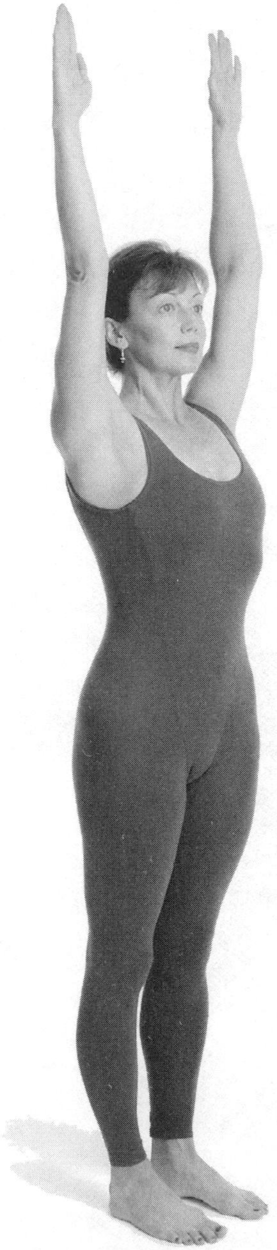

EXHALE

INHALE

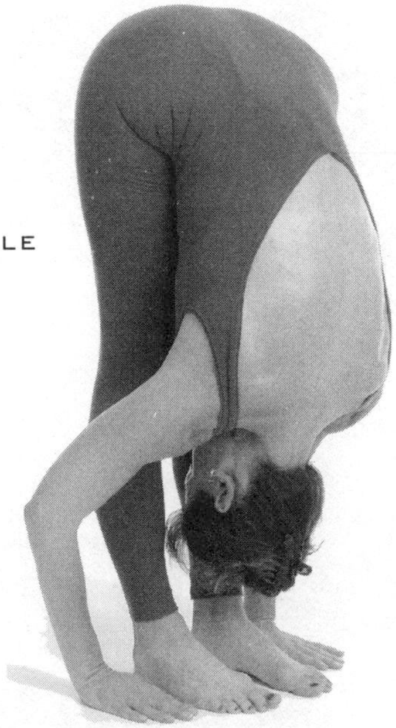

B: From the *uttānāsana* position, place fingers under balls of feet.

On inhale: Lift chest up and away from thighs, flattening upper back.

On exhale: Return to starting position.

Number: Repeat A and B four times each.

DETAILS:

On exhale: Bend knees to facilitate stretching lower back, and bring belly and chest to thighs. Move chin down toward throat.

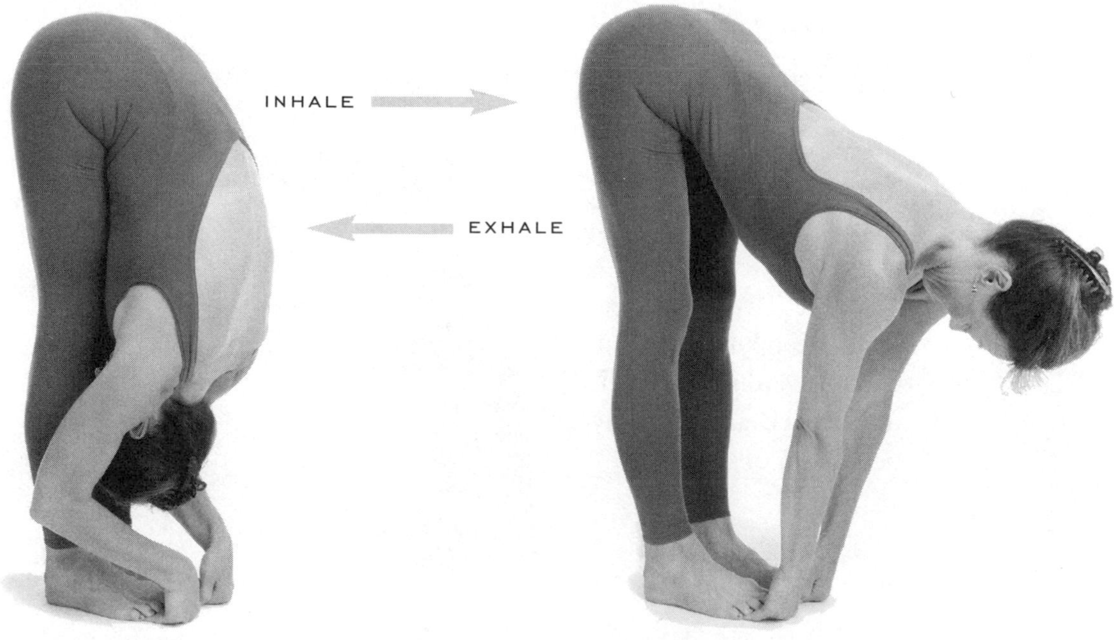

5.

POSTURE: *Adho Mukha Śvānāsana*

EMPHASIS: To extend upper back.
To stretch shoulders.
To transition from standing to supine position.
To prepare for inversion.

TECHNIQUE:
Stand on hands and knees.

On exhale: Push buttocks upward, lifting knees off ground, and pushing chest toward feet.
Stay in position one breath longer with each successive repetition, from one to four breaths.

On inhale: Return to starting position.

Number: Four times.

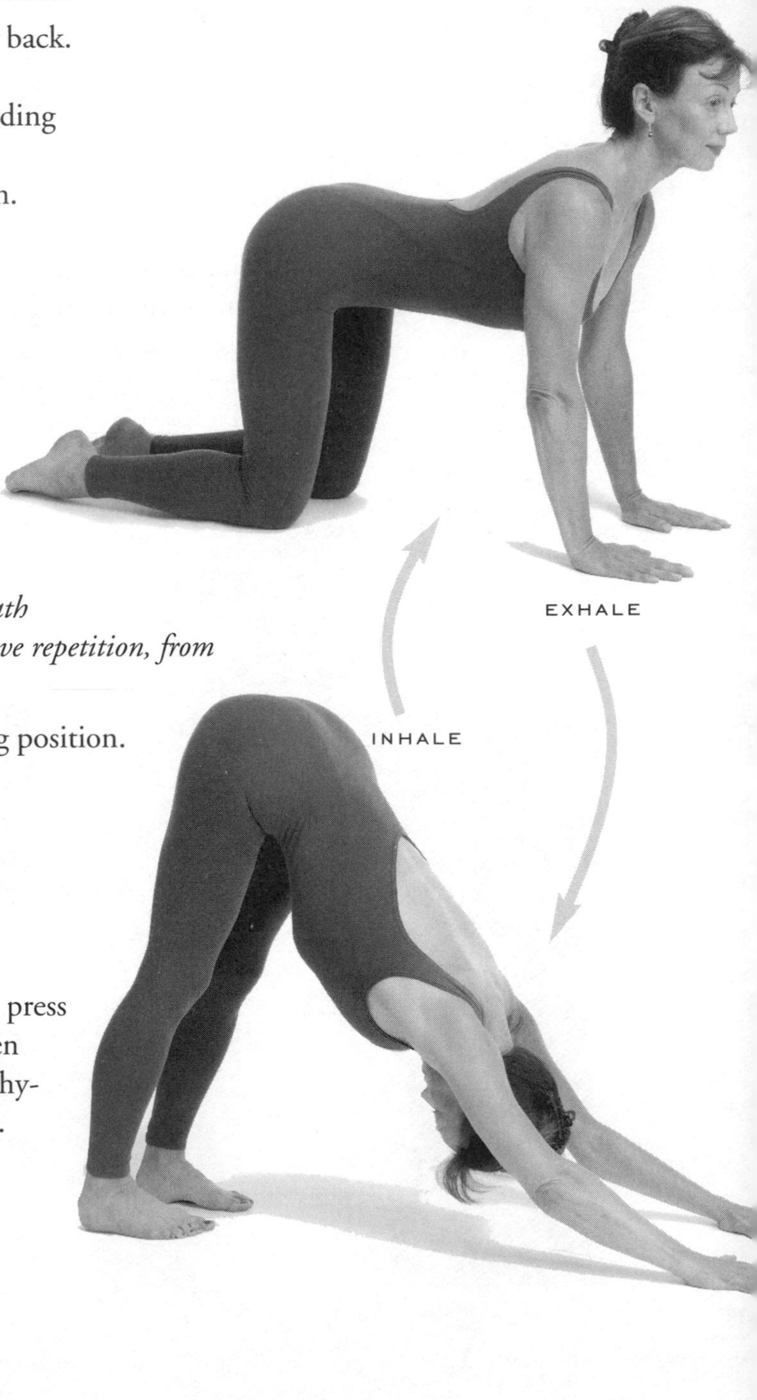

DETAILS:

On exhale: Keep knees bent, press chest toward feet, flatten upper back, and avoid hyperflexion of shoulders.

6.

POSTURE: *Dvipāda Pīṭham*

EMPHASIS: To stretch upper back and neck in preparation for headstand.

TECHNIQUE: Lie on back with arms down at sides, knees bent, and feet on floor, slightly apart and comfortably close to buttocks.

On inhale: Pressing down on feet and keeping chin down, raise pelvis until neck is gently flattened on floor, while raising arms up over head to floor behind.

Stay in position one breath longer with each successive repetition, from one to four breaths.

On exhale: Return to starting position.

Number: Four times.

DETAILS:

On inhale: Lift spine, vertebra by vertebra, from bottom up.

On exhale: Unwind spine, coming down vertebra by vertebra.

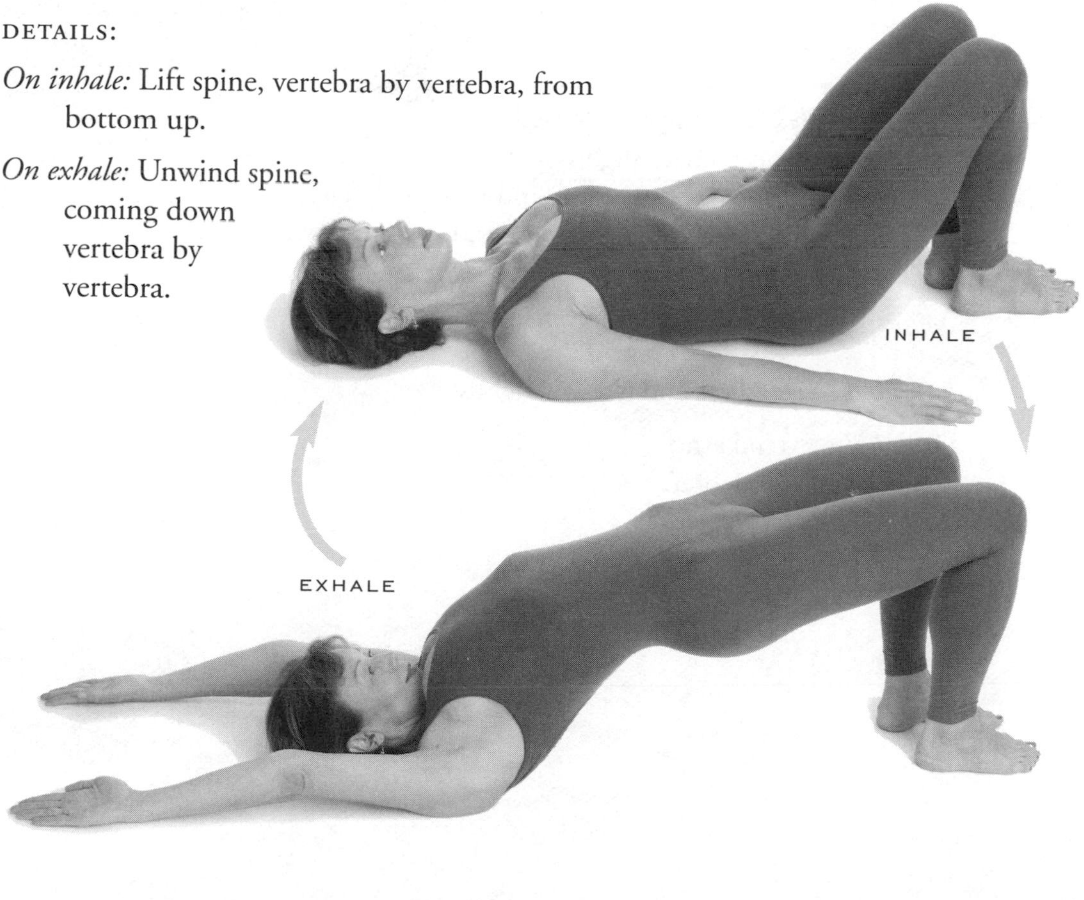

7.

POSTURE: *Ūrdhva Prasṛta Pādāsana*

EMPHASIS: To extend spine and flatten it onto floor.
To stretch legs.
To prepare for inversion.

TECHNIQUE: Lie on back with arms down at sides, legs bent, and knees lifted toward chest.

On inhale: Raise arms upward all the way to floor behind head, and legs upward toward ceiling.
Stay in position one breath longer with each successive repetition, from one to four breaths.

On exhale: Return to starting position.

Number: Four times.

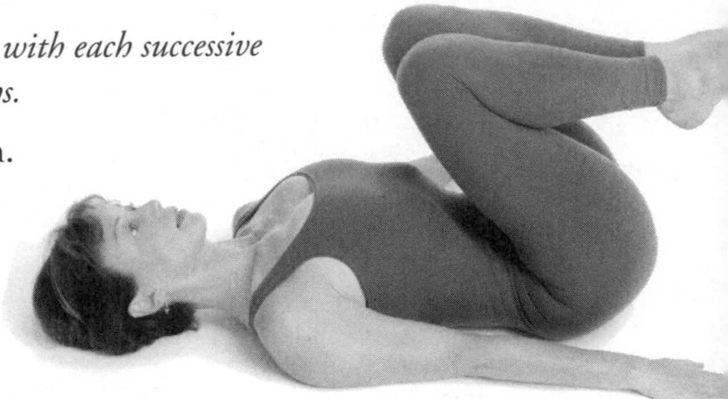

DETAILS:

On inhale: Flex feet as legs are raised upward. Keep knees slightly bent, and keep angle between legs and torso less than ninety degrees. Push lower back and sacrum downward. Bring chin down.

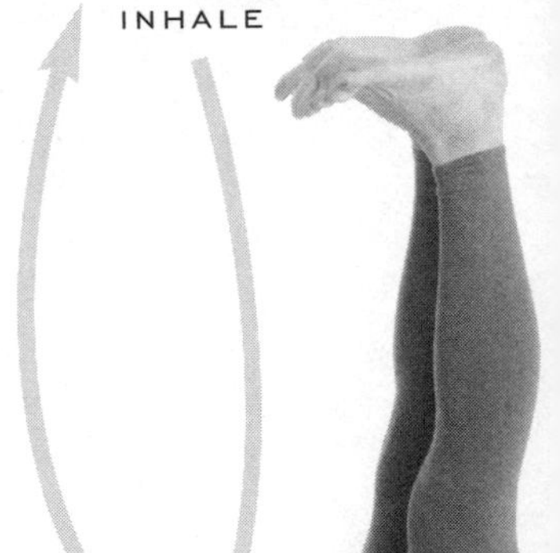

While staying in position:

On exhale: Flex knees and elbows slightly.

On inhale: Extend arms and legs straighter.

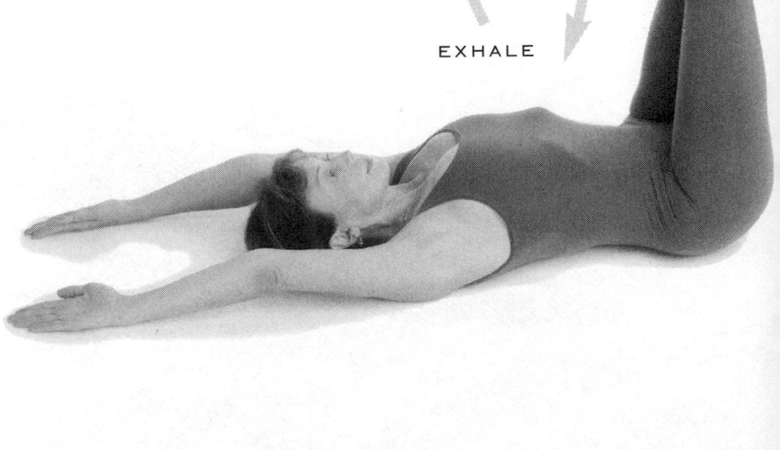

8.

POSTURE: *Śirṣāsana* (practice with caution)

EMPHASIS: To strengthen spinal musculature.
To deepen respiratory rhythms.
To reverse effects of gravity.

TECHNIQUE: From hands and knees, interlock fingers with elbows, forearm's length apart. Cupping head in hands, stand on toes, lifting knees off floor. Walk forward with toes until hips are vertically above shoulders.

On inhale: Lift legs to vertical position.
Stay sixteen breaths.

On exhale: Return to starting position.
Rest for a few moments.

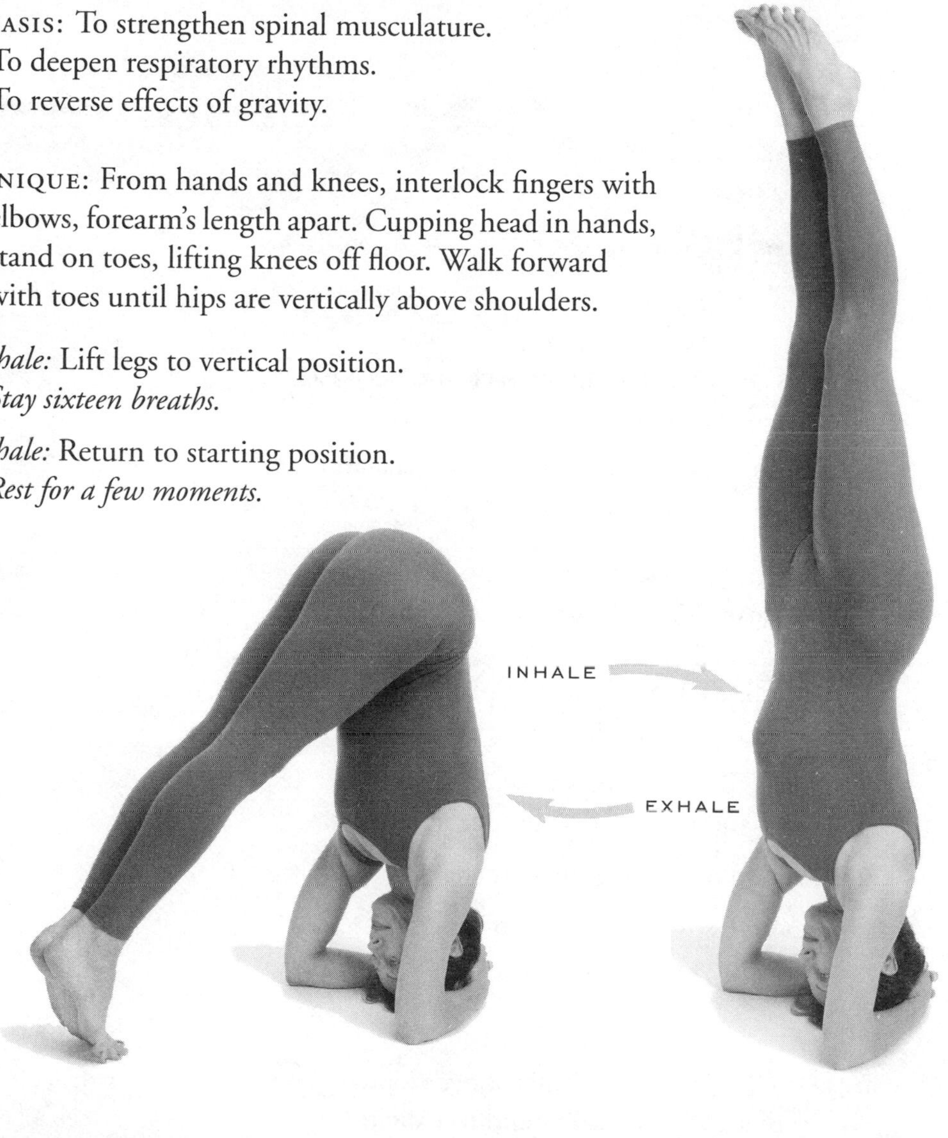

DETAILS: Position should be comfortable. If there is neck stress, come down. Focus on long and smooth inhalation and exhalation, of approximately equal length.

9.

POSTURE: *Sarvāṅgāsana*

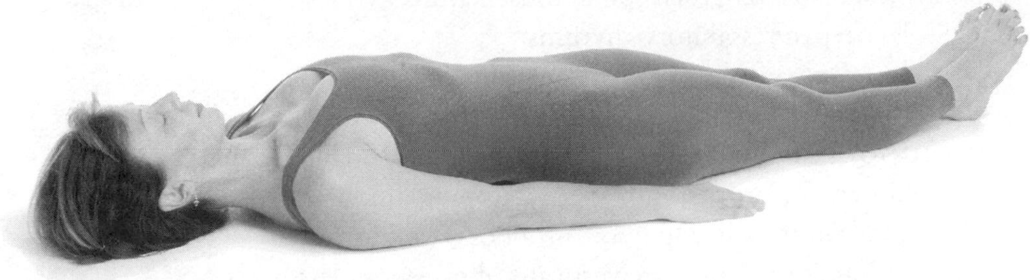

EMPHASIS: To stretch upper back and neck to counter effects of headstand.

Combination: To strengthen musculature of lower back. To deepen inversion effect.

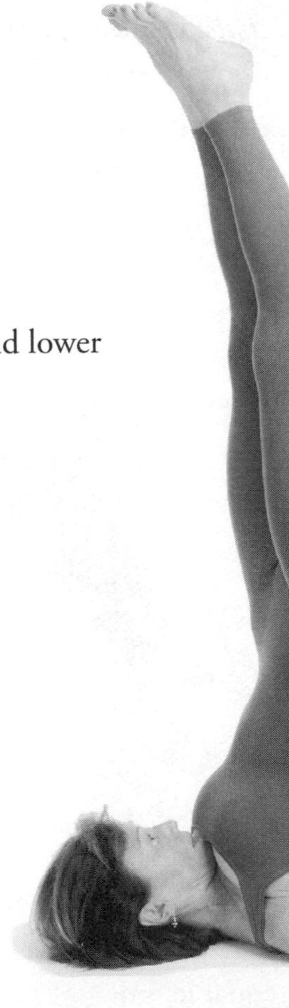

TECHNIQUE: Lie on back.

On exhale: Flip legs up over head, lifting buttocks and lower to midback off floor, and placing palms on middle of back.

On inhale: Raise legs upward.
Stay and breathe deeply sixteen breaths.

On exhale: Lower knees toward chest.

On inhale: Return to starting position.
Rest for a few moments.

DETAILS: Place hips vertically above elbows, rather than shoulders, and feet slightly beyond head. Focus on long and smooth inhalation and exhalation, of approximately equal length.

10.

POSTURE: *Bhujaṅgāsana*

EMPHASIS: To arch upper back and neck while mobilizing arms, as a counterpose to shoulderstand.

TECHNIQUE: Lie on belly, forehead on floor, with arms behind back, hands crossed over sacrum, and palms up.

On inhale: Lift chest, sweeping arms wide and forward.

On exhale: Return to starting position.

Number: Eight times.

DETAILS:

On inhale: Lead with chest, and let arms and head follow. Lift chin slightly at end of inhale.

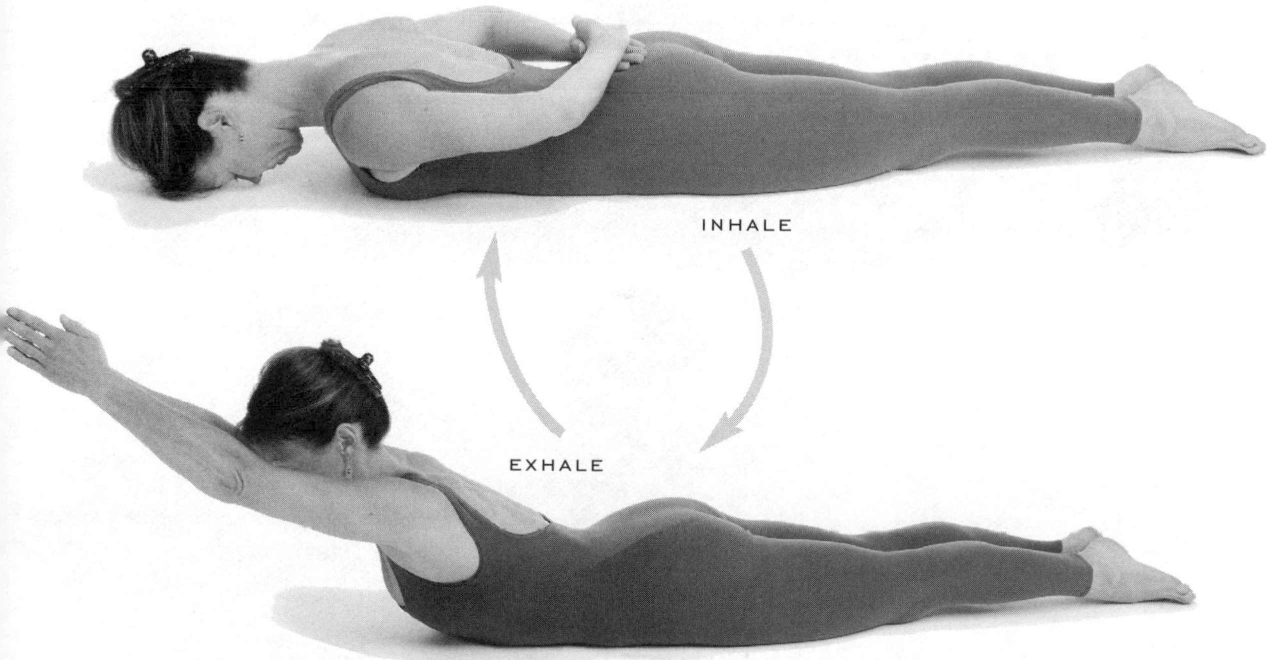

11.

POSTURE: *Dhanurāsana*

EMPHASIS: To expand chest, stretch front of torso, flatten upper back, and strengthen back and legs.

TECHNIQUE: Lie on stomach, resting on forehead, with knees bent and hands grasping ankles.

On inhale: Simultaneously press feet behind you, pull shoulders back, lift chest, and lift knees off ground.
Stay in position one breath longer with each successive repetition, from one to four breaths.

On exhale: Return to starting position.

Number: Four times.

DETAILS: While staying in position, lift chest slightly higher on inhale.

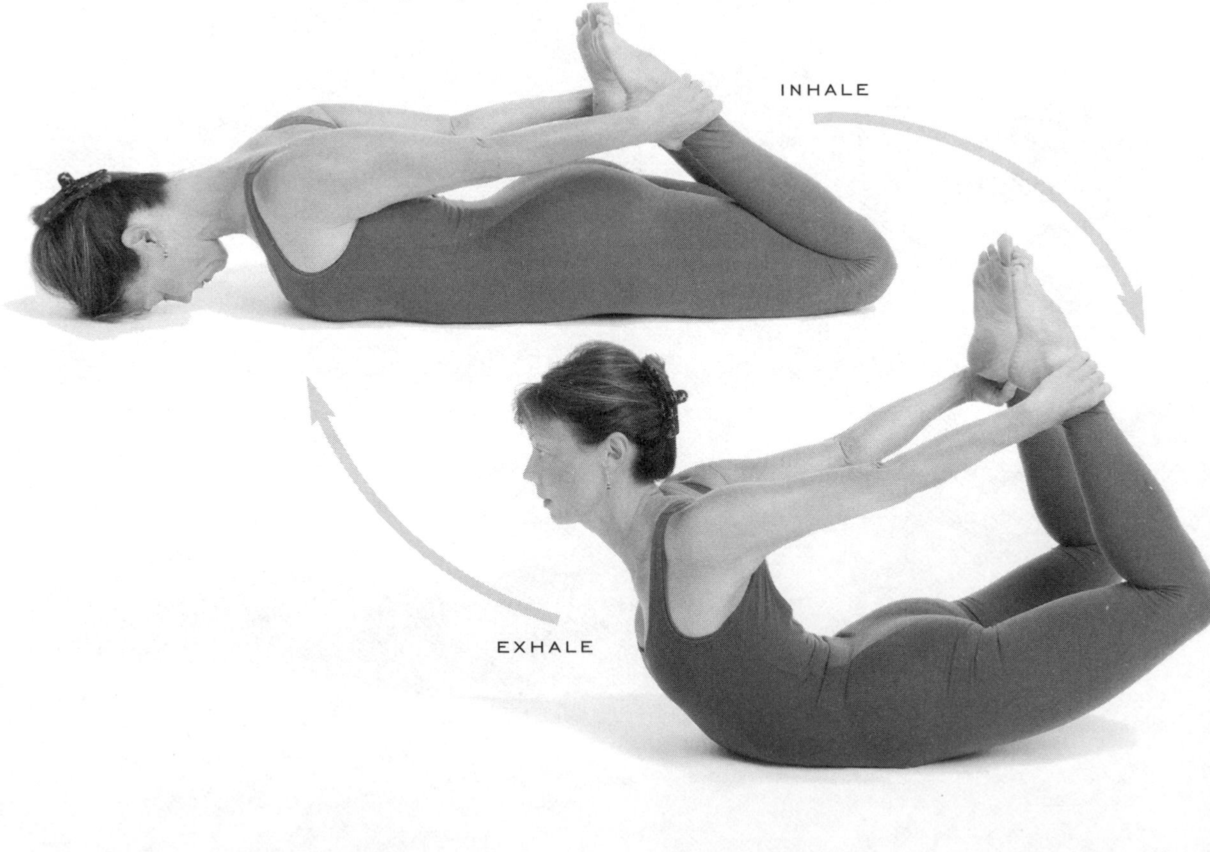

12.

POSTURE: *Apānāsana*

EMPHASIS: To gently stretch and relax lower back.

TECHNIQUE: Lie on back with both knees bent toward chest and feet off floor. Place each hand on its respective knee.

On exhale: Pull thighs gently but progressively toward chest.

On inhale: Return to starting position.

Number: Eight times.

DETAILS:

On exhale: Pull gently with arms, keeping shoulders relaxed and on floor. Press lower back down into floor and drop chin slightly toward throat.

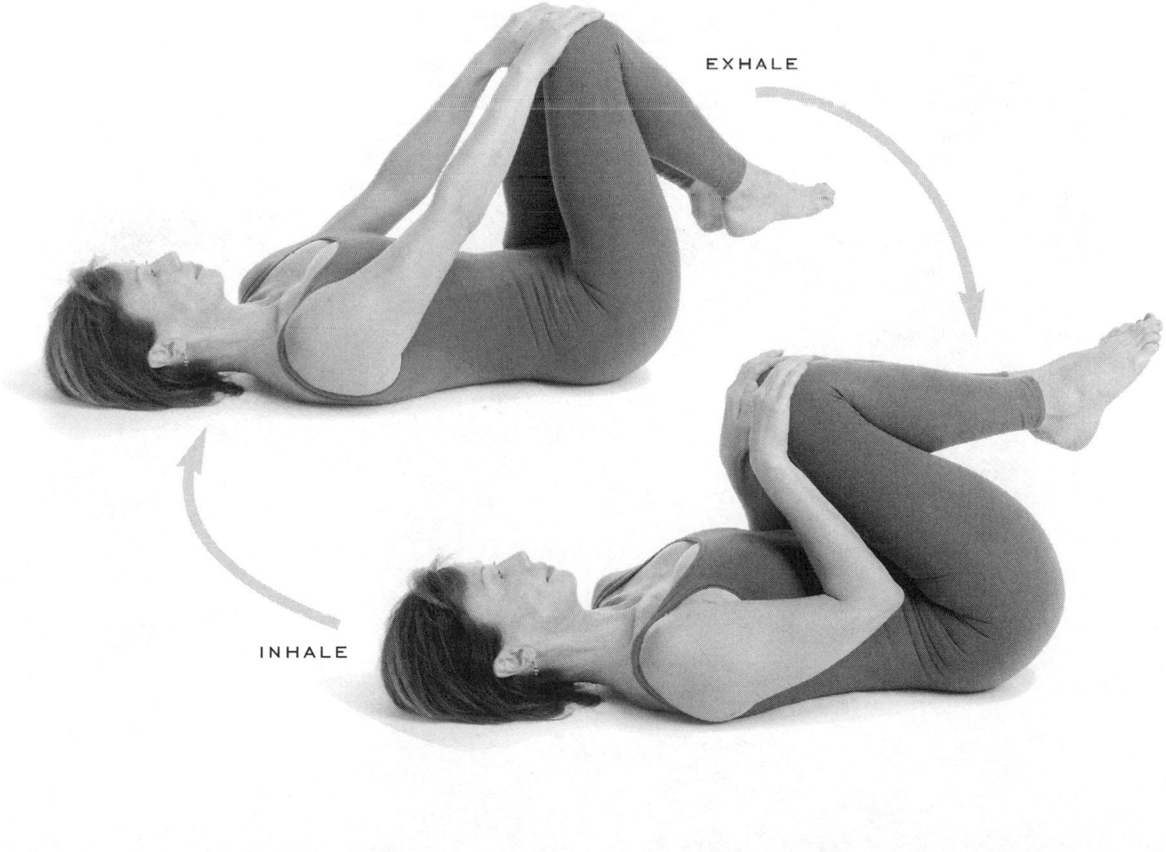

13.

POSTURE: *Paścimatānāsana*

EMPHASIS: To stretch back to compensate for backward bend.

TECHNIQUE:

A: Sit with legs forward, back straight, and arms raised over head.

On exhale: Bending knees slightly, bend forward, bringing chest to thighs, and palms to balls of feet.

On inhale: Return to starting position.

Repeat.

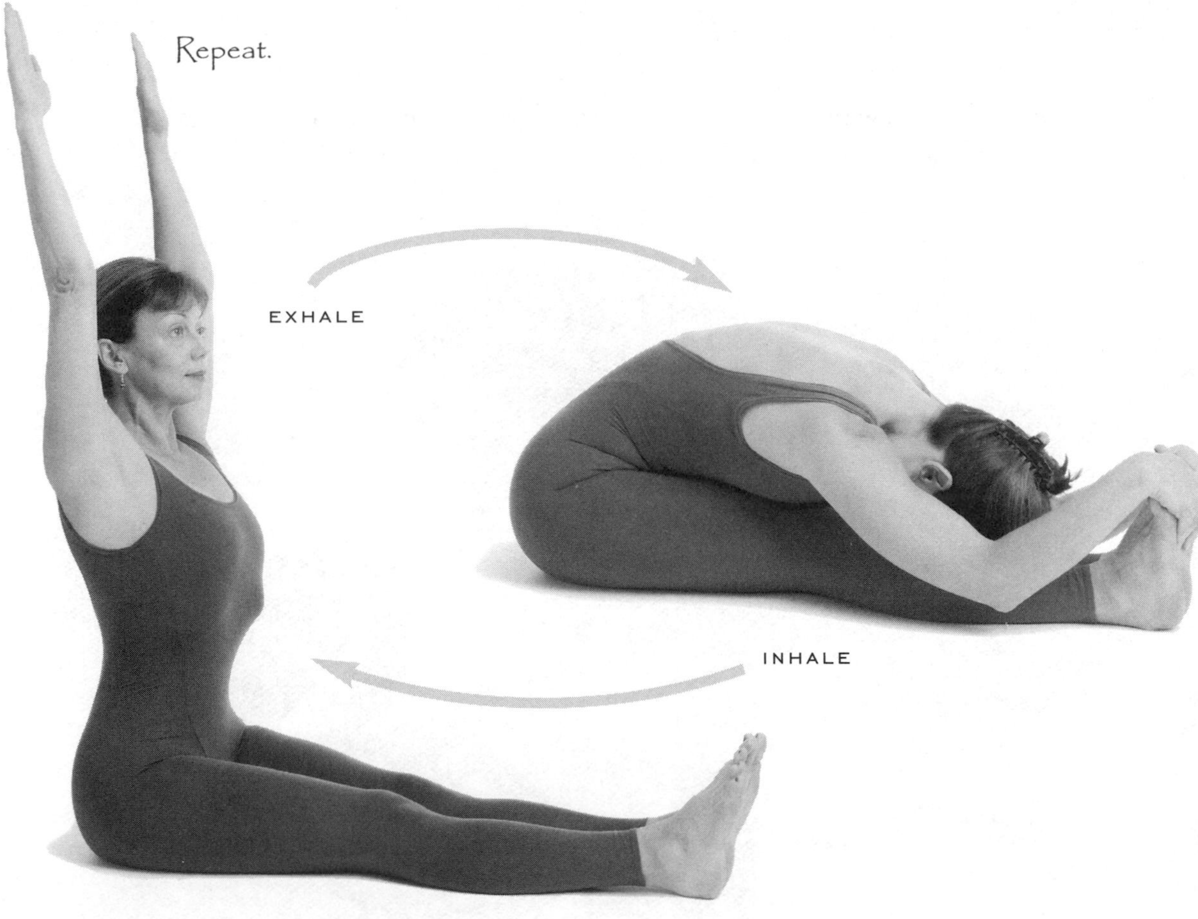

TECHNIQUE:

B: From forward bend position, palms holding balls feet.

On inhale: Lift chest up and away from thighs, flattening upper back.

On exhale: Return to starting position.

Number: Repeat A and B four times each.

DETAILS:

On exhale: Bend knees to facilitate stretching lower back, and bring belly and chest to thighs. Move chin down toward throat.

On inhale: Lift chest up and away from thighs, flattening upper back.

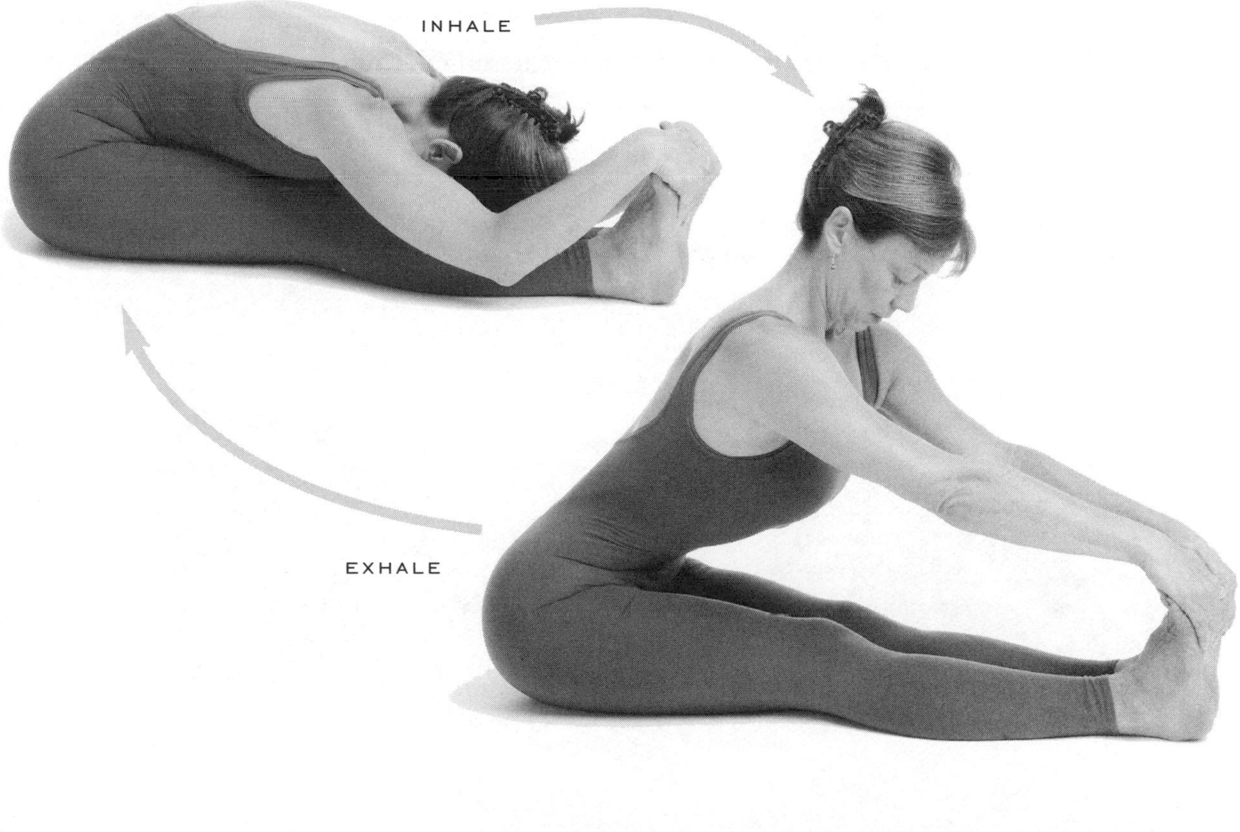

14.

POSTURE: *Ardha Matsyendrāsana*

EMPHASIS: To twist spine.
To help balance neck and shoulders after headstand.

TECHNIQUE: Sit with right leg bent beneath left leg, right foot by left hip, and left knee bent and straight up, left foot crossing over on outside of right knee, left arm behind back with palm down on floor by sacrum, and right arm across outside of left thigh, right hand on left hip.

On inhale: Extend spine upward.

On exhale: Twist torso and look over left shoulder.

Number: Eight breaths each side.

DETAILS:

On exhale: Control torsion from deep in belly, using arm leverage only to augment twist.

On inhale: Subtly untwist body to facilitate extension of spine.

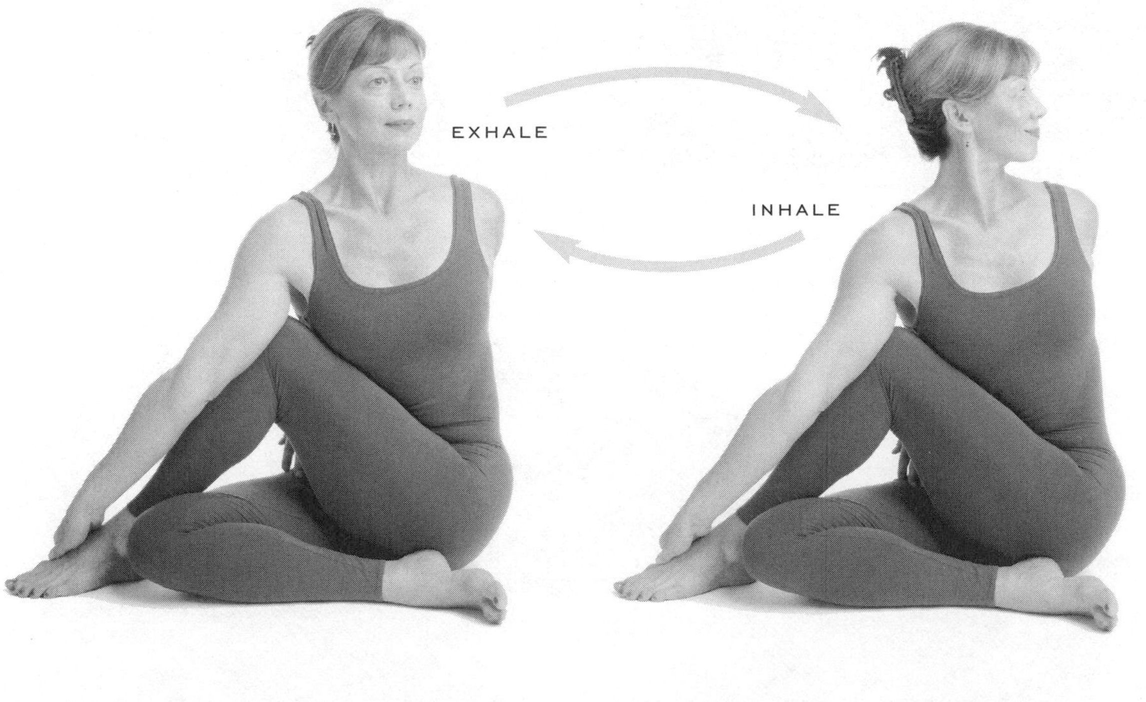

15.

POSTURE: *Vajrāsana*

EMPHASIS: To stretch back gently and symmetrically, as a counterpose for the seated twist.

TECHNIQUE: Stand on knees with arms over head.

On exhale: Bend forward, sweeping arms behind back, and bringing hands to sacrum, keeping palms up, forehead to the floor.

On inhale: Return to starting position.

Number: Eight times.

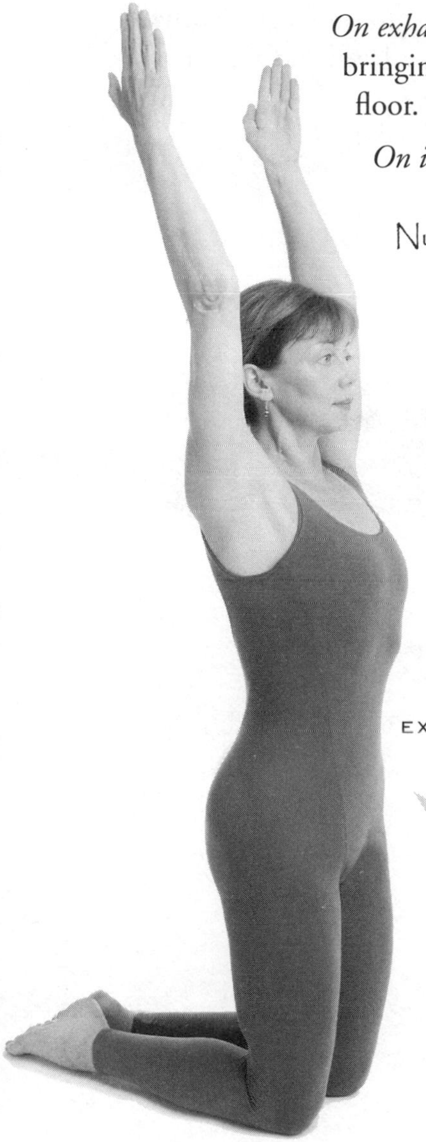

DETAILS:

On exhale: Bring chest to thighs before bringing buttocks to heels. Rotate arms so palms are up and hands are resting on sacrum.

On inhale: Expand chest and lift it up off of knees as arms sweep wide.

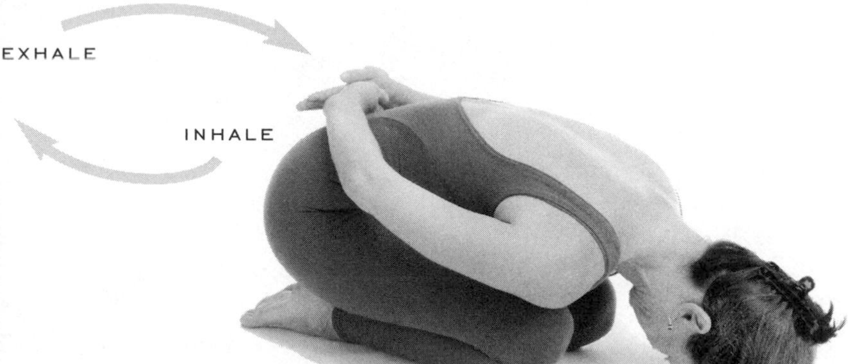

16.

POSTURE: *Śavāsana*

EMPHASIS:

To rest.

TECHNIQUE: Lie flat on back, with arms at side, palms up, and legs slightly apart. Close eyes. Relax body fully, keeping mind relaxed and alert to sensations in body.

Duration: Eight minutes.

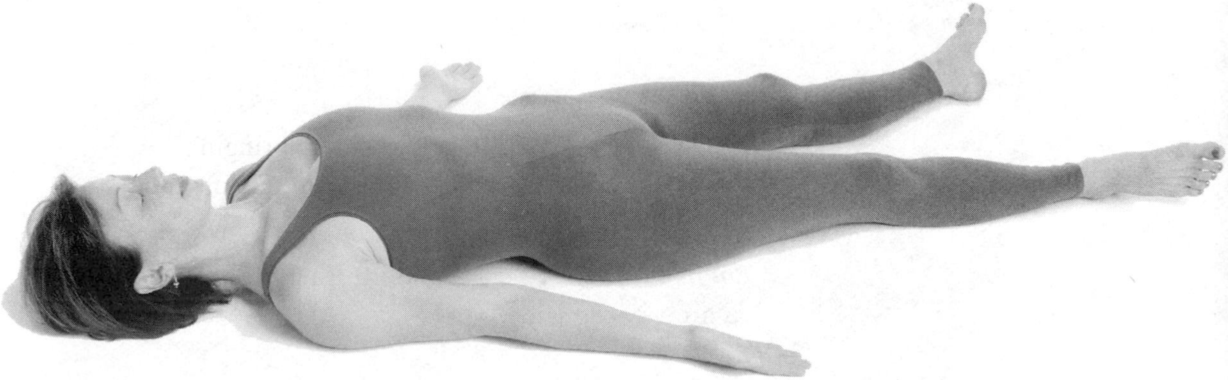

CHAPTER FIVE

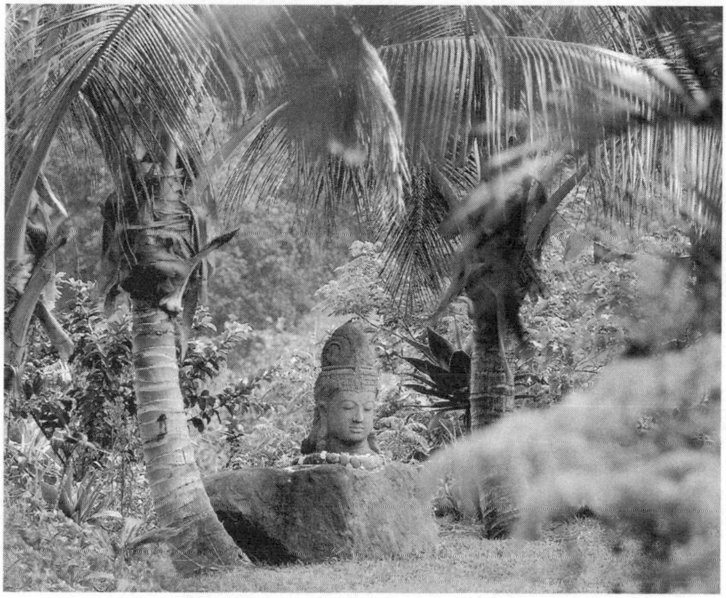

Energizing the Vital

LIGHTNESS AND LUMINOSITY: WORKING THROUGH THE BREATH THE *PRĀṆAMAYA* LEVEL

PRĀṆĀYĀMA AND PERSONAL PRACTICE

AS *ANNAMAYA* REPRESENTS THE PHYSICAL BODY, *prāṇamaya* represents the vital body. It is the "energy department" of our human system, in relation to which the ancients identified five aspects: *prāṇa, apāna, vyāna, udāna,* and *samāna.*

THE FIVE ASPECTS OF THE VITAL BODY

Prāṇa or "that which goes everywhere" is responsible for reception or input, including that of breath, food, and sensory input.

Apāna or "that which takes away" is responsible for elimination: what should be eliminated, what should not be eliminated, and when to eliminate.

Vyāna or "that which makes things distinct" is responsible for sensation, as well as for lifting, grasping, and throwing.

Udāna or "that which leads up" is responsible for our ability to speak, as well as for our ability to move our bodies.

Samāna or "that which takes what is required to where it is required" is responsible for distributing nourishment throughout the body.

We have considered how *āsana* can be adapted to positively influence our physical structure. We can also adapt *āsana* to influence our systems energetically and to address our constitutional needs. The primary means of adapting *āsana* to support our constitutional needs involves the appropriate selection of postures and the adaptation of the breath throughout our practice. In this context, *āsana* can be used to support a deeper constitutional work that is achieved through *prāṇāyāma*.

EXPLORING THE BREATH

The breath is considered to be the link between body, mind, and spirit. Conscious control of the breath—*prāṇāyāma*—helps us to identify subtle mechanisms of contraction in the body and mind, and to release them at their root. It is a means of purifying the subtle channels of energy underlying the physical structure, through which flow both our awareness and our vital energy. It not only builds the breath capacity, it vitalizes and stimulates the whole system.

In this chapter we will develop the *Viniyoga* principles concerning inhalation and exhalation, the science of ratio (the proportional lengths of inhale, hold after inhale, exhale, and hold after exhale), and various other techniques for controlling the breath, as they relate to the practices of *āsana* and meditation. We will show that, through *prāṇāyāma*, our sense of stillness deepens, our attention turns inward without dullness or agitation, our mind feels light and luminous, and we become ready for meditation.

Exploring Your Inhale and Exhale

The starting point for developing a *prāṇāyāma* practice is to familiarize yourself with your inhalation and exhalation. In order to do this, we recommend that you simply sit in a comfortable position and begin to progressively deepen your inhale and lengthen your exhale. In this initial process, you are simply examining your ability to lengthen the breath.

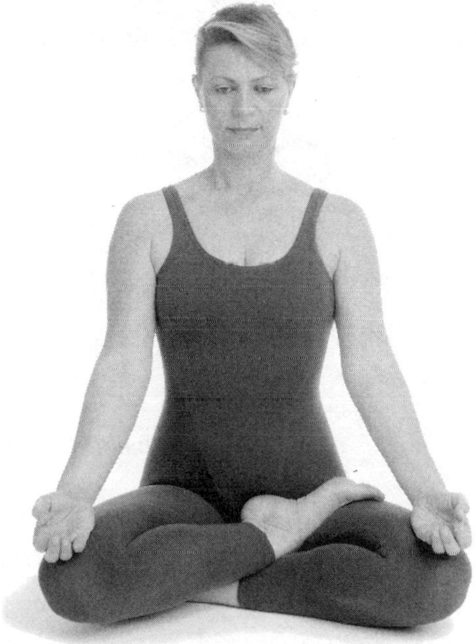

Sit in a comfortable posture. Start with normal comfortable breathing (the average rate for a healthy person is between twelve and eighteen breaths per minute), then, every second or third breath, increase the length of inhale and exhale by one or two seconds. Continue with this process until you reach a comfortably maximum length of inhale. For most people the exhalation will naturally be longer. You can continue to increase the length of your exhale when you have reached your comfortable maximum inhale. When you have reached a comfortable and sustainable length of inhalation and exhalation, maintain that ratio for another eight to twelve breaths, then begin to progressively shorten the inhale and exhale until you return to normal breathing.

How to Inhale and Exhale

There are a variety of ways to control the flow of inhalation and exhalation. And, in fact, it is this discussion that has become the subject of some controversy—a controversy that is never a question of right or wrong and that can only be solved by recognizing that different methods have different effects. The fundamental principle of *Viniyoga* is the application of the appropriate method for each context. In order to better understand this principle, we will examine several types of inhalation and exhalation.

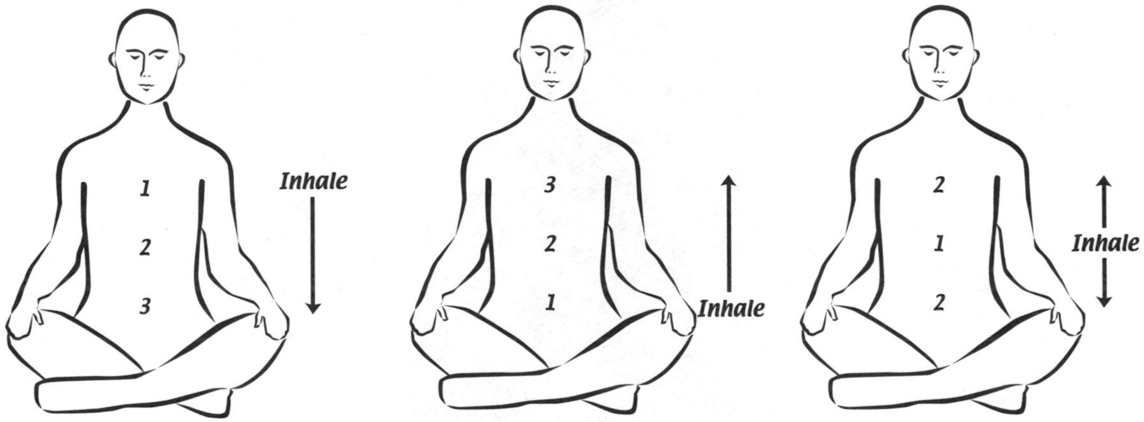

FIVE TYPES OF INHALATION

- Chest
- Belly
- Chest to belly (continuous flow with no hold)
- Belly to chest (continuous flow with no hold)
- Solar plexus, radiating out; and, on the exhalation, allowing everything to return to the solar plexus

The biomechanics of inhalation is basically consistent no matter which method we are emphasizing. Like all movement in the body, breathing is related to muscular contraction; inhalation is specifically initiated as a result of the contraction of the intercostal muscles (the muscles between the ribs) and the diaphragm. This process is as follows: the intercostals contract; the rib cage elevates; the diaphragm contracts downward. The elevation of the rib cage, combined with the downward movement of the diaphragm, creates a negative density in the thoracic cavity, allowing air to be sucked into the lungs; the result is an expansion of the thoracic cavity. Other muscles involved in the process include the erector spinae, the semispinalis, the multifidus, the serratus posterior group, and the interspinalis—all of which contribute to the elevation of the rib cage, expansion of the chest, flattening of the thoracic curve, and vertical extension of the spine.

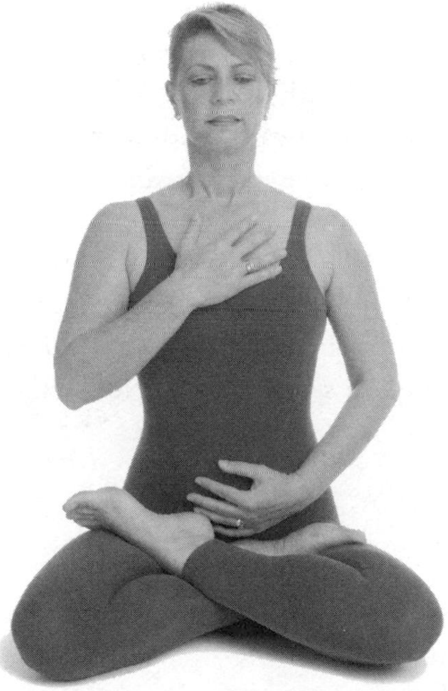

EXPAND CHEST

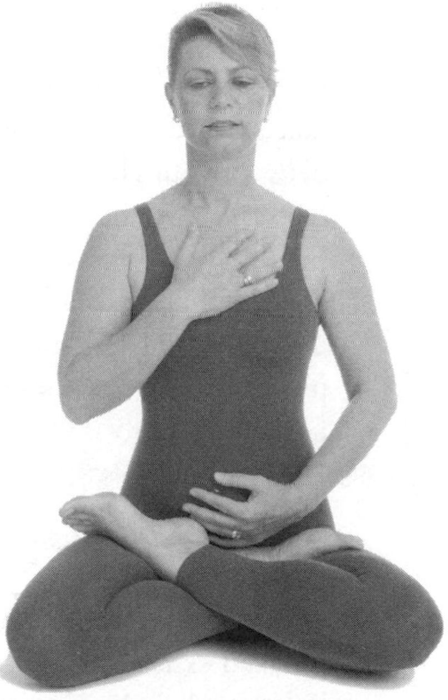

EXPAND BELLY

It is important to emphasize that these various techniques have more to do with both the movement of awareness and the control of the auxiliary muscles of respiration than they do with the movement of the air.

As a means of personal observation, let's explore each of these types of inhalation.

Sit in a comfortable position.

- Place your right hand on your chest and your left hand on your lower abdomen. With your awareness in your chest, inhale, expanding the chest and noticing the right hand rising. Repeat several times. Notice the effects.
- Then, with your awareness in your belly, inhale, expanding the belly and noticing the left hand rising. Repeat several times. Notice the effects.
- Now expand the chest and, for the first half of the inhale, notice the right hand rising; then expand the belly and, for the second half of the inhale, notice the left hand rising. Repeat several times. Notice the effects.
- Now expand the belly and, for the first half of the inhale, notice the left hand rising; then expand the chest and, for the second half of the inhale, notice the right hand rising. Let your awareness flow from your belly to your chest as you inhale. Repeat several times. Notice the effects.
- Finally, with your awareness at your solar plexus, try expanding your chest and belly simultaneously. Notice the simultaneous rising of both the right and left hands. Let your awareness move from your solar plexus up and down as you inhale. Repeat several times. Notice the effects.

THREE TYPES OF EXHALATION

Sit in a comfortable position.

- Relaxed exhale without contraction.

  Where inhalation is a function of muscular contraction, normal unconscious exhalation is the result of the relaxation of the muscles responsible for inhalation. This process is as follows: as the intercostal muscles relax, the rib cage returns from its elevated position; as the diaphragm relaxes, it raises up; and the result is the expulsion of air from the lungs.
- Exhale with contraction of the abdomen.

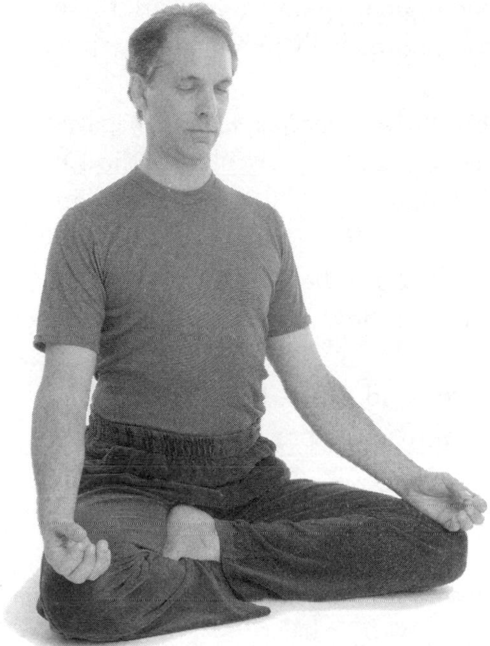

EXPAND BELLY

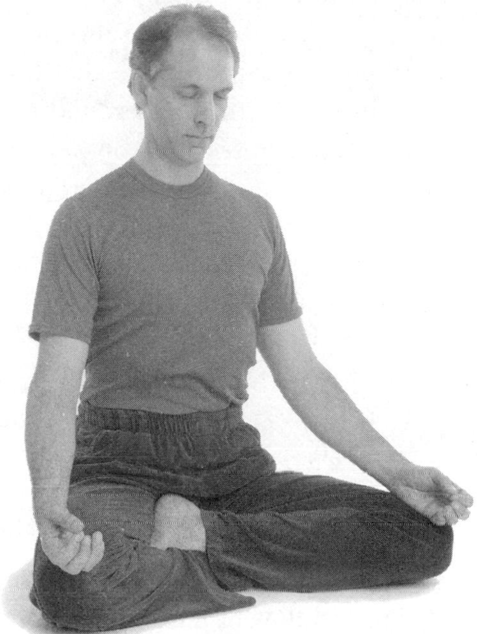

EXPAND CHEST

In the practice of *prāṇāyāma,* however, rather than simply relaxing the muscles contracted to create the inhalation, we may intentionally contract the abdominal muscles progressively from the pubic bone to the navel to the sternum.

- Exhale, pulling up from the muscles of the perineal floor, including the anal sphincter muscle, to the sternum.

  In certain circumstances, we may also intentionally contract the superficial and deep musculature of the perineal floor.

Each of these different ways of controlling the flow of inhalation and exhalation has slightly different structural and energetic effects. It would be wrong to suggest that one of these methods is correct and the others are incorrect—one or another of these methods would be more appropriate in a particular context.

As we have seen, chest inhalation is the most effective technique for straightening the spine and improving the posture. Therefore, as indicated earlier, unless otherwise contraindicated, in *āsana* practice, we emphasize inhalation in the area of the chest, above the diaphragm. Exhalation, instead, is adapted to keep the belly firm and the pelvic lumbar spine stable. And, therefore, in *āsana* practice, we also emphasize pulling the belly in toward the spine throughout the process of exhalation.

In one of the greatest and most authoritative Yoga texts, the Bhagavad Gitā, there is a teaching on *prāṇāyāma* that suggests a particular method of controlling the flow of inhalation and exhalation (4:28). It suggests that inhalation is a downward flow in which we "offer" or link *prāṇa* (which is symbolically located in the chest) to *apāna* (which is symbolically located in the lower abdomen), and that exhalation is an upward flow in which we "offer" or link *apāna* to *prāṇa*.

This is the method we generally recommend for a developmental approach to *prāṇāyāma* practice. When the approach is preventative or therapeutic, we may adopt one or another of the above-mentioned methods, depending upon the condition to be addressed.

The following practice utilizes breath control in *āsana* as a support for the practice of two different *prāṇāyāma* techniques, both designed to illustrate the downward flow of inhalation and the upward flow of exhalation. This practice also illustrates how to adapt *āsana* to prepare for *prāṇāyāma*.

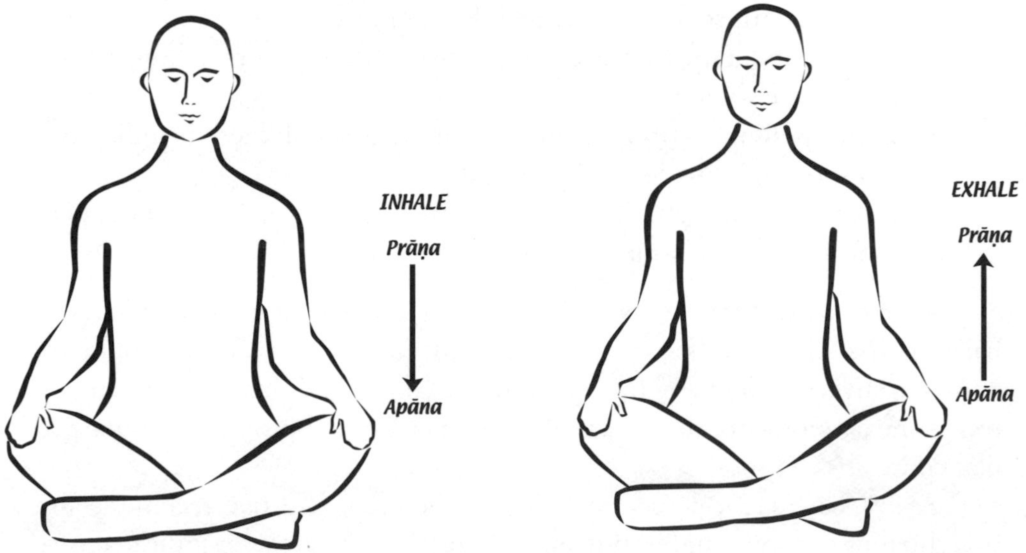

PRĀṆAMAYA PRACTICE

1.

POSTURE: *Siddhāsana*
EMPHASIS: Seated breath awareness

TECHNIQUE:

A: Progressively deepen inhalation and exhalation to a comfortable maximum length of inhalation. Let exhalation pace inhalation.
B: Sustain this breathing.
C: Progressively reduce length of inhalation and exhalation to normal breathing.

Number: Repeat A, B, and C six times each.

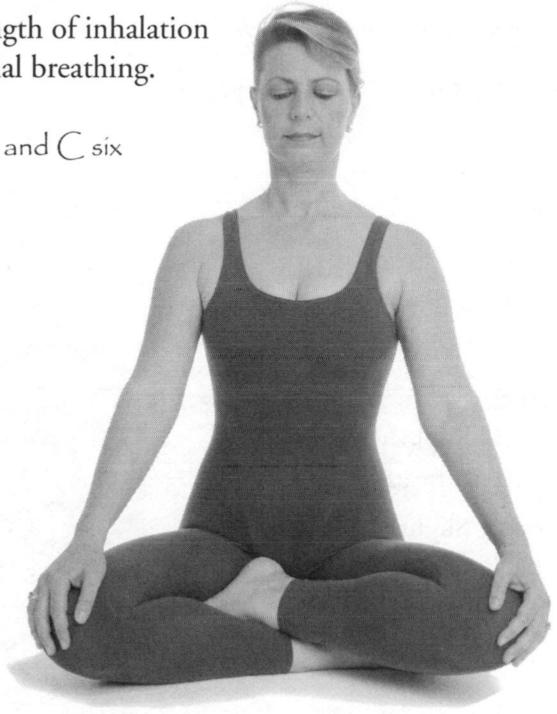

DETAILS:

On inhale: Follow the downward flow of inhalation, expanding progressively from chest to belly.

On exhale: Follow the upward flow of exhalation, contracting progressively from pubic bone to navel.

2.

POSTURE: *Tāḍāsana*
EMPHASIS: To extend the spine.
To introduce retention of the breath after inhalation.

TECHNIQUE: Stand with arms at side, feet parallel.

On inhale: Raise up on toes while simultaneously raising arms up over head, fingers interlocked, palms up.

Retain breath after inhalation two seconds, four seconds, six seconds, two times each.

On exhale: Return to starting point.

Number: Six times.

DETAILS:
On inhale: Slightly arch back and lift head.

On exhale: Slightly flatten lower back, chin down.

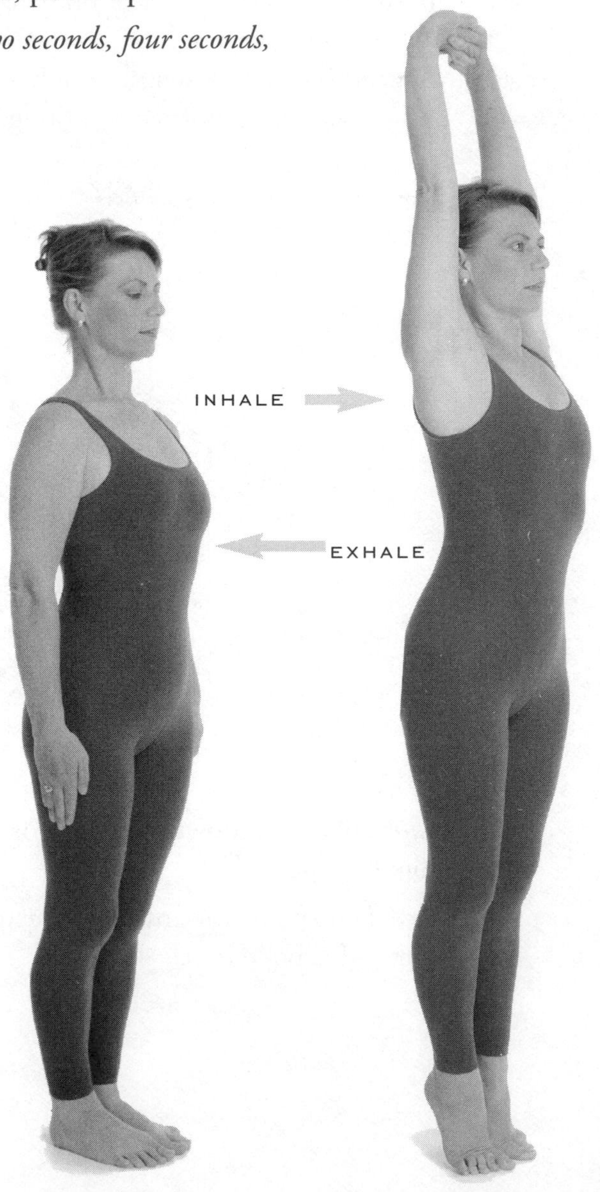

3.

POSTURE: *Vīrabhadrāsana*

EMPHASIS: To expand chest and enhance inhalation.
To continue retention of the breath after inhalation.

TECHNIQUE: Stand with left foot forward, feet as wide as hips, and arms at sides.

On inhale: Simultaneously bend left knee, displace chest slightly forward and hips slightly backward, and bring arms forward and up over head, fingers interlocked, palms up. Arch upper back.

Retain breath after inhalation two seconds, four seconds, six seconds, two times each.

On exhale: Return to starting position.

Number: Six times each side.

DETAILS:
On inhale: Feel expansion of chest. Avoid compressing lower back.

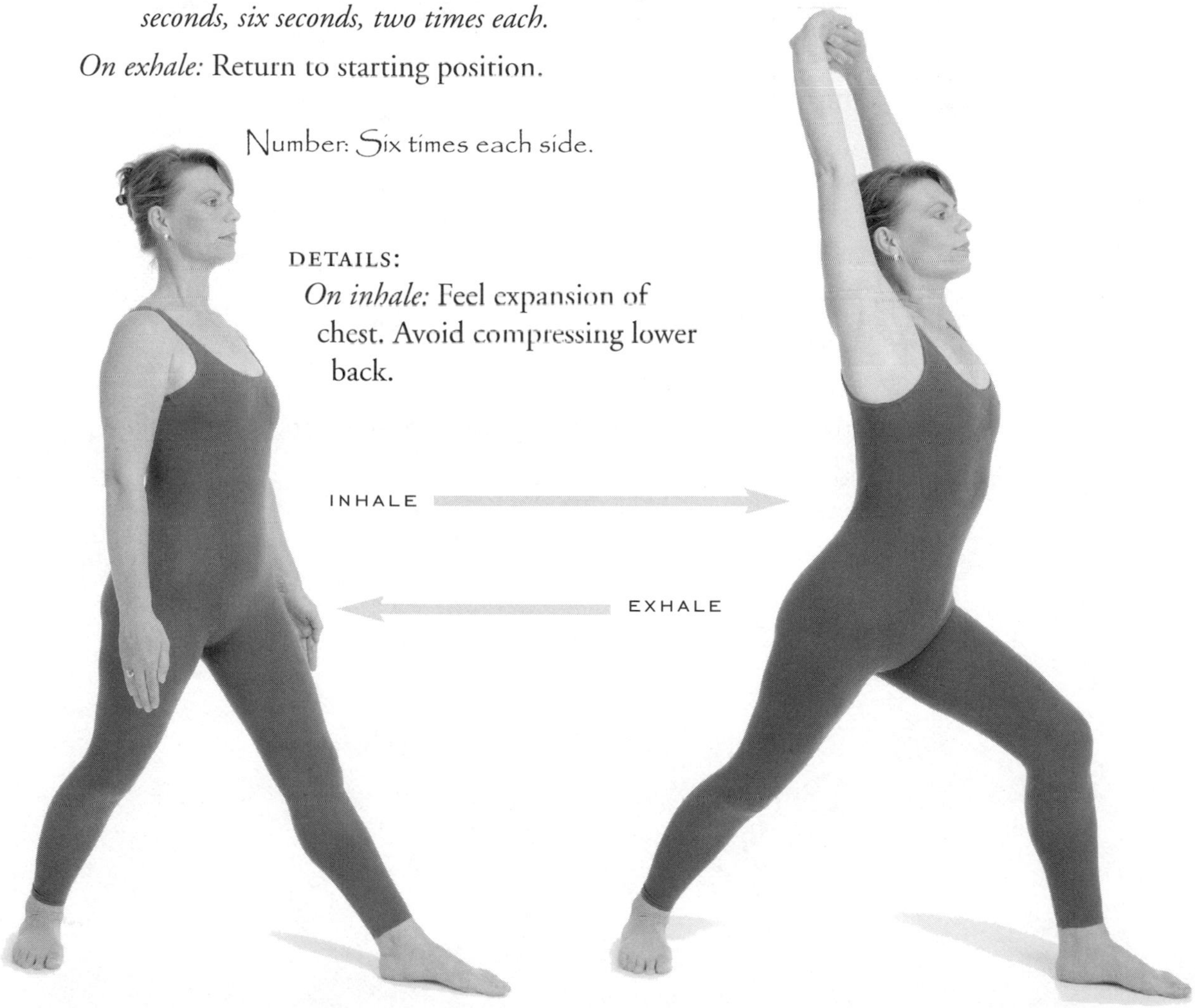

4.

POSTURE: *Vajrāsana/Ūrdhva Mukha Śvānāsana* combination

EMPHASIS: To continue expanding chest and further enhance inhalation. To continue retention of the breath after inhalation.

TECHNIQUE: Stand on knees with arms over head.

On exhale: Bend forward, bringing arms to floor in front of you.

On inhale: Stretch body forward and arch back, keeping only hands and from knees to feet on floor.

Retain breath after inhalation two seconds, four seconds, six seconds, two times each.

On exhale: Return to previous position.

On inhale: Return to starting position.

Number: Six times.

DETAILS:

On inhale: Expand chest, stretch belly, and avoid compressing lower back.

On exhale: End in forward bend position.

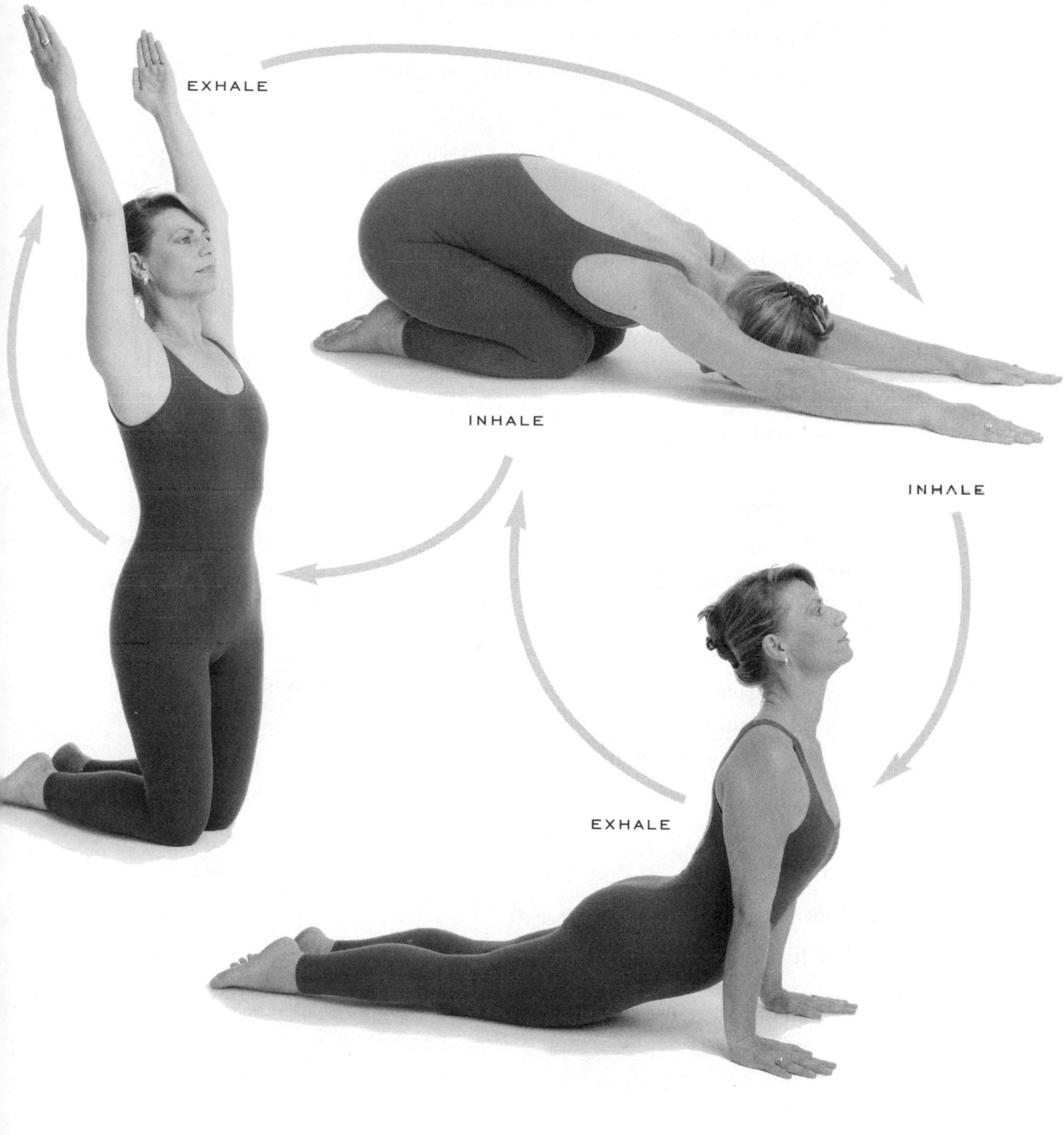
EXHALE
INHALE
INHALE
EXHALE

5.

POSTURE: *Siddhāsana Prāṇāyāma: Anuloma Krama*—
two stage inhale; three-stage inhale

EMPHASIS: To experience the downward flow of inhale.

TECIINIQUE: A:

Exhale deeply and fully.

Inhale first half of breath in five seconds.

Pause five seconds.

Inhale remainder of breath in five seconds.

Pause five seconds.

Exhale slowly and fully.

Number: Six times.

DETAILS:

On first stage of inhale: Expand chest from pit of throat to sternum.

On second stage of inhale: Expand abdomen from sternum to pubic bone.

On exhale: Contract abdomen progressively from pubic bone to navel to sternum.

TECHNIQUE: B:

Exhale deeply and fully.

Inhale first third of breath in four seconds.

Pause four seconds.

Inhale second third of breath in four seconds.

Pause four seconds.

Inhale last third of breath in four seconds.

Pause four seconds.

Exhale slowly and fully.

Number: Six times.

DETAILS:

On first stage of inhale: Expand chest from pit of throat to sternum.

On second stage of inhale: Expand abdomen from sternum to navel.

On third stage of inhale: Expand abdomen from navel to pubic bone.

On exhale: Contract abdomen progressively from pubic bone to navel to sternum.

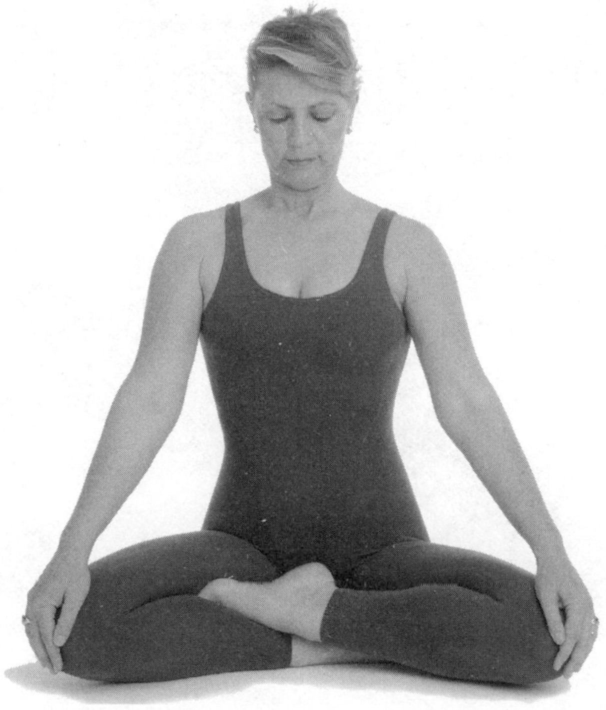

6.

POSTURE: *Dvipāda Pīṭham*

EMPHASIS: To relax neck and upper and lower back.
To gently stretch between belly and thighs.

TECHNIQUE: Lie on back with arms down at sides, knees bent, feet slightly apart on floor, and comfortably close to buttocks.

A:

On inhale: Press down on feet, raising pelvis, keeping chin down until neck is gently flattened on floor.

On exhale: Return to starting position.

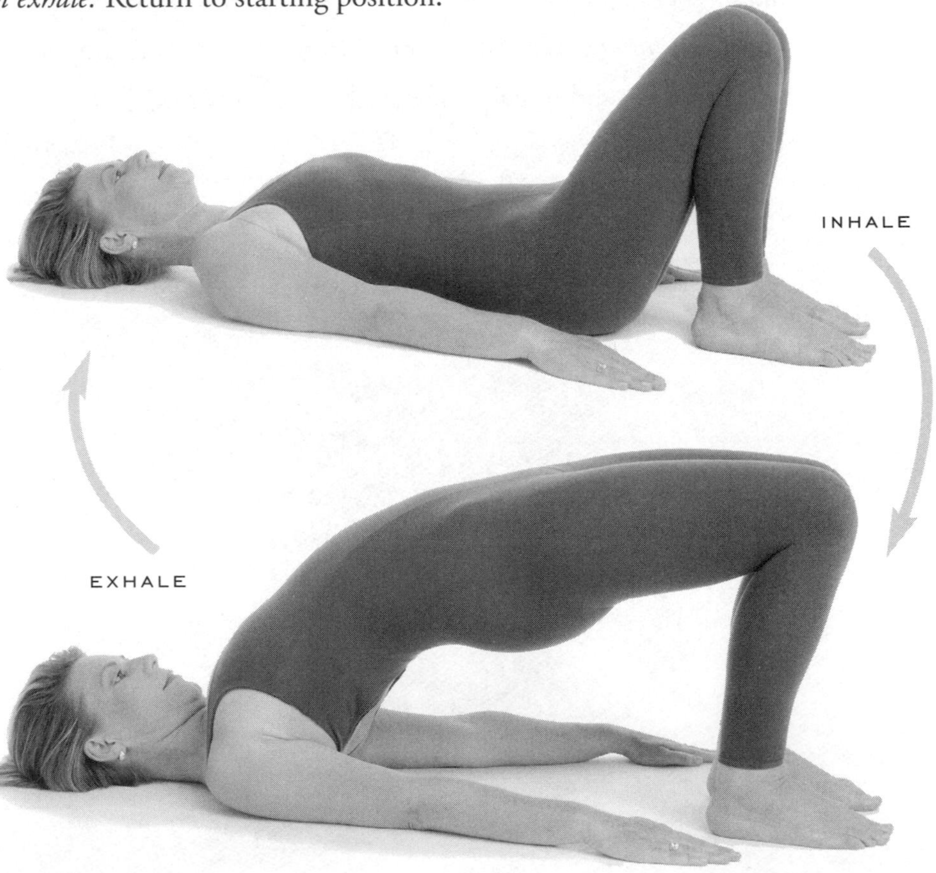

B:

On inhale: Press down on feet, raising pelvis, keeping chin down until neck is gently flattened on floor, while raising arms over head to floor behind.

On exhale: Return to starting position.

Number: Repeat A and B three times each.

DETAILS:

On inhale: Lift spine, vertebra by vertebra, from bottom up.

On exhale: Unwind spine, coming down vertebra by vertebra.

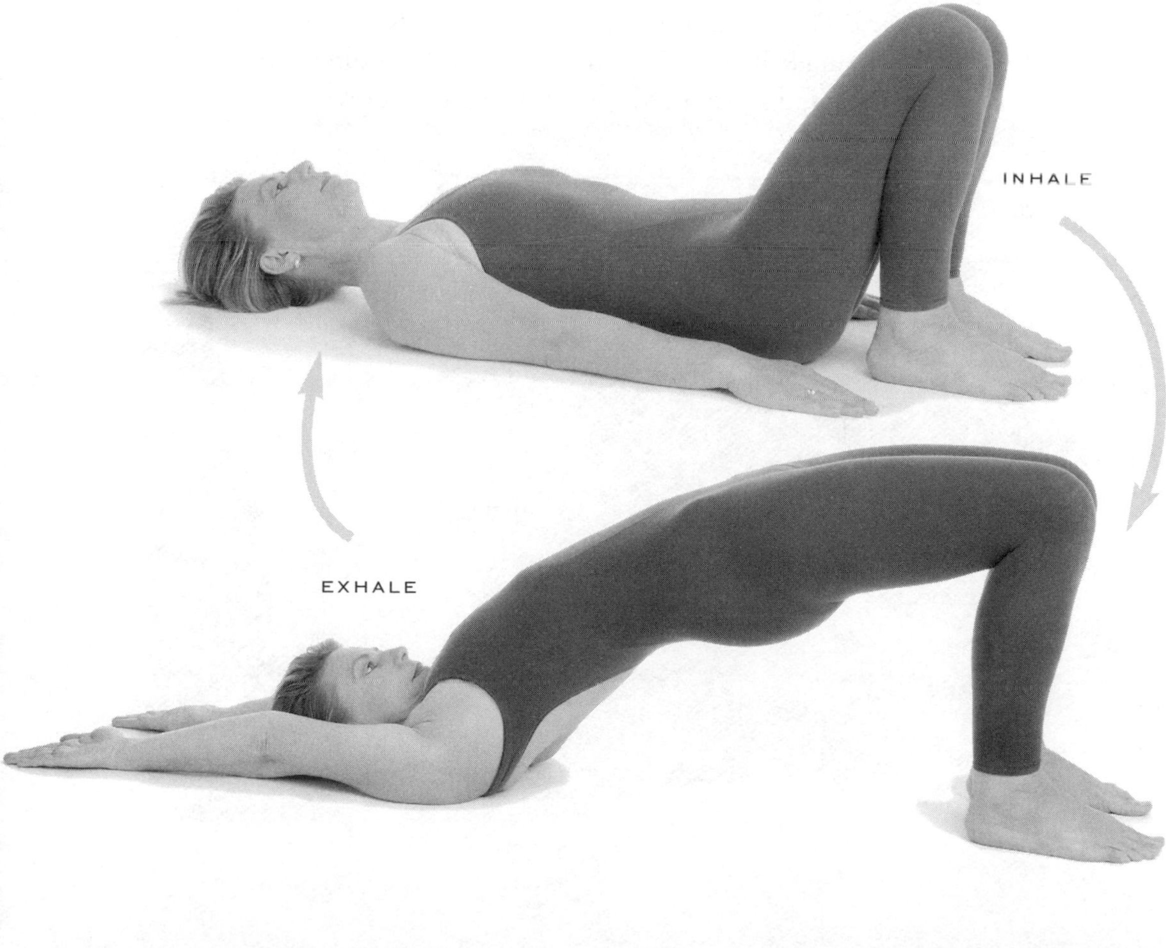

7.

POSTURE: *Ūrdhva Prasṛta Pādāsana*

EMPHASIS: To extend spine and flatten it onto floor.
To stretch legs.

TECHNIQUE: Lie on back with arms down at sides, legs bent, and knees lifted toward chest.

On inhale: Raise arms upward all the way to floor behind head and legs upward toward ceiling.

On exhale: Return to starting position.

Number: Six times.

DETAILS: *On inhale:* Flex feet as legs are raised upward. Keep knees slightly bent, and keep angle between legs and torso less than ninety degrees. Push lower back and sacrum downward. Bring chin down.

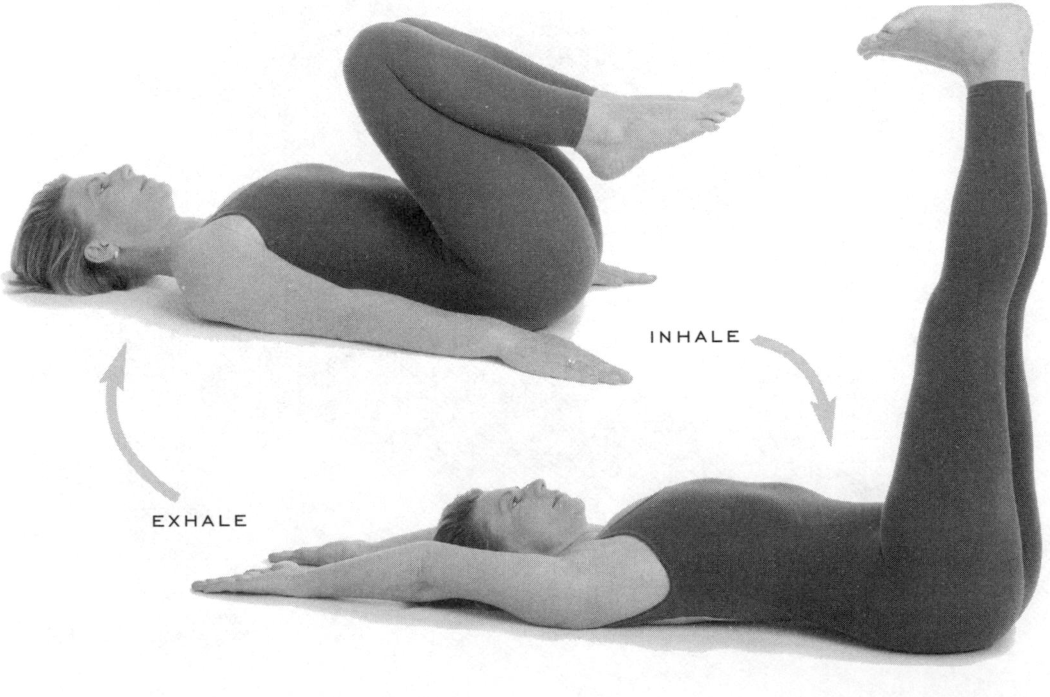

8.

POSTURE: *Jaṭhara Parivṛtti*

EMPHASIS: To gently twist and compress belly, and stretch hips.
To facilitate exhalation and introduce suspension of the breath after exhalation.

TECHNIQUE: Lie on back with both knees bent, thighs lifted toward chest, and both feet off the ground. Arms out to sides, slightly less than right angles to torso, palms down.

On exhale: Bring both knees toward floor on right side of body, twisting abdomen while simultaneously turning head to left.

Suspend breath after exhalation two seconds, four seconds, six seconds, two times each.

On inhale: Return to starting position.

Repeat six times each side, alternating sides.

DETAILS: *On exhale:* Throughout movement, keep knees at an angle to torso that is less than ninety degrees.

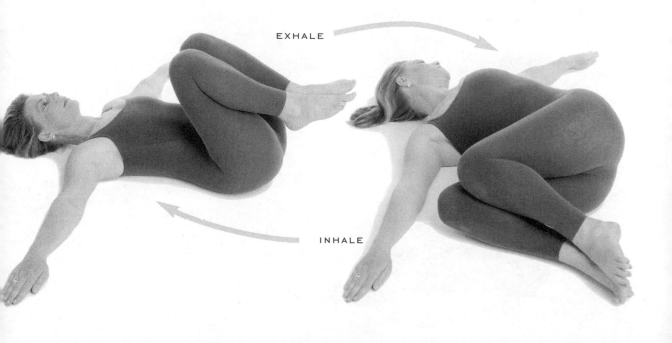

9.

POSTURE: *Ardha Matsyendrāsana*

EMPHASIS: To twist abdomen and spine.
To continue suspension of the breath after exhalation.

TECHNIQUE: Sit with left leg straight, and right knee bent and straight up, right foot crossing over on outside of left knee, right arm behind back with palm down on floor by sacrum, and left arm across outside of right thigh, left hand holding the arch of the right foot.

On inhale: Extend spine upward.

On exhale: Twist torso and look over right shoulder.

Suspend breath after exhalation two seconds, four seconds, six seconds, two times each.

Number: Six breaths each side.

DETAILS:

On exhale: Control torsion from deep in belly, using arm leverage only to augment twist.

On inhale: Slightly untwist body to facilitate extension of spine.

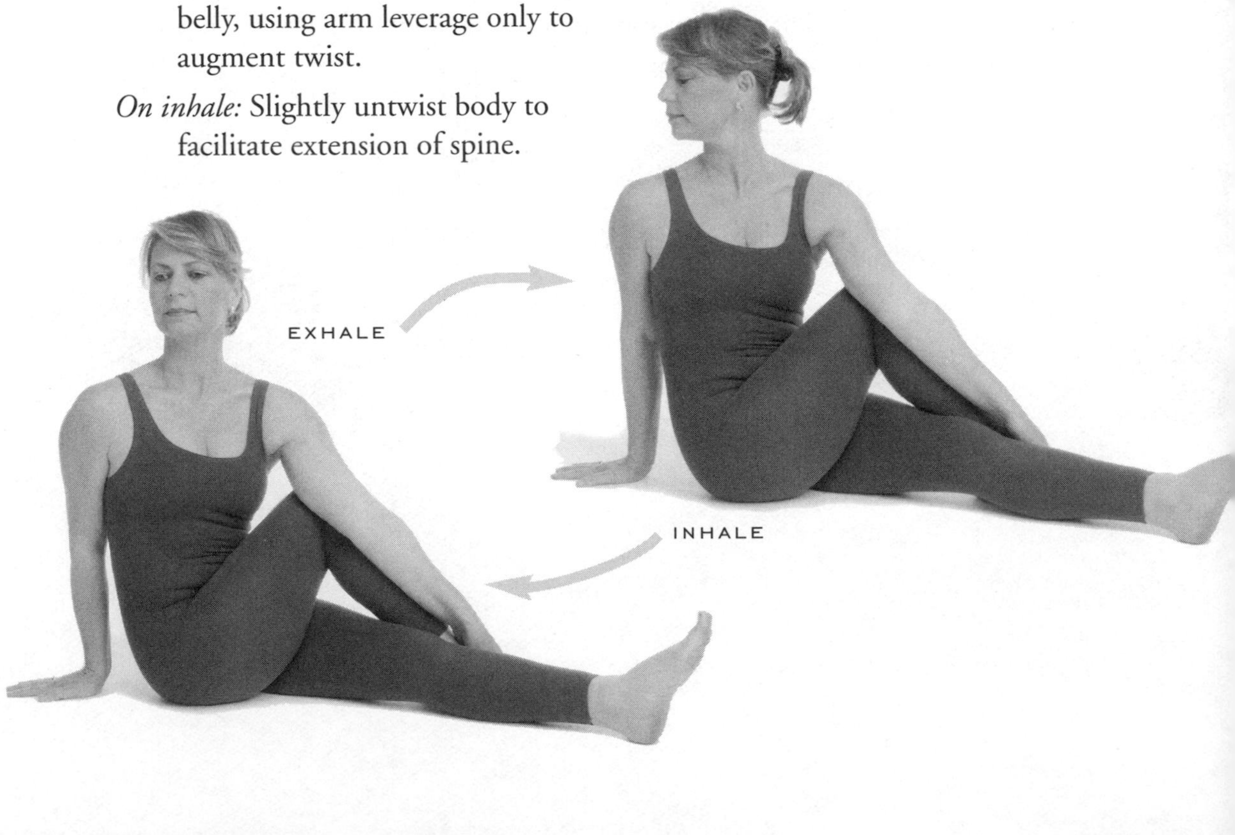

10.

POSTURE: *Paścimatānāsana*

EMPHASIS: To stretch back after twist.

To continue suspension of the breath after exhalation.

TECHNIQUE: Sit with legs forward, back straight, and arms raised over head, fingers interlocked, palms up.

On exhale: Bending knees slightly, bend forward, bringing chest to thighs, and interlocked fingers to balls of feet, palms out.

Suspend breath after exhalation two seconds, four seconds, six seconds, two times each.

On inhale: Return to starting position.

Number: Repeat six times.

DETAILS:

On exhale: Bend knees to facilitate stretching lower back, and bring belly and chest to thighs. Move chin down toward throat.

On inhale: Lift chest up and away from thighs, flattening upper back.

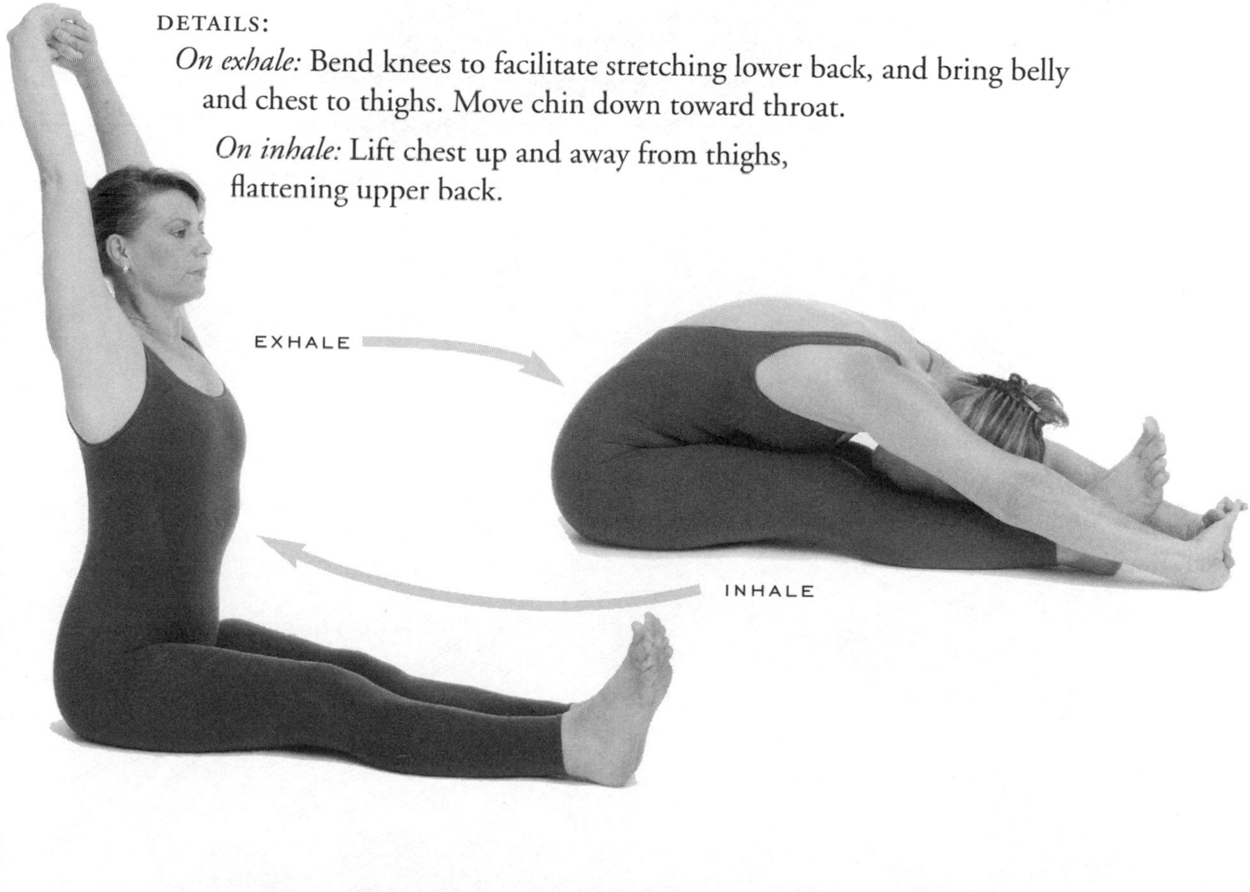

11.

POSTURE: *Śavāsana*

EMPHASIS: To rest.

TECHNIQUE: Lie flat on back, arms at side, palms up, and legs slightly apart. Close eyes. Relax body fully, keeping mind relaxed and alert to sensations in body.

Duration: Minimum five minutes.

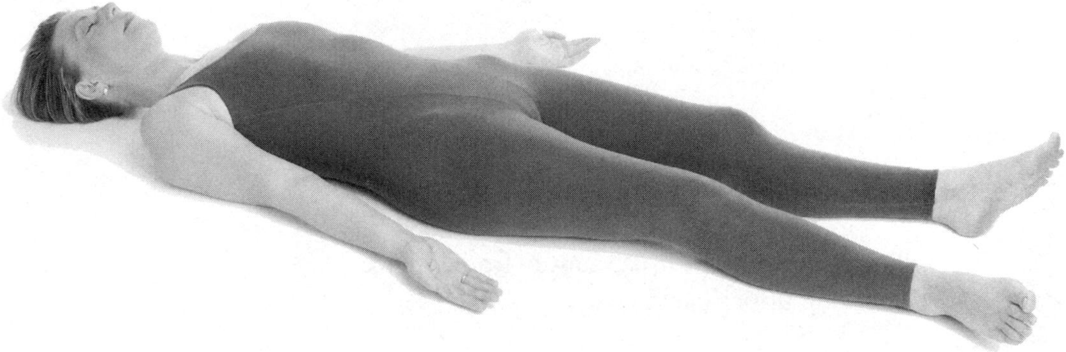

12.

POSTURE: *Siddhāsana Prāṇāyāma: Viloma Krama*—two-stage exhale; three-stage exhale

EMPHASIS: To experience the upward flow of exhale.

TECHNIQUE: A:

Inhale deeply and fully.

Exhale first half of breath in six seconds.

Pause six seconds.

Exhale remainder of breath in six seconds.

Pause six seconds.

Inhale slowly and fully.

Number: Six times.

DETAILS:

On first stage of exhale: Contract abdomen from pubic bone to navel.

On second stage of exhale: Contract abdomen from navel to sternum.

On inhale: Expand chest, then relax abdomen progressively from sternum to pubic bone.

TECHNIQUE: B:

Inhale deeply and fully.

Exhale first third of breath in five seconds.

Pause five seconds.

Exhale second third of breath in five seconds.

Pause five seconds.

Exhale last third of breath in five seconds.

Pause five seconds.

Inhale slowly and fully.

Number: Six times.

DETAILS:

On first stage of exhale: Contract muscles from perineal floor to pubic bone.

On second stage of exhale: Contract abdomen from pubic bone to navel.

On third stage of exhale: Contract abdomen from navel to sternum.

On inhale: Expand chest, then relax abdomen progressively from sternum to pubic bone, and then relax muscles of the perineal floor.

TECHNIQUE:

C: Sit quietly, resting with breathing relaxed.

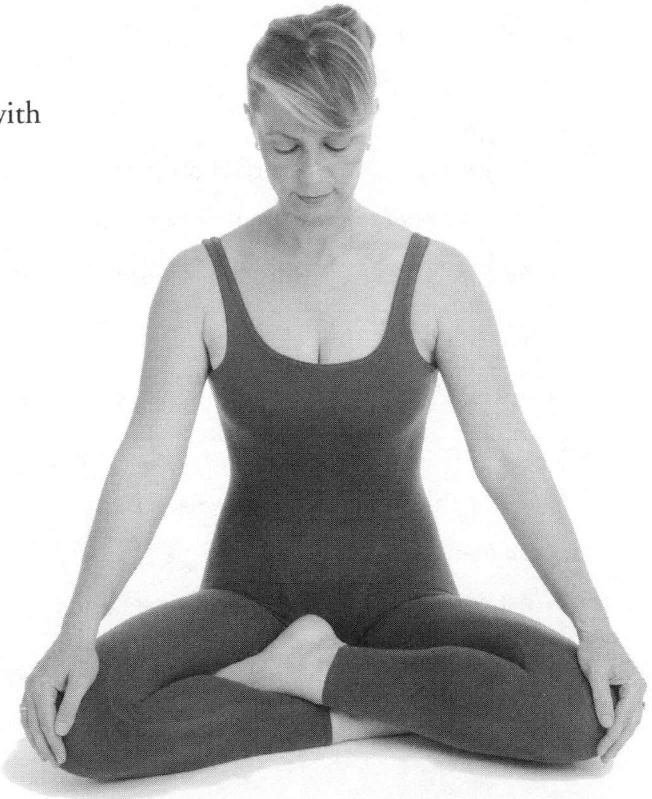

EXPLORING RATIO

Understanding Ratio

Once we become comfortable with extending the length of inhale and exhale over a period of time, and have explored the various ways of controlling both the inhale and the exhale, we can then begin to study the science of ratio. In this science, the flow of the breath is considered in four parts:

- the flow of inhalation,
- retention of the breath after inhalation,
- the flow of exhalation, and
- suspension of the breath after exhalation.

The science of ratio considers the proportional relationship between these four parts of the breath. To make this complex topic more easily understood, consider the following drawing.

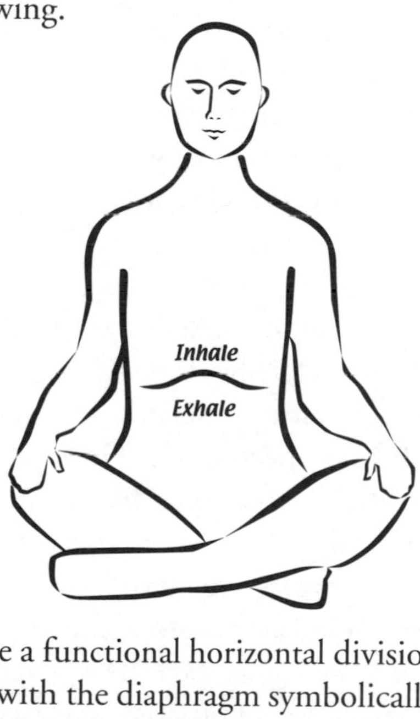

Here we have made a functional horizontal division of the body in the region of the diaphragm, with the diaphragm symbolically representing the floor of the thoracic cavity and the roof of the abdominal cavity. For the sake of introducing the science of ratio, let's consider that inhalation symbolically affects what is above the diaphragm, and that exhalation symbolically affects what is below the diaphragm.

We have seen that there are a variety of ways in which we can control the inhalation. In general, no matter which technique we are applying, the effects of inhalation are considered to be energizing, vitalizing, and expanding. This effect is augmented when the primary emphasis during the inhalation is expanding the chest. If, on the other hand, the emphasis during inhalation is more on expanding the belly, then the effect will be more grounding.

The retention of the breath after inhalation extends, prolongs, and deepens the effects of inhalation. A long retention after inhale needs to be used with **caution**. You can use your will to retain the breath longer than you should. This increases pressure in the thoracic cavity, which can increase pressure on the heart. It can also create neck tension and even dizziness.

As we have seen with inhalation, there are also a variety of ways in which we can control exhalation. No matter which technique we are applying, the effects of exhalation are generally considered to be more calming, grounding, and stabilizing. This effect is augmented by the contraction of the lower abdominal wall. If the exhalation occurs with no added abdominal or perineal contraction, the "letting go" quality of the exhalation will be augmented.

In general, the suspension of the breath after exhalation prolongs and deepens the effects of exhalation. It is very calming and very grounding. Because we are emptying our system, and we can't depend on anything from the outside, we must rely on our inner resources. Therefore, suspension of the breath after exhale is **challenging** for most people, and requires training. If we hold a little too long, an uncontrolled and shortened inhale is provoked, and the calming effect may be lost. Though this technique is particularly challenging for those who have respiratory problems, it is relatively safe because the body will automatically inhale when needed. However, extended suspension of the breath should be **avoided** in conditions like asthma.

Initially, suspension of the breath after exhalation can bring up repressed emotions. Often students report feeling inexplicably angry or anxious after this kind of practice. In one such incident, a student reported that she suddenly remembered a near-drowning incident when she was very young, which her parents, much to their surprise at her recall, were able to confirm.

As we continue to work with suspension after exhalation over time, however, it creates deeper levels of silence. Memories can arise without the accompanying negative emotional charge. If any emotions emerge, they move more in the direction of gratitude. That is why I like to call this technique the "open secret of *prāṇāyāma*."

Developing Ratio

Classically, ratios were classified as either *samavṛtti,* where the lengths of all four parts of the breath are equal, or *viṣamavṛtti,* where the lengths of the four parts of the breath are not equal. There are many possible variations that can be developed. In the classical tradition, the lengths of the breath were measured by the mental recitation of *mantra.* It must be remembered that these practices evolved as part of a holistic process, which included not only *āsana* and *prāṇāyāma* but chanting, meditation, prayer, and ritual as well.

If we are not working with particular *mantra-s,* we may measure the length of our breath by simply counting. The use of a metronome may be helpful at the beginning, especially when exploring more complex ratios. For a brief discussion on the differences and benefits of these different ratios, please see "The Basic Paradigm," on page 131. Beyond this brief theoretical explanation, the subtleties of this complex science can be best understood through practice under the guidance of a competent teacher.

The table below shows some examples of useful ratios—demonstrated at varied levels of duration—that can be explored in personal practice. **These ratios should be explored cautiously, preferably with the guidance of a trained teacher, within the boundaries of our established thresholds (see page 118), and after reading and understanding the cautions for the practice of *prāṇāyāma* listed on page 119.**

All numbers represent seconds. All ratios are written in this order:

INHALATION	RETENTION AFTER INHALATION	EXHALATION	SUSPENSION AFTER EXHALATION

THE CLASSIC *SAMAVṚTTI* RATIO

The ratio where the lengths of inhalation, retention of the breath after inhalation, exhalation, and suspension of the breath after exhalation are all equal:

1-1-1-1
6-6-6-6
8-8-8-8
12-12-12-12

Ratios where the lengths of inhalation and exhalation are equal, and where the lengths of retention of the breath after inhalation and suspension of the breath after exhalation are equal:

1-0-1-0	**2-1-2-1**	**3-1-3-1**	**3-2-3-2**
8-0-8-0	8-4-8-4	9-3-9-3	9-6-9-6
10-0-10-10	10-5-10-5	12-4-12-4	12-8-12-8
12-0-12-0	12-6-12-6	15-5-15-5	15-10-15-10

Viṣamavṛtti Ratios

Ratios where the length of inhalation and exhalation, and/or the lengths of retention of the breath after inhalation and suspension of the breath after exhalation are not equal:

2-2-3-1	**2-3-3-1**	**2-3-3-2**
6-6-9-3	6-9-9-3	6-9-9-6
8-8-12-4	8-12-12-4	8-12-12-8
10-15-15-5	10-15-15-5	10-15-15-10

Ratios in which there is either no retention of the breath after inhalation or no suspension of the breath after exhalation:

1-1-1-0	**1-0-1-1**	**2-3-3-0**	**3-0-3-2**
6-6-6-0	6-0-6-6	6-9-9-0	9-0-9-6
8-8-8-0	8-0-8-8	8-12-12-0	12-0-12-8
10-10-10-0	10-0-10-10	10-15-15-0	15-0-15-10

VINYĀSA IN *PRĀṆĀYĀMA*: PROGRESSIVE STEPS IN BUILDING A RATIO DURING PRACTICE

Just as appropriate steps must be taken to prepare our body to perform a challenging *āsana,* we must prepare progressively to perform a challenging *prāṇāyāma* ratio.

For example, as the goal of the practice, we will consider a *viṣamavṛtti* ratio, 2-3-3-1, in which the exhalation is longer than the inhalation.

Even though the goal of the practice will be this ratio, we would begin at an easy pace, establishing the relationship between inhale and exhale, without fixing either the retention of the breath after inhale or the suspension of the breath after exhale. From here we would build up the holding of the breath in stages. An example of one progression would be:

8-0-12-0—four times
8-4-12-0—four times
8-4-12-4—four times
8-8-12-4—four times
8-12-12-4—twelve times
8-0-12-0—eight times

This practice has a total of thirty-two breaths, and would take just over fifteen minutes. The peak threshold for this practice is thirty-six seconds per complete breath. Notice that we took several stages to arrive at the peak of the practice, sustained the peak twelve breaths, and then returned to the first stage at the end. We always prepare for the peak, and take some time to come down off the peak.

The following examples of a *samavṛtti* ratio demonstrate two different approaches to developing the same ratio:

10-0-10-0—five times
10-5-10-5—five times
10-10-10-5—five times
10-10-10-10—ten times
10-0-10-0—ten times

4-4-4-4—four times
6-6-6-6—six times
8-8-8-8—eight times
10-10-10-10—ten times
8-8-8-8—eight times
6-6-6-6—six times
4-4-4-4—four times

We can see by these examples that not only are there a variety of steps that can be taken to prepare for a given ratio, there are also a variety of steps that can be taken to return to normal breathing. The first example would take just over fifteen minutes; the second just over twenty-two minutes.

Finding Our Threshold

Our threshold is the total duration of one full breath that we can sustain for a number of breaths in succession, usually a minimum of twelve breaths. Of course, within any given threshold there are a variety of possibilities. The peak threshold of the examples above is forty seconds per complete breath. Other examples of a forty-second threshold that could be the goal of a particular practice include:

15-5-15-5 15-10-15-0 20-0-20-0 10-5-20-5 10-10-15-5 10-5-15-10

In the development of your capacity in *prāṇāyāma,* we recommend that you explore a variety of possibilities within a given threshold before you move to the next step. In the above example, once you are able to do each of these ratios for a **minimum of twelve breaths**, you could then progress to a **forty-five-second threshold**, such as:

15-10-15-5 10-15-15-5

It is important to remember, however, that **the goal in *prāṇāyāma* is not necessarily to continually expand your capacity**. If you currently can practice comfortably at a thirty-second threshold, then, to be sure, expanding your capacity to a fifty-second threshold or beyond would have significant impact on your condition. If you are able to practice at a fifty-second threshold for twelve breaths, however, it may still be more useful to practice at a thirty-second threshold for twenty-four breaths.

It is also important to have a clear intention in personal practice.

Remember that we can come to our practice with a developmental, preventative, therapeutic, or transcendental orientation. With a developmental orientation, it would be useful to explore and expand our threshold capacity as illustrated above. As our intention changes, we shift the emphasis from simply exploring and expanding our capacity to adapting practices to serve particular needs or interests. We will explore some principles of application after we introduce the techniques of *prāṇāyāma* and their symbolism below.

Some cautions in ratio development. We recommend the following guidelines:

- **Make exhalation equal to or longer than inhalation. Never make inhalation longer than exhalation.**
- **Make exhalation equal to or longer than retention of the breath after inhalation. There is a famous Habha Yoga ratio: 1-4-2-1, for example: 8-32-16-8. This ratio was given to adepts by their gurus as part of their intensive personal practice. Such a powerful ratio has risks and, in our view, should not be practiced without personal guidance.**
- **Let the focus of your practice be the smooth-flowing quality of inhalation and exhalation. This can be measured by the sound and feel of the breath at the valve point. If the breath gets strained or jerky, then reduce the threshold.**
- **Retention of the breath after inhalation and suspension of the breath after exhalation must not compromise the smooth flow of inhalation and exhalation.**
- **Never force the breath.**

CLASSIC *PRĀṆĀYĀMA* TECHNIQUES

There are many classic techniques of *prāṇāyāma*. These techniques are distinguished primarily by the location of the valve used to regulate the flow of the breath. In the main techniques, this valve is established in one of the following locations: in the throat, at the right or left nostril, at the tongue, alternately at the throat and either or both nostrils, or alternately between the nostrils. These techniques create a slight vibration at the site of the valve. This vibration can be used to measure how the body is responding to the practice. When the ratio is appropriate, the flow of the breath will be long, smooth, and subtle. If the body becomes stressed, it will be seen in the vibration, which may become rough and jumpy. In addition to serving as a way of measuring the body's response to the breath, these valves can also serve as a point of focus for the mind during the practice.

Specific differences between these various techniques will be further elaborated in the brief discussion that follows.

UJJĀYĪ

In this technique the valve is established by a partial contraction of the glottis. This contraction is used during inhale and exhale. The sound of the vibration at the throat can be so subtle as to be inaudible even to the practitioner or loud enough to be heard by others nearby. The general effect of this technique is said to be heating. The heating effect is intensified as the sound at the throat becomes louder.

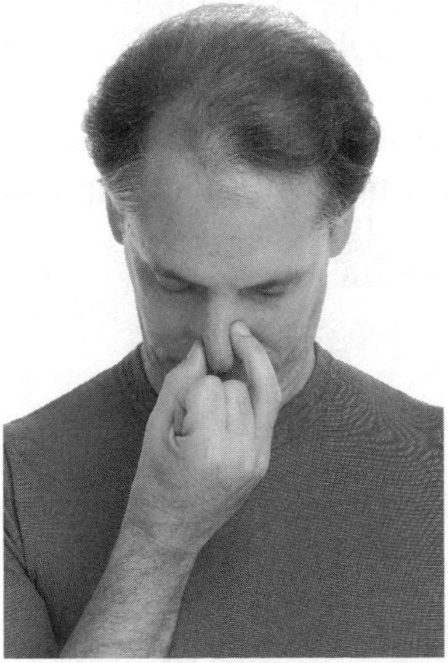

INHALE LEFT

The method of controlling the flow of breath at the nostril is often not understood. In the classical hand position (*mṛgī mudrā*), we use the thumb and ring finger of the right hand to regulate airflow. When we are using nostril control, we are not using the partial glottal contraction used in *ujjāyī*. The throat is left relaxed. Instead, the valve is created at the nostril. One nostril is sealed completely, usually at the soft part of the nostril flap below the cartilage of the nose. The nostril through which we are either inhaling or exhaling is **partially sealed** by pressing slightly just below the cartilage, with either the thumb or ring finger.

ANULOMA *(WITH THE GRAIN)* UJJĀYĪ

In this technique, we inhale using the *ujjāyī* glottal contraction, and we exhale through alternate nostrils.

VILOMA *(AGAINST THE GRAIN)* UJJĀYĪ

In this technique, we exhale using the *ujjāyī* glottal contraction, and we inhale through alternate nostrils.

As we have seen, exhalation tends to have a more calming effect, whereas inhalation tends to have a more stimulating effect. Therefore, alternate nostril exhalation (*anuloma ujjāyī*) tends to be more calming, while alternate nostril inhalation (*viloma ujjāyī*) tends to be more energizing.

PRATILOMA UJJĀYĪ

This technique is carried out as follows:

First we

- inhale, using the *ujjāyī* glottal contraction,
- exhale through the left nostril,
- inhale through the left nostril, and
- exhale, using the *ujjāyī* glottal contraction.

Then we

- inhale, using the *ujjāyī* glottal contraction,
- exhale through the right nostril,
- inhale through the right nostril,
- exhale, using the *ujjāyī* glottal contraction.

CANDRABHEDANA

In this technique, we inhale through the left nostril and exhale through the right nostril.

SŪRYABHEDANA

In this technique, we inhale through the right nostril and exhale through the left nostril.

NĀḌĪ ŚODHANA

In this technique, we inhale through the left nostril and exhale through the right nostril. Then we inhale through the right nostril and exhale through the left nostril.

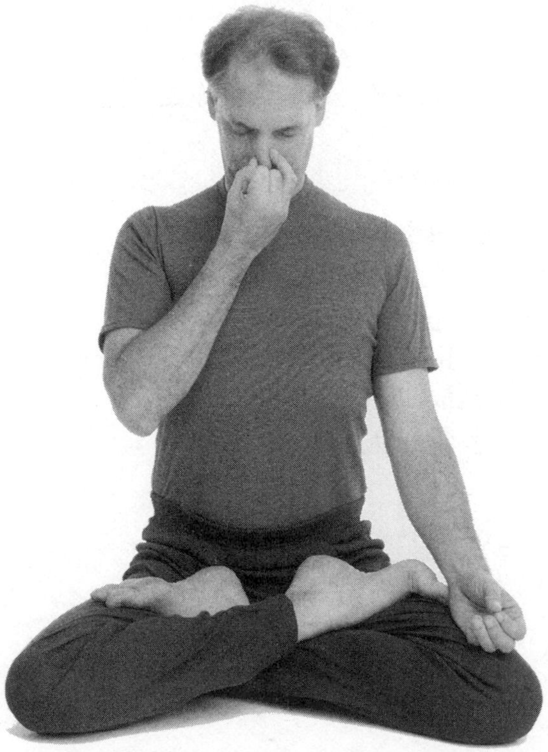

Śītalī

This technique is carried out as follows:
On inhale:

- Begin with the chin down and the tongue curled and fully extended.
- Throughout inhale, raise chin to just beyond level.
- At end of inhale, fold back tongue on itself so that the bottom of it touches the palate; close the mouth; and drop the chin.

Then exhale through alternate nostrils.

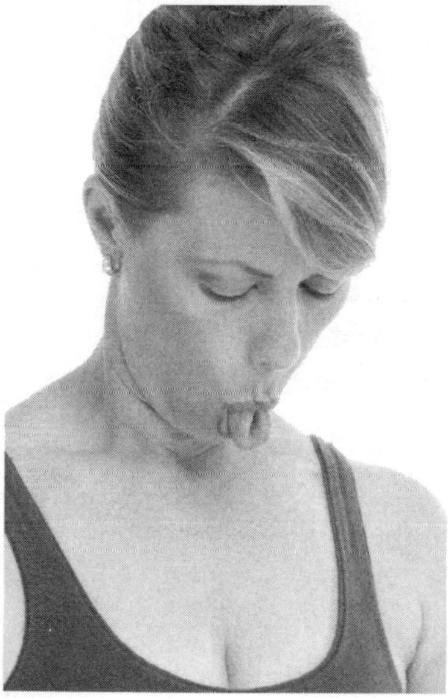

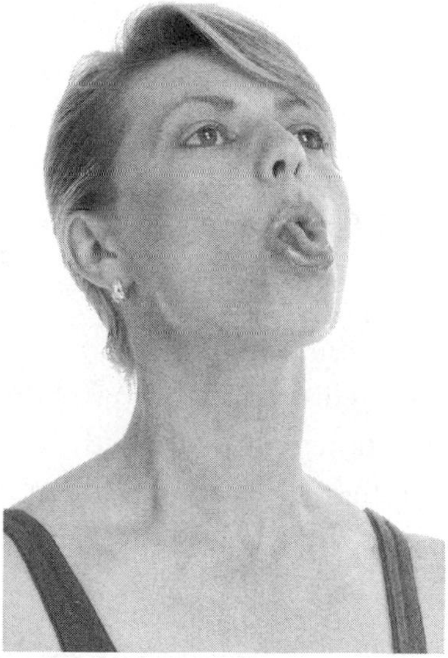

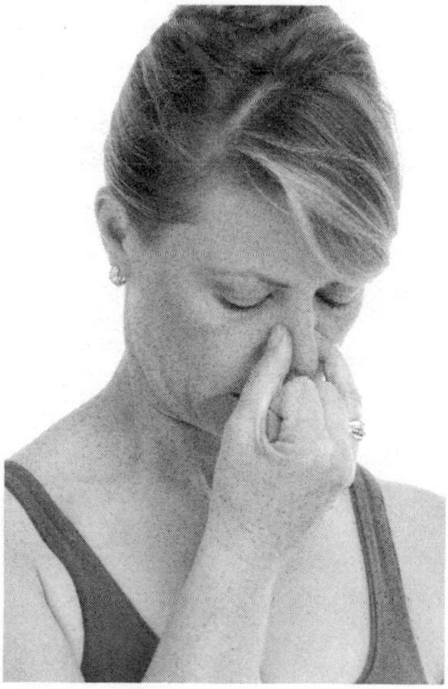

śītalī

Sītkārī

This technique is much like *śītalī,* with a similar effect. The difference, however, lies in the placement of the tongue on inhale, as follows:

On inhale:

- Begin with the chin down and the tongue placed on the palate, with its tip touching the back of the front teeth.
- Throughout the inhale, draw the breath in between the tongue and the palate.
- At the end of inhale, drop the head.

On exhale (as with *śītalī*):

- fold the tongue back on itself, and
- exhale through alternate nostrils.

Kapālabhāti

Patañjali's teaching on *prāṇāyāma* suggests the conscious extension and regulation of the flow of inhalation and exhalation. In each of the previous techniques, we have applied a valve for this purpose, either in the throat, tongue, or at the nostril.

However, *kapālabhāti*—perhaps more correctly called a cleansing exercise (*kriyā*)—involves rapid breathing with no control valve and, in this sense, is not classically considered a *prāṇāyāma.* In this technique, we focus on rapid and vigorous exhalation through repeated lower abdominal contraction. The inhalation is taken rapidly following each forced exhalation. Both exhalation and inhalation are taken through the nose with the mouth closed.

Bhastrikā

This technique is much like *kapālabhatī,* except that the rapid breathing is done through alternate nostrils. In the classic form, we alternate nostrils after each inhalation. In an adaptation that I have found particularly useful, the forced exhalation and the rapid inhalation are done through one nostril rapidly for a number of breaths, followed by the same rapid exhalation and inhalation through the other nostril.

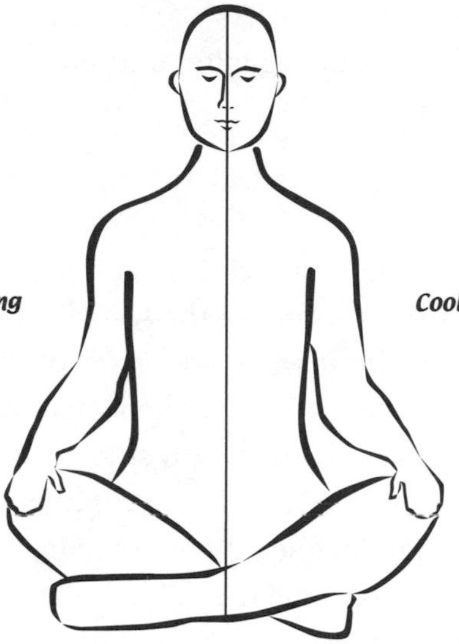

THE DEEPER SYMBOLISM OF *PRĀṆĀYĀMA*

Whereas in our consideration of ratio, we drew an imaginary horizontal line through the body at the level of the diaphragm, in considering Yoga techniques, we draw an imaginary vertical line through the body, beginning at the crown and extending down through the body to the perineal floor.

For the sake of making the complexity of *prāṇāyāma* techniques understandable, let's consider the classic symbolism given by the tradition.

IḌĀ

Iḍā, the main channel on the left side of the body, is symbolically identified as the lunar channel (*candra nāḍī*). This channel has a cooling quality. Like the moon, it is also said to have a changing character. It represents materiality (*prakṛti*), which is always changing. It symbolically represents the feminine quality.

PINGALĀ

Pingalā, the main channel on the right side of the body, is symbolically identified as the solar channel (*sūrya nāḍī*). This channel has a heating quality. Like the sun, it is said to have a steady, unchanging character. It represents consciousness (*puruṣa*), which is unchanging and eternal. It symbolically represents the masculine quality.

Suṣumnā

Suṣumnā is the central channel. It is said to be located in the center of the body and to extend from the root of the spinal column up to the top of the head. It is known as the *mokṣa mārga*—the "path of freedom."

According to this symbolic system, when there is either too much or too little energy in the left or right channels, our system will be unbalanced. For example, defects of character are related to conditions of excess or deficiency in either the lunar or the solar channels. More specifically, insecurity, instability, depression, grief, and disillusionment may be related to defects in the lunar channel; while anger, arrogance, impatience, and fanaticism may be related to defects in the solar channel. These defects are the result of blockages that obstruct the flow of *prāṇa* in the central channel (*suṣumnā*), and that keep *prāṇa* out of balance in the lunar and solar channels. The purpose of Yoga practice, from this perspective, is to bring the system into balance, and remove the obstacles that prevent *prāṇa* from entering *suṣumnā*.

According to the symbolism of this system, the lunar and solar channels (*nāḍī-s*) terminate in the left and right nostrils, respectively. When the valve that is used to control the flow of air is placed at the left or right nostril, the particular qualities of that *nāḍī* are emphasized. For example, stimulating the lunar channel (*candra nāḍī*) is said to cool the system down, whereas stimulating the solar channel (*sūrya nāḍī*) is said to increase the heat in the system.

THE CLASSIC *BANDHA-S*

The ancients proposed three particular practices, developed in the context of *prāṇāyāma,* to accelerate the action of transforming the human vessel. These practices are called *bandha-s,* which can be translated as "locks."

The Deeper Symbolism of *Bandha-s*

The ancients explained the esoteric purpose of the psychophysical practices of *āsana, prāṇāyāma,* and *bandha* symbolically. They said that when we are born there is a source, essence, or nectar (known variously as *amṛta* or *soma*) that is said to be contained in the "spring-fed lake of the mind," symbolically located in the region of the head.

In the newborn, this lake is full. If we look at the glow in the eyes of very young children, we perceive a sign of what they are referring to. In any case, the symbolism suggests that at puberty there is a descent of a large quantity of this essence to the level of the genitals, where it becomes known as *vīrya,* and we become fertile. The rest of this *amṛta* drips slowly down from its source and is consumed in the fire (*agni* or *sūrya*) that is symbolically placed in the region of the navel. And when that lake or spring is emptied, we have reached the end of our lives.

Below the fire, in the region of our intestines, is the place where impurities (*mala*) accumulate. Over time, these impurities poison our systems and, according to the esoteric model, prevent our vital energy (*prāṇa*) from fully entering the central channel (*suṣumnā*), which is its proper resting place.

Therefore, to understand the purpose of practice from this perspective, we can think of this in terms of a mountain spring, which becomes the source for a river that ultimately goes to the ocean. The ocean water, due to evaporation, gets back to the mountain spring through rain. The sun, as it were, pulls it back up. The ancients conceived the esoteric purpose of practice to model the action of the sun. Through the heat of these practices, we evaporate, as it were, the descended essence which thus rises and, as rain, replenishes that "lake of the mind."

The Bandha Techniques

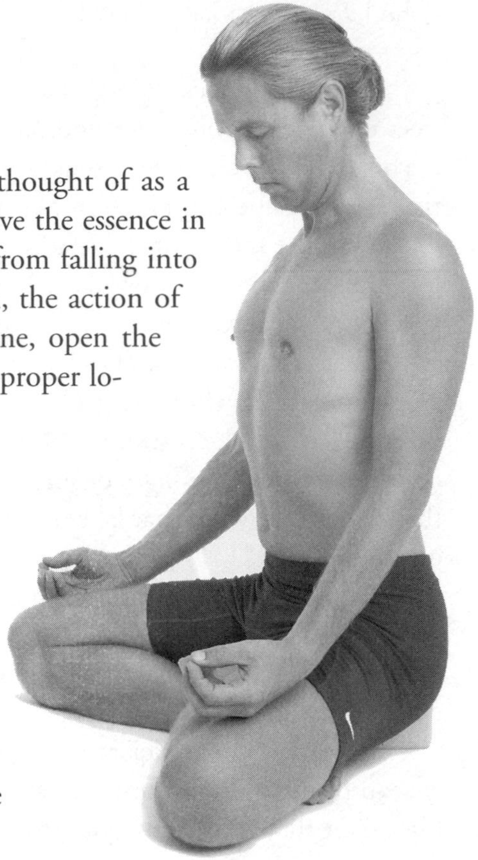

JĀLANDHARA BANDHA

Jālandhara bandha is commonly thought of as a chin lock. Its esoteric purpose is to preserve the essence in the "lake of the mind," by preventing it from falling into the fire and being consumed. In addition, the action of *jālandhara bandha* helps to align the spine, open the channels, and bring the *cakra-s* into their proper locations (see Part II, Chapter 3).

TECHNIQUE:

- On inhalation, vertically align the head, neck, and upper and lower back.
- *On retention of the breath, after inhalation,* while displacing the head slightly backward and straightening the neck, lower the chin toward the notch between the collarbones.

UDDĪYĀNA BANDHA

The esoteric purpose of *uddīyāna bandha* is to hold the impurities (*mala*) up closer to the fire—the fire in the navel—so that they can be reduced to ashes. In this context, inhalation fans the fire downward toward the impurities, as gently blowing on a candle directs the flame and also heats the fire and as blowing on a fire intensified its heat.

TECHNIQUE:

- On exhalation, progressively pull the abdomen in from the pubic bone to the sternum at the base of the ribs.

- At the end of the exhalation, *while suspending the breath out after exhalation,* continue pushing the belly in and up. Gently lift the ribs. This will create a concavity in the abdomen.
- After sustaining this concavity for a few seconds, gently release the concavity from the sternum to the navel and then take the next inhalation.

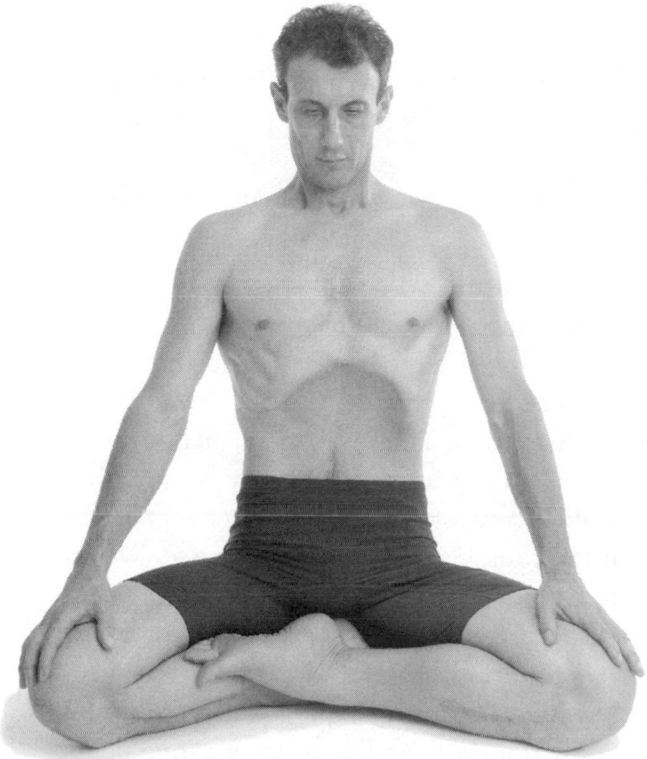

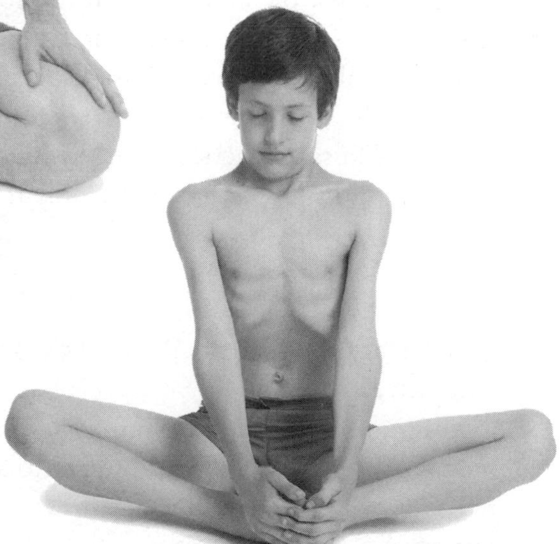

MŪLA BANDHA

The esoteric purpose of *mūla bandha* is to hold the impurities up and thereby sustain the effect of *uddīyāna bandha*. In addition, it lifts the *mūlādhāra cakra,* the root support of the entire system (see Part II, Chapter 3), to its proper location, which, when it drops downward, indicates a loss of energy.

TECHNIQUE:

- After *uddīyāna bandha* is lifted and *while suspending the breath out after exhalation,* gently contract the muscles from the perineal floor upward to the navel.
- After *uddīyāna bandha* is released, *mūla bandha* is maintained for the duration of the practice.

These techniques have value beyond their use in this esoteric system of practice. *Jālandhara bandha* helps with the alignment of the spine and in correcting postural problems. *Uddīyāna bandha* can be helpful for certain digestive and menstrual disorders, as well as for a prolapsed uterus. *Mūla bandha* can be helpful for certain reproductive disorders, as well as for hemorrhoids.

However, these techniques are strong and should not be practiced without proper instruction and guidance. Moreover, this classic presentation, if practiced, must be understood in the context of *prāṇāyāma* practice. We can see by the description above that, in order to practice *uddīyāna bandha* correctly, we will need to be able to suspend the breath after exhalation for at least ten seconds, for a minimum of twelve breaths, before we can even begin its practice. Thus, to practice these techniques correctly requires a degree of training and conditioning that comes only from regular practice over a long period of time.

THE CLASSICAL THEORY OF PRACTICE

From the above discussion it becomes apparent that the way we practice *prāṇāyāma* will depend on several factors, including our intention for the practice, our breathing capacity, our structural needs, our constitutional needs, and our psycho-emotional state.

The Basic Paradigm

From a structural perspective, we can say that an emphasis on inhale will have particular benefit for the chest and upper back, while emphasis on exhale will have particular benefit for the abdomen and lower back.

Beyond structural considerations and a purely exploratory and developmental orientation, the basic paradigm for understanding how to choose a particular ratio for our personal practice can be understood in the paradigm of ***bṛhmana*** and ***langhana***.

Bṛhmana, coming from a Sanskrit root meaning "expand," refers to practices that build or nourish the system. Theoretically, *bṛhmana* practices include inhalation, holding after inhalation, backward-bending, fast movements, and chanting loudly and/or in a higher pitch.

Langhana, coming from a Sanskrit word meaning "light" (as in weight), refers to practices that calm or pacify the system and that emphasize reduction. Theoretically, *langhana* practices include exhalation, short hold after exhalation, forward-bending, slow movements, and chanting softly and/or in a lower pitch.

Perhaps the primary factor to consider is your constitutional needs. If you want to use your practice to address low morning energy, for example, we might recommend a *bṛhmana* practice, using ratios that emphasize inhalation and retention of the breath after inhalation, or techniques that utilize alternate nostril inhalation. If, on the other hand, you want to use your practice to help soothe an agitated mind, we might recommend a *langhana* practice, using ratios that emphasize progressively lengthening exhalation, short suspension of the breath after exhalation, or techniques that utilize alternate nostril exhalation.

The information offered here is not meant to be a substitute for working with a qualified teacher when developing a personal practice, but rather as an attempt to share the breadth and complexity of this beautiful, subtle, and powerful practice.

The Relationship Between Ratio and Technique

The next step is to consider how to link particular ratios with particular techniques. Although there are no hard-and-fast rules, we encourage the use of long flowing ratios, where the valve used to control the flow of the breath is placed at either or both nostrils. This extension of the length of the flow of inhale and/or exhale allows more time for the subtle effects of the nostril control to be realized.

To explore the technique know as *nāḍī śodhana,* for example (where we inhale through the left nostril and exhale through the right nostril, then inhale through the right nostril and exhale through the left nostril), we would **initially** recommend something like a *3-1-3-1* ratio, rather than a *1-1-1-1* ratio:

9-3-9-3
12-4-12-4
15-5-15-5

Depending on the development of your breath, you could pick any of these thresholds and simply sustain the ratio for a minimum of twelve breaths. Another possibility would be to sustain each threshold a minimum of six breaths, beginning with 9-3-9-3. And, of course, once you are familiar with the various nostril techniques, you can use them with any ratio.

Application

If you'd like to explore this complex practice, we recommend that you begin by observing the natural flow of your breath. You may sit in a comfortable posture with your spine erect and simply watch the natural flow of inhale and exhale. Then, in the process described at the beginning of this chapter, gradually increase the length of inhale and exhale. Over time your goal should be to be to extend the flow of both inhale and exhale, to equalize their flow, and to sustain long-flowing breath over a period of time.

After exploring your breath in this way for some time, you can begin the exploration of ratio. To work with ratio, you must bring your full attention to the subtle effects achieved by varying the lengths of inhalation, the retention of the breath after inhalation and exhalation, and the suspension of the breath after exhalation.

Āsana practice is considered the primary and essential preparation for *prāṇāyāma.* Using *āsana* practice as preparation for *prāṇāyāma,* however, requires a different approach than using *āsana* practice for the sake of the structure. When we use *āsana* in the service of *prāṇāyāma,* we select a limited number of specific postures linked to the goal of the practice, and we carefully develop the breath work in the *āsana* practice in order to facilitate the breath work in the *prāṇāyāma* practice that follows.

The next practice is specifically designed to further illustrate how *āsana* practice can be adapted in the service of *prāṇāyāma.* In this practice, we introduce the principles of building ratio and preparing for *bandha* practice. **However, because *banda-s* are strong, we recommend that they be practiced only after being initiated by a qualified teacher.** And we suggest that when this is not the case that the sequence below be carried out by merely bringing awareness to the areas involved rather than by actually applying the *bandha-s.*

Finally, for the sake of simplicity in an otherwise complex practice, we use the *ujjāyī* technique. In all cases **where the breath becomes short or rough, release the *bandha* technique**. Remember that the length of the breath in the *prāṇāyāma* practice is measured in seconds. And feel free to shorten the lengths if they are too long, trying always to experience the ratio. Thus, for example, 10-10-10-10 could be practiced at 8-8-8-8 or 6-6-6-6.

PRĀṆAMAYA PRACTICE

1.

POSTURE: *Uttānāsana*

EMPHASIS: To warm up back and legs.

TECHNIQUE: Stand with arms over head.

On exhale: Forward bend, bringing belly and chest toward thighs, and hands to feet.

On inhale: Return to starting position.

Number: Five times

DETAILS:

On exhale: Bend knees to facilitate stretching of lower back. Move chin *down toward* throat.

On inhale: Lift chest up and away from thighs, flattening upper back. Keep knees bent until end of movement.

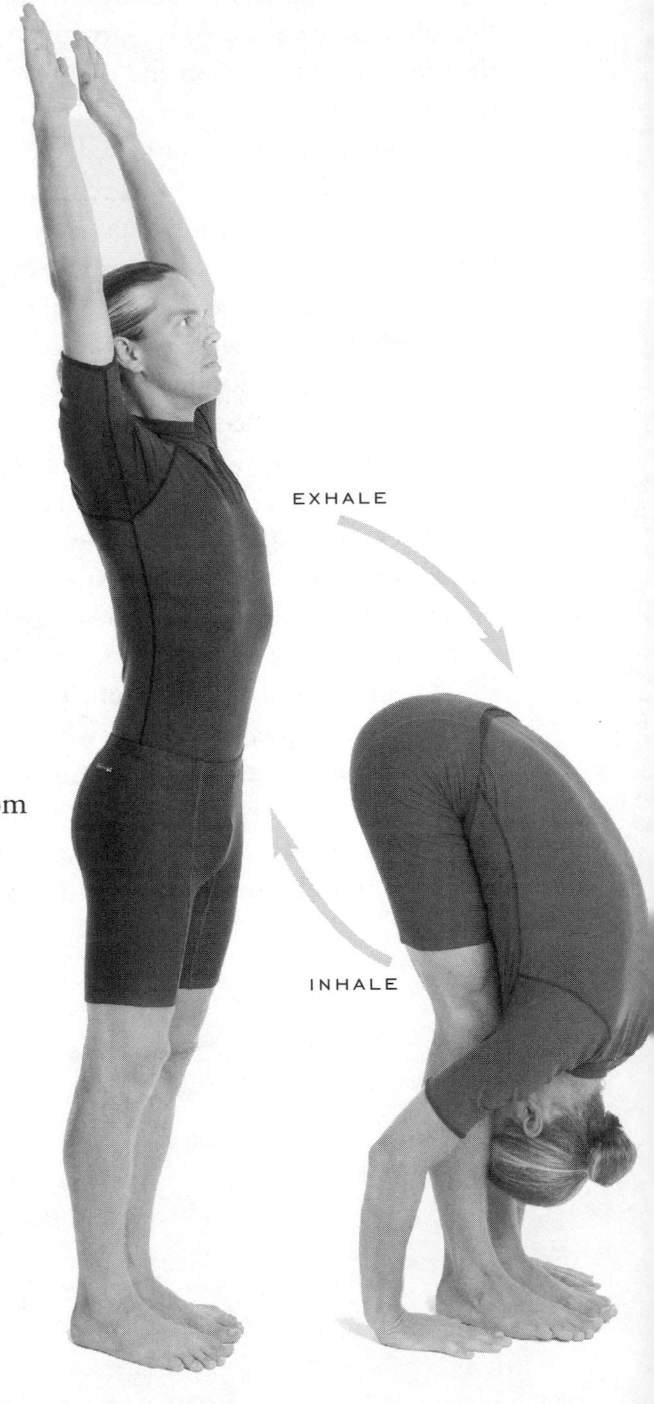

2.

POSTURE: *Vīrabhadrāsana*

EMPHASIS: To strengthen muscles of back and legs, expand chest, and flatten upper back. To introduce retention of the breath after inhalation in preparation for the *prāṇāyāma* practice.

TECHNIQUE: Stand with left foot forward, feet as wide as hips, and arms at sides.

On inhale: Simultaneously bend left knee, displace chest slightly forward and hips slightly backward, and bring arms forward and up over head. Arch upper back.

Retain breath after inhale five seconds.

On exhale: Return to starting position.

Number:
Five times each side.

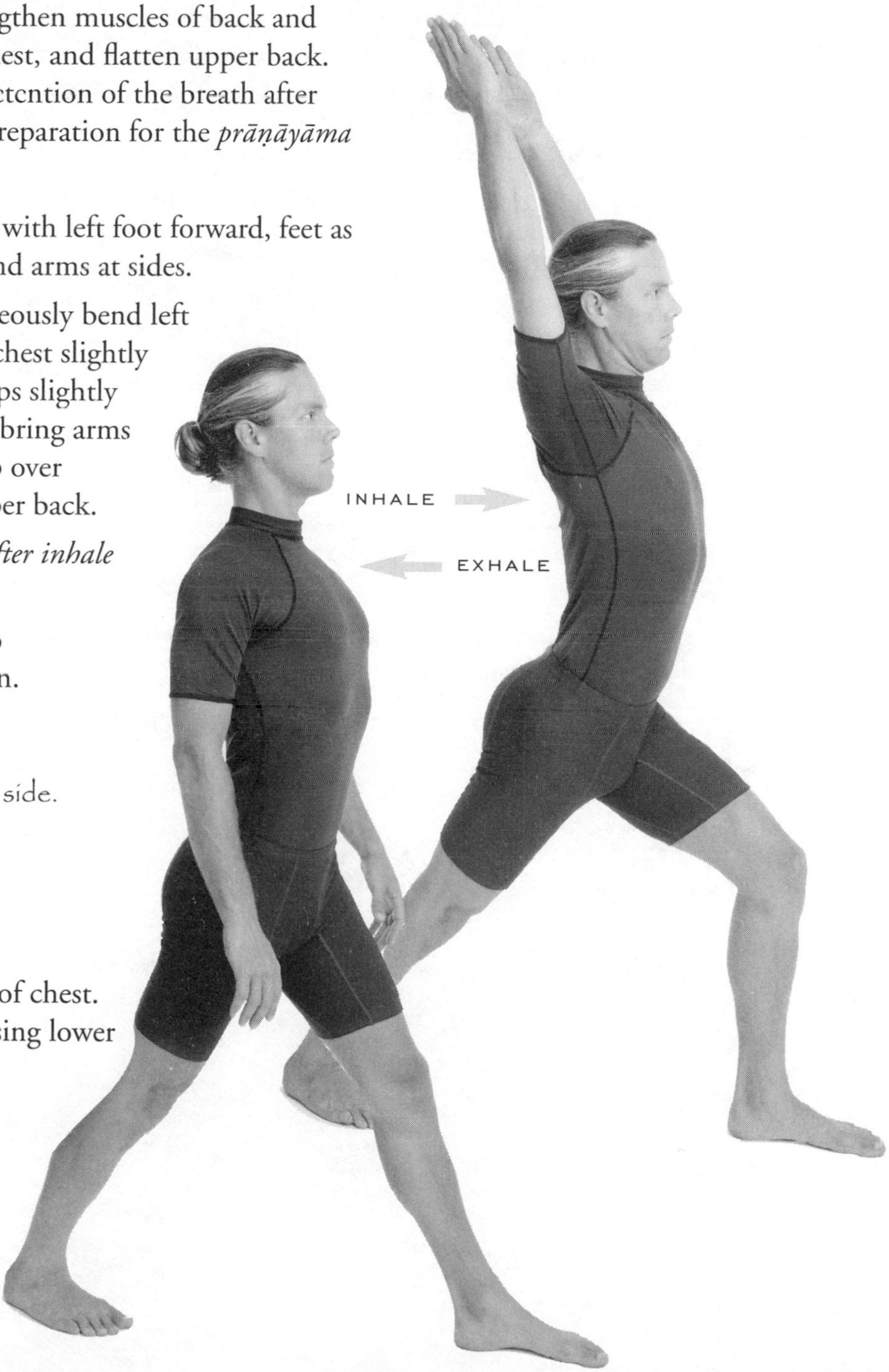

DETAILS:

On inhale:

Feel expansion of chest. Avoid compressing lower back.

3.

POSTURE: *Vajrāsana/Ūrdhva Mukha Śvānāsana* combination

EMPHASIS: To energize system by engaging musculature of upper body, expanding chest, and stretching belly. To introduce suspension of the breath after exhalation in preparation for the *prāṇāyāma* and *bandha* practice.

TECHNIQUE: Stand on knees with arms over head.

On exhale: Bend forward, bringing arms to floor in front of you.

Suspend breath after exhale five seconds.

On inhale: Stretch body forward and arch back, keeping only hands and from knees to feet on floor.

On exhale: Return to previous position.

Suspend breath after exhale five seconds.

On inhale: Return to starting position.

Number: Five times.

DETAILS: *On inhale:* Expand chest, stretch belly, and avoid compressing lower back.

On exhale: End in forward bend position.

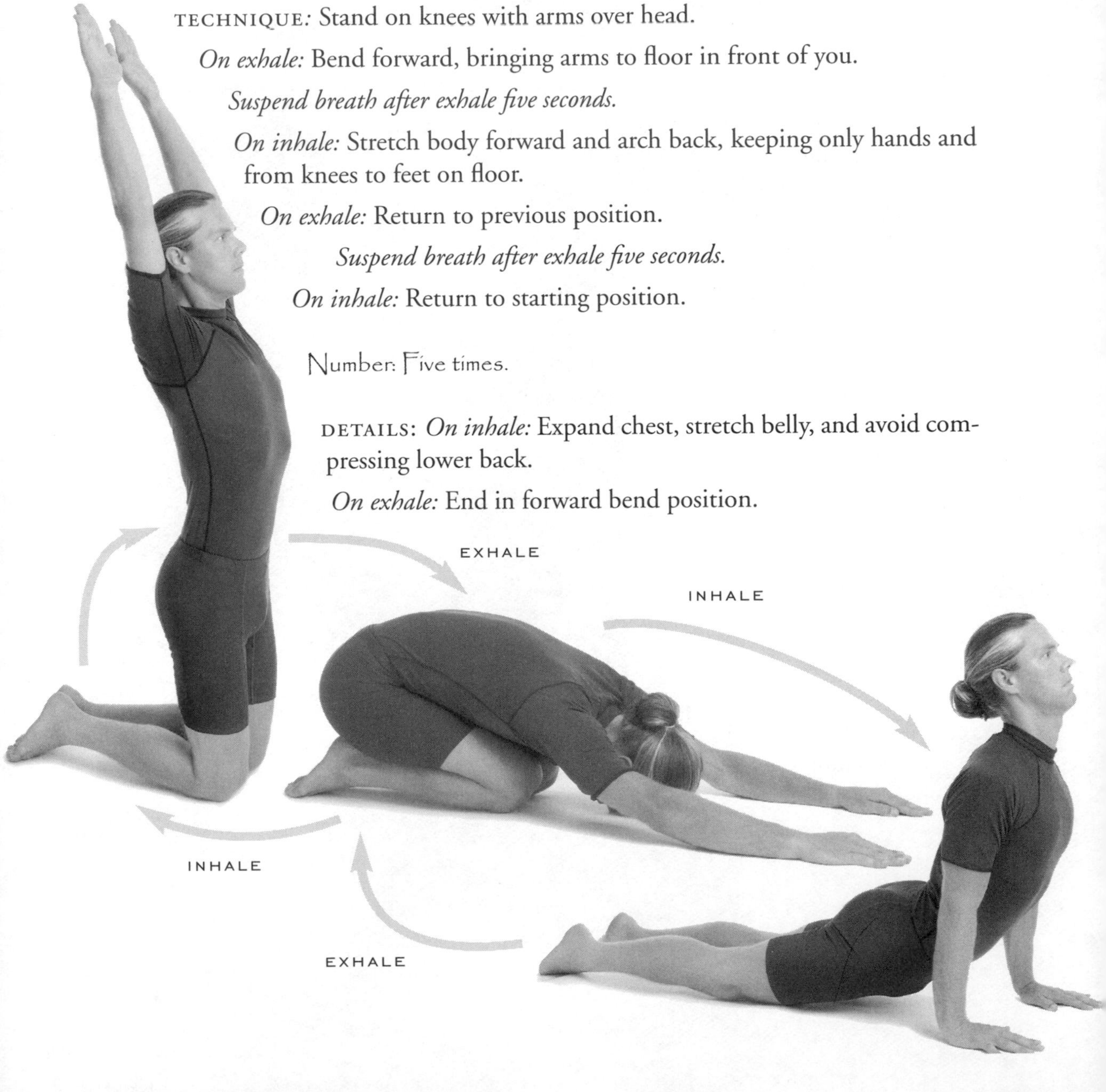

4.

POSTURE: *Ardha Śalabhāsana*

EMPHASIS: To strengthen back while mobilizing shoulders and arms.

TECHNIQUE: Lie on stomach, with head turned to left, hands crossed over sacrum, and palms up.

On inhale: Lift chest, left arm, and right leg, turning head to center.

On exhale: Lower chest and leg, while sweeping arm behind back and turning head to right.

Repeat on other side.

Number: Five times each side, alternately.

DETAILS:

On inhale: Lift chest slightly before leg, and emphasize chest height. Keep pelvis level.

On exhale: Turn head opposite arm being lowered.

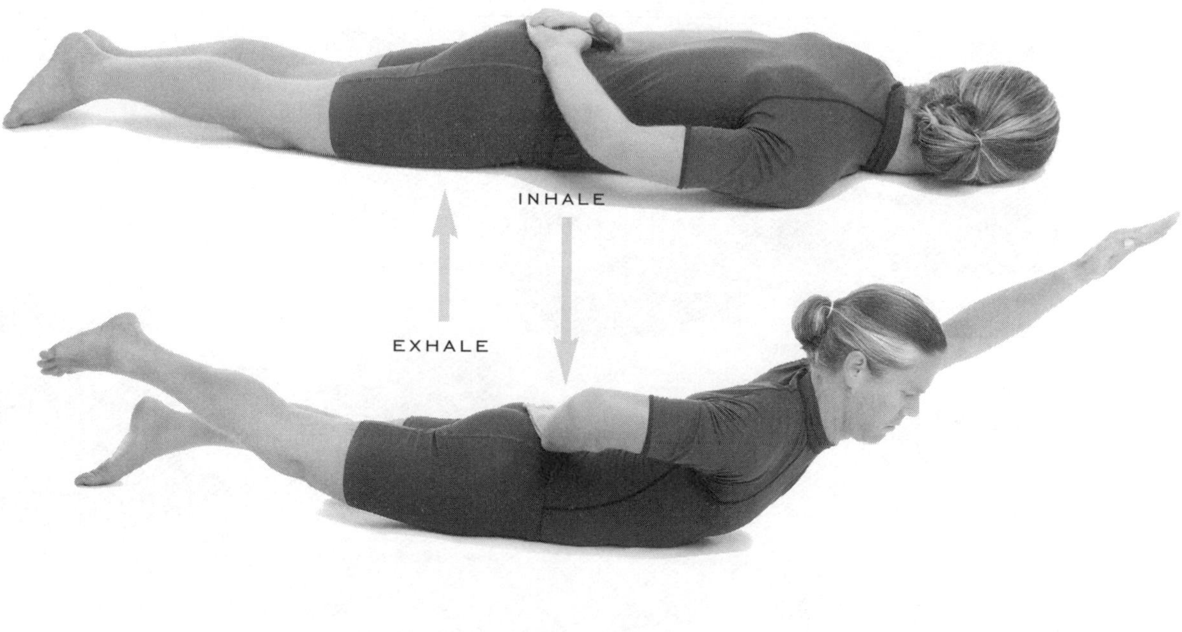

5.

POSTURE: *Supta Pādāṅguṣṭhāsana* adaptation

EMPHASIS: To stretch and relax lower back after back bend. To continue retention of the breath after inhalation and suspension of the breath after exhalation in preparation for the *prāṇāyāma* and *bandha* practice.

TECHNIQUE: Lie on back with legs bent, knees lifted toward chest, hands holding thighs behind knee, and arms bent.

On inhale: Extend legs upward, straightening arms. *Retain breath after inhalation five seconds.*

On exhale: Return to starting position. *Suspend breath after exhalation five seconds.*

Number: Five times.

DETAILS:

On inhale: Flex feet as legs are raised upward.
Slightly bend knees. Push lower back and sacrum downward.
Keep chin down.

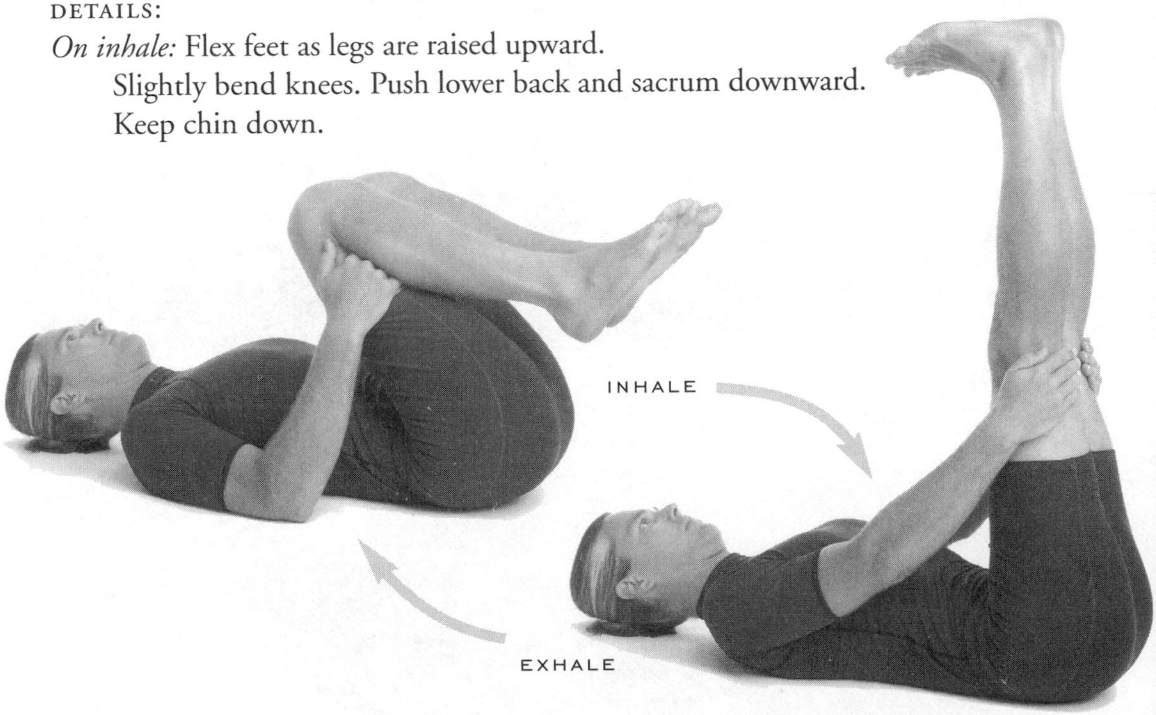

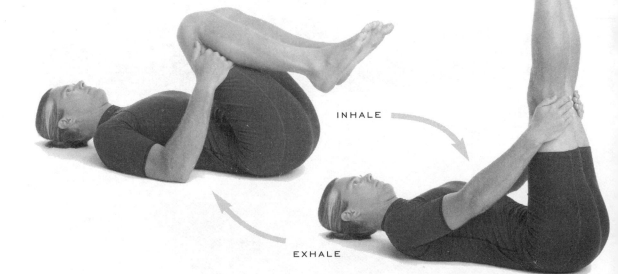

6.

POSTURE: *Jaṭhara Parivṛtti*

EMPHASIS: To gently twist and compress belly, and stretch hips. To facilitate exhalation and continue suspension of the breath after exhalation in preparation for the *prāṇāyāma* and *bandha* practice.

TECHNIQUE: Lie on back with right leg fully extended and left knee bent, left thigh lifted toward chest, and left foot off the ground. Arms out to sides, slightly less than right angles to torso.

On exhale: Bring left knee toward floor on right side of body, twisting abdomen while simultaneously turning head to left. *Suspend breath after exhale five seconds.*

On inhale: Return to starting position.

Repeat five times each side, one side at a time.

DETAILS: *On exhale,* throughout movement, keep knees at an angle to torso that is less than ninety degrees.

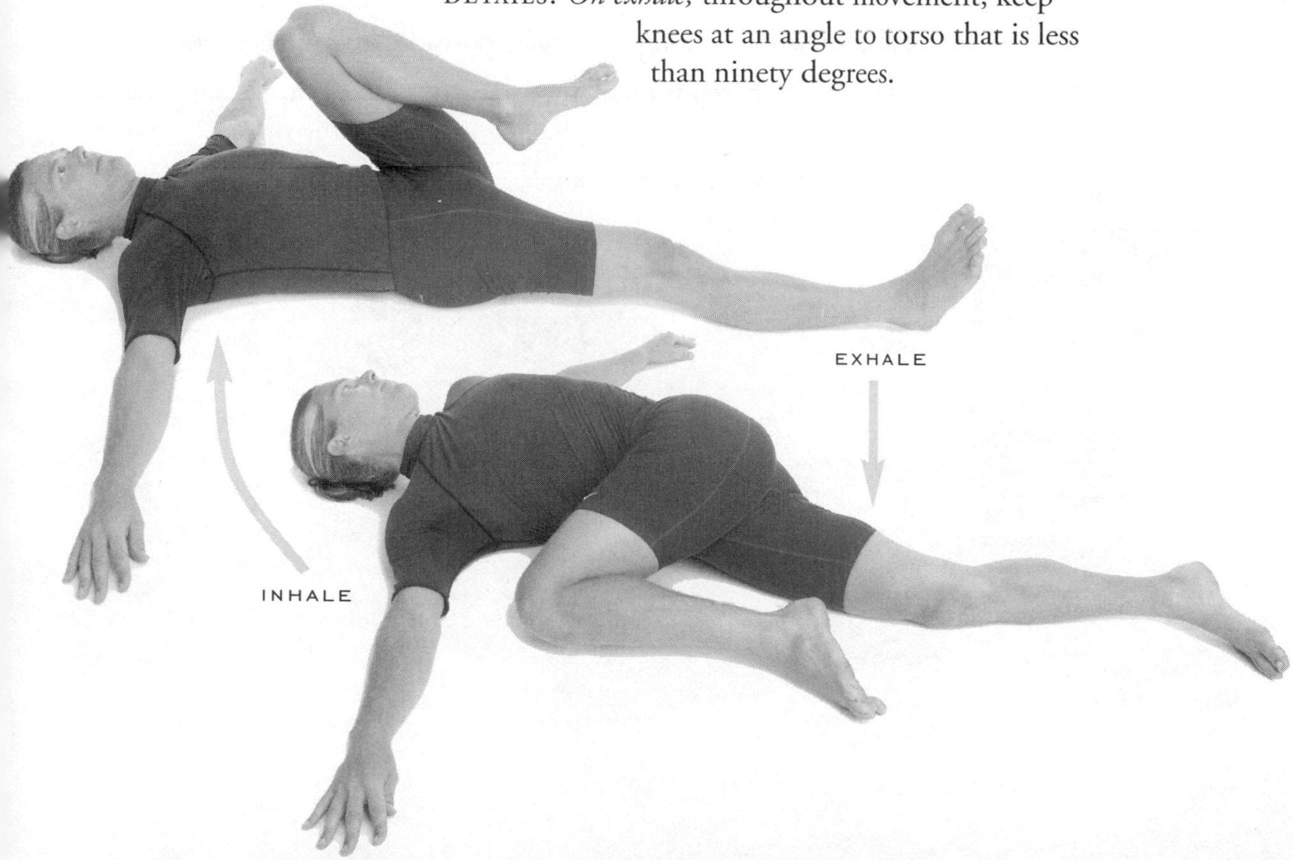

7.

POSTURE: *Jānu Śirṣāsana* and *Mahāmudrā* combination

A: *Jānu Śirṣāsana*

EMPHASIS: To stretch lower back and legs. To prepare for *mahāmudrā*.

TECHNIQUE: Sit with right leg folded in, heel to groin, left leg extended forward, and arms over head.

On exhale: Bend forward, bringing belly and chest toward left leg and bringing hands to left foot.

On inhale: Return to starting position.

Number: Repeat five times on one side, then:

B: *Mahāmudrā*

EMPHASIS: To strengthen musculature of torso. To establish a breathing ratio in preparation for *bandha* practice.

TECHNIQUE: From *jānu śirṣāsana* position, holding left foot:

On inhale: Extend spine upward, expanding chest, flattening upper back, and lengthening in front of the torso.

Retain the breath after inhale.

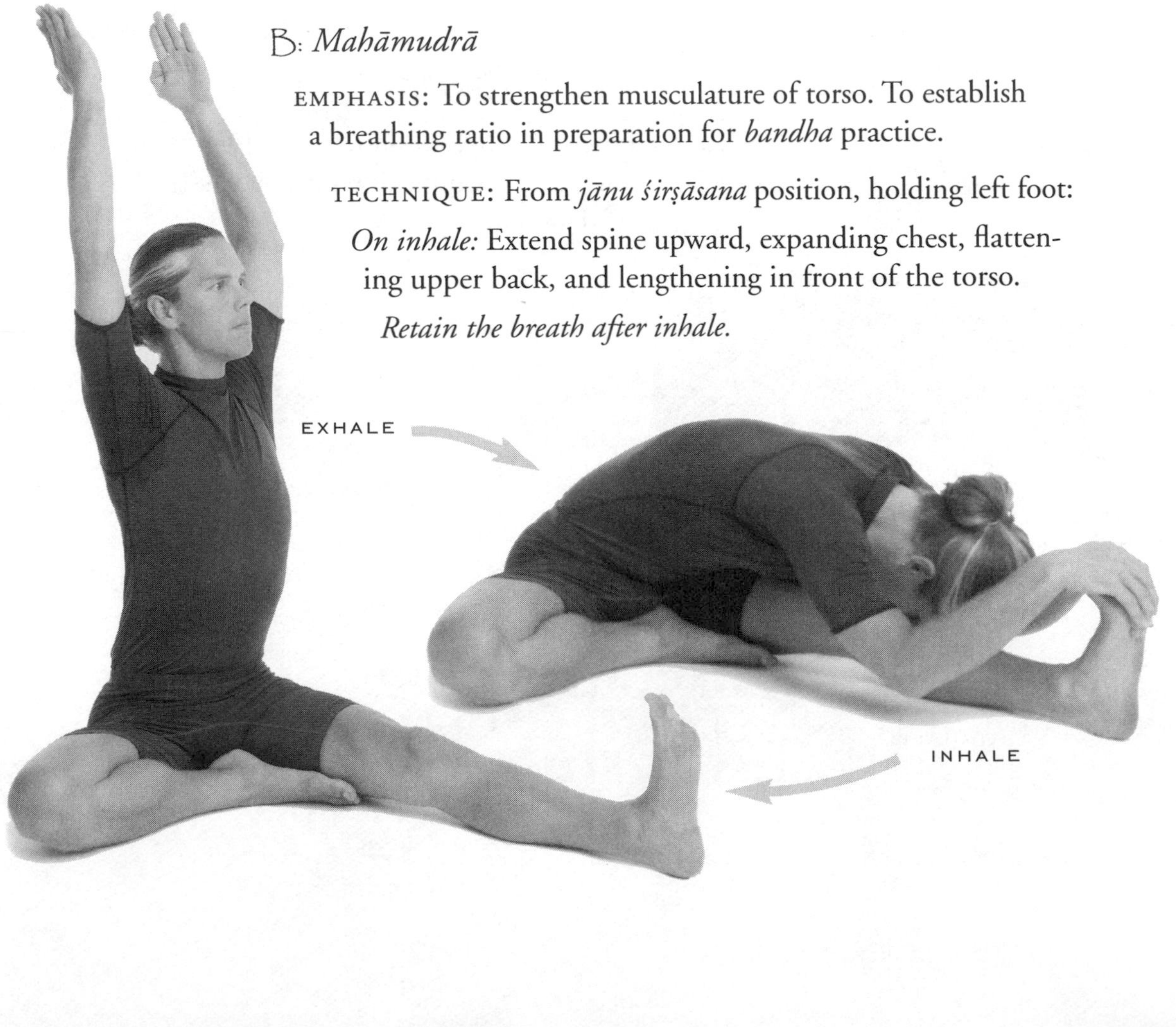

On exhale: Maintain posture while pulling upward from perineal floor, and pulling belly firmly in. *Suspend the breath after exhale.*

Ratio: 10-5-10-5

Number: Stay in position ten breaths on one side, then:

DETAILS:

On inhale: Lift chest slightly, extending spine.
On exhale: Tighten belly, *maintaining* extended spine.

C: *Jānu Śirṣāsana*

EMPHASIS: To relax back and neck.

TECHNIQUE: From *jānu śirṣāsana* position, holding left foot:

Number: Stay down in forward bend position for five breaths.
Then repeat A, B, and
C on other side.

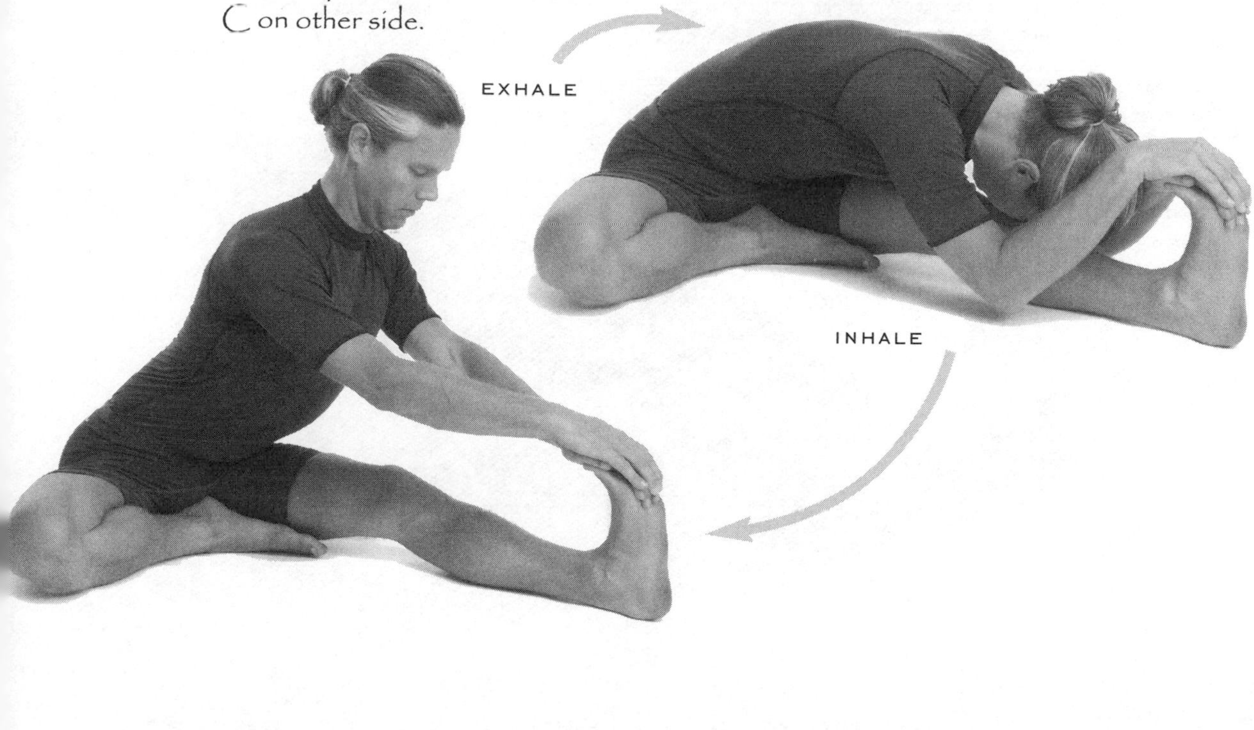

8.

POSTURE: *Dvipāda Pīṭham*

EMPHASIS: To relax neck and upper and lower back, and to gently stretch between belly and thighs.

TECHNIQUE*:* Lie on back with arms down at sides, knees bent, feet slightly apart on floor, and comfortably close to buttocks.

A:

On inhale: Press down on feet, raising pelvis and arms up toward ceiling, keeping chin down until neck is gently flattened on floor.

On exhale: Return to starting position.

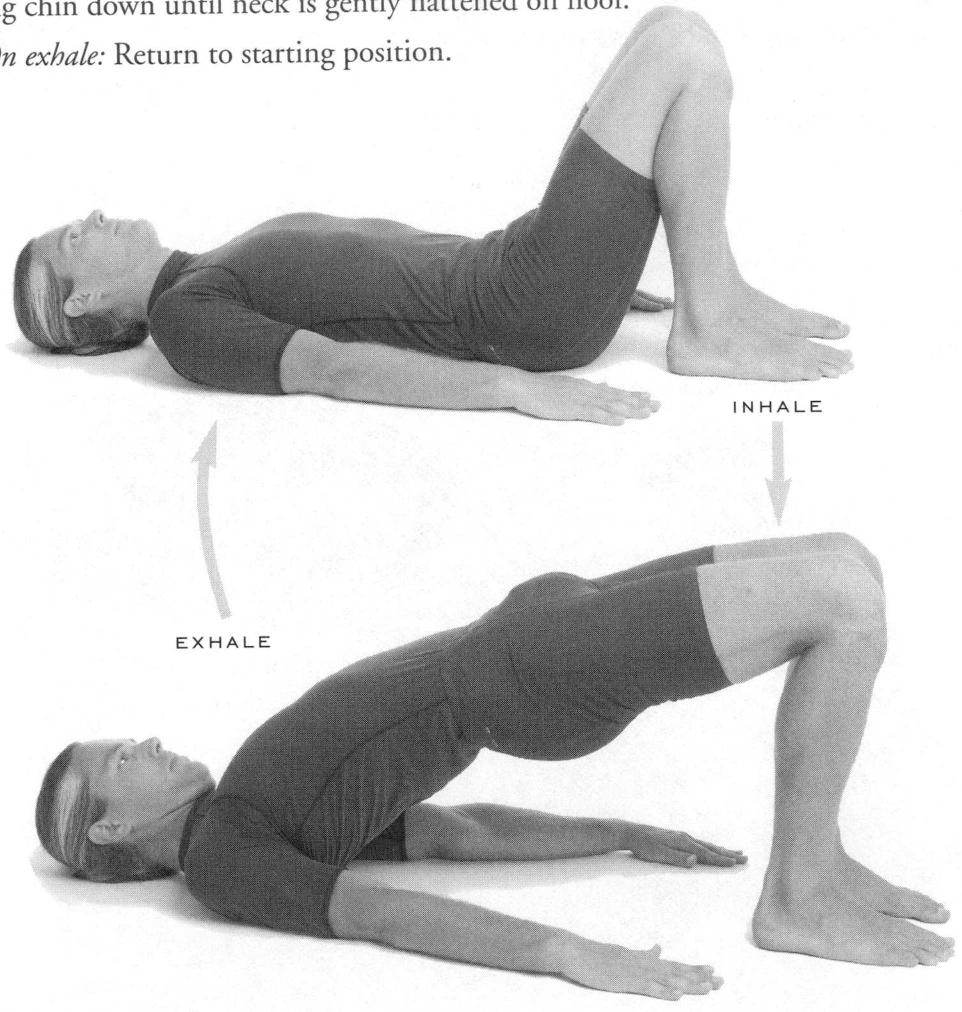

B:

On inhale: Press down on feet, raising pelvis and arms up toward ceiling, keeping chin down until neck is gently flattened on floor, while raising arms over head to floor behind.

On exhale: Return to starting position.

Number: Repeat A and B five times each.

DETAILS:

On inhale: Lift spine, vertebra by vertebra, from bottom up.

On exhale: Unwind spine, coming down vertebra by vertebra.

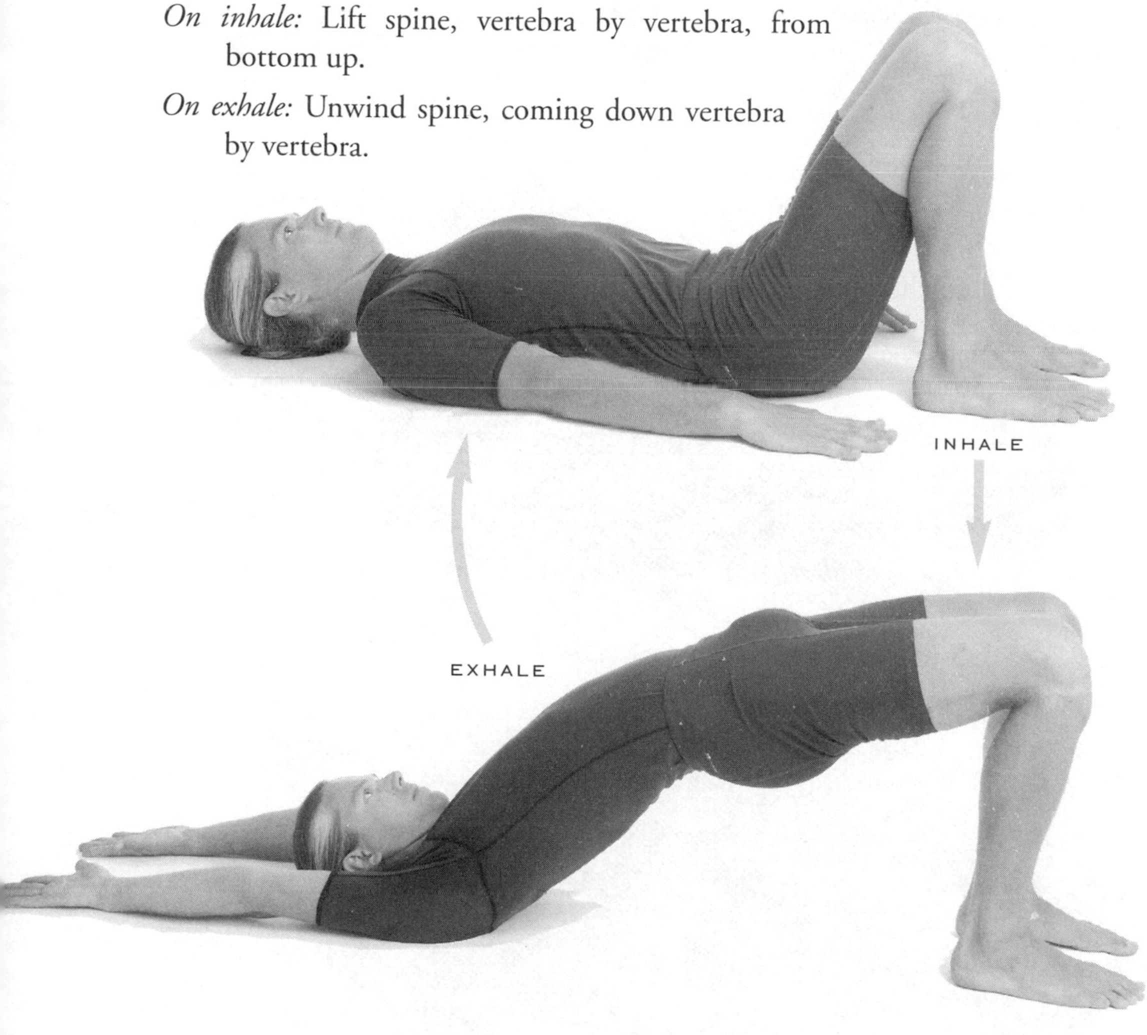

9.

POSTURE: *Apānāsana*

EMPHASIS: To gently stretch and relax lower back.

TECHNIQUE: Lie on back with both knees bent toward chest and feet off floor. Place each hand on its respective knee.

On exhale: Pull thighs gently but progressively toward chest.

On inhale: Return to starting position.

Number: Five times.

DETAILS:

On exhale: Pull gently with arms, keeping shoulders relaxed and on floor. Press lower back down into floor and drop chin slightly toward throat.

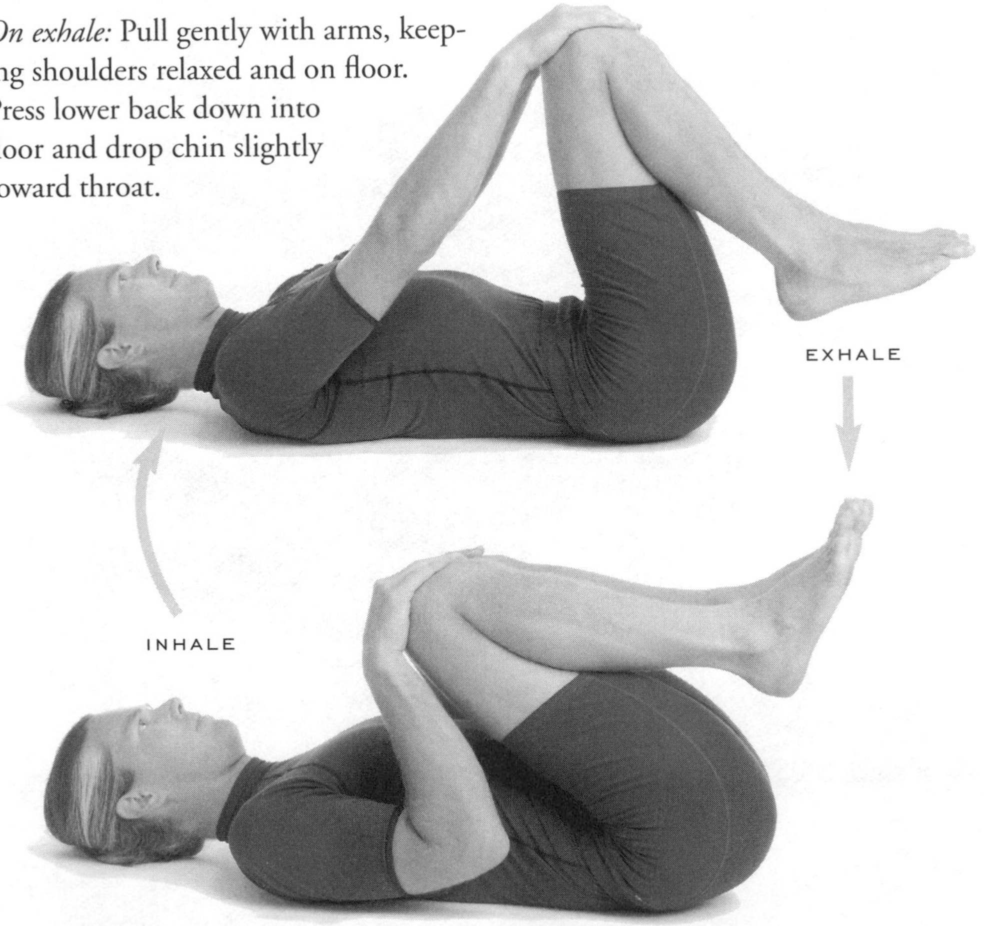

10.

POSTURE: *Śavāsana*

EMPHASIS: To rest.

TECHNIQUE: Lie flat on back, arms at side, palms up, and legs slightly apart. Close eyes. Relax body fully, keeping mind relaxed and alert to sensations in body.

Duration: Minimum five minutes.

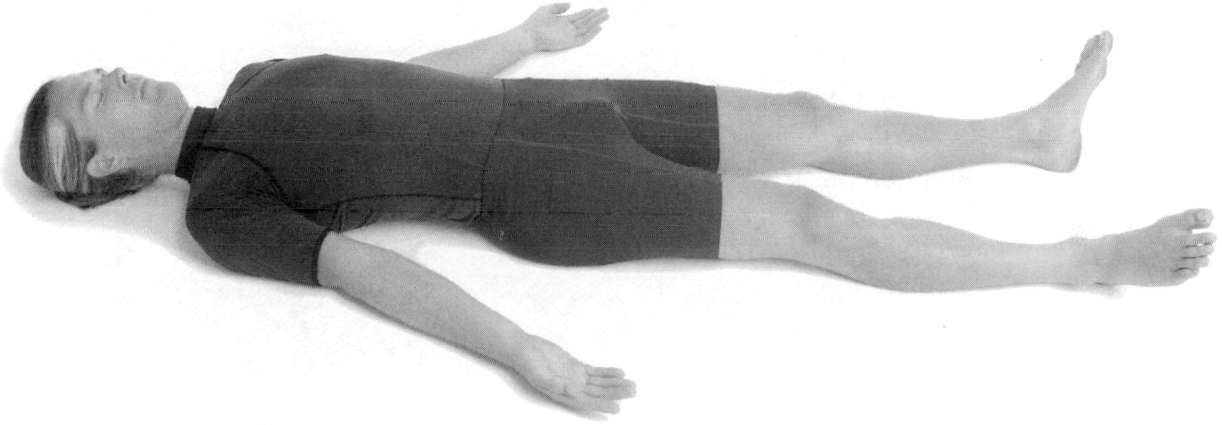

11.

POSTURE: *Siddhāsana*

EMPHASIS: *Prāṇāyāma* with *bandhas.*

TECHNIQUE: *Ujjāyī*

A: Establish a deep and equal inhale and exhale, with no breath retention.

B: Initiate retention after inhale and suspension of the breathafter exhale.

C: Increase retention after inhale and establish *jālandhara bandha* (see page 128).

D: Increase suspension of the breath after exhale.

E: Establish *uddīyāna bandha* (see pages 128–129).

F: Establish *mūla bandha* (see page 130).

G: Deep inhale and exhale, no *bandha-s,* no breath retention.

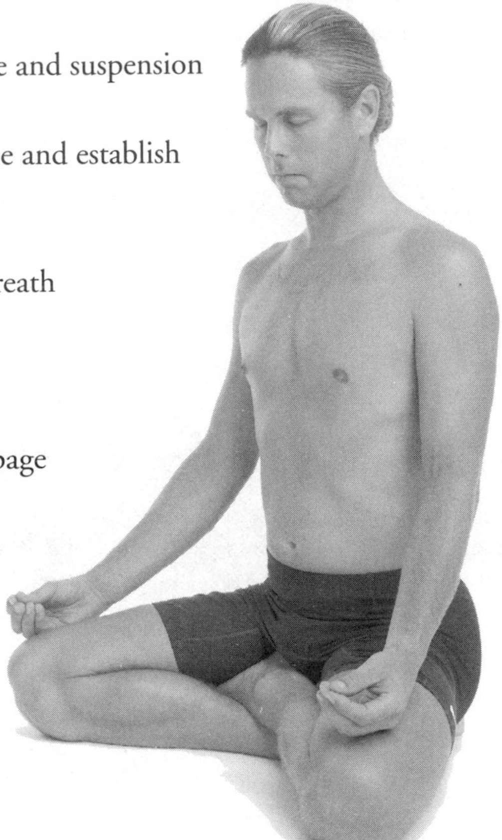

Round:	*Inhale*	*Hold*	*Exhale*	*Hold*	*Number*	*Technique*
A.	10	0	10	0	5	*on inhale:* lift head *on exhale:* lower head
B.	10	5	10	5	5	*on inhale:* lift head *on hold after inhale:* lower head

Round:	*Inhale*	*Hold*	*Exhale*	*Hold*	*Number*	*Technique*
C.	10	10	10	5	5	*on hold after inhale:* sustain *jālandhara bandha,*
D.	10	10	10	10	5	maintain *jālandhara bandha*

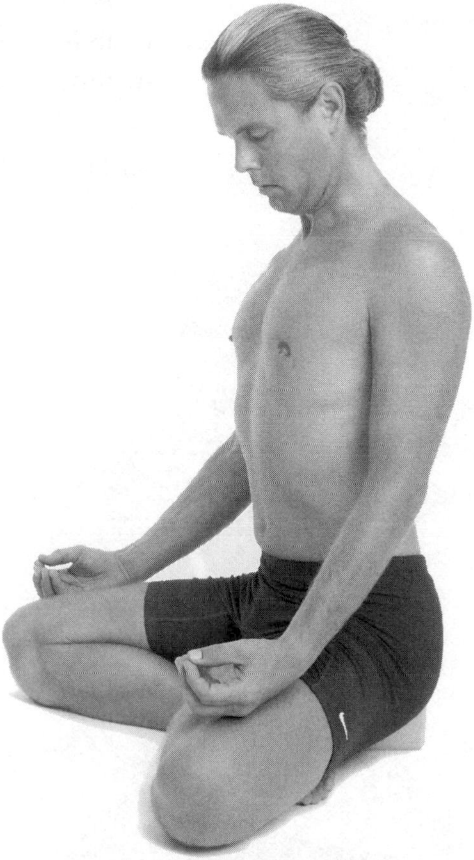

Round:	*Inhale*	*Hold*	*Exhale*	*Hold*	*Number*	*Technique*
E.	10	10	10	10	5	maintain *jālandhara bandha* *on hold after exhale:* establish *uddīyāna bandha,* sustain, then release *uddīyāna bandha*
F.	10	10	10	10	10	maintain *jālandhara bandha* *on hold after exhale:* establish *uddīyāna bandha,* establish *mūla bandha,* release *uddīyāna bandha*
G.	10	0	10	0	5	*on inhale:* lift head *on exhale:* lower head

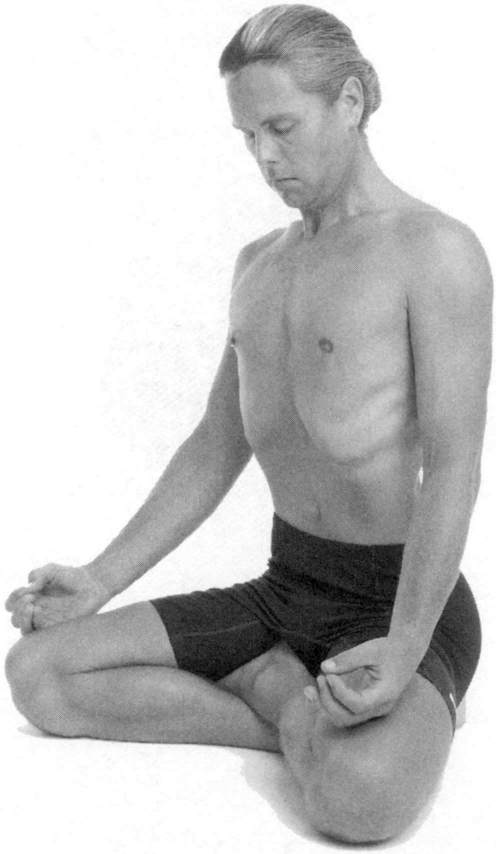

12.

POSTURE: *Siddhāsana*

EMPHASIS: Sit quietly.

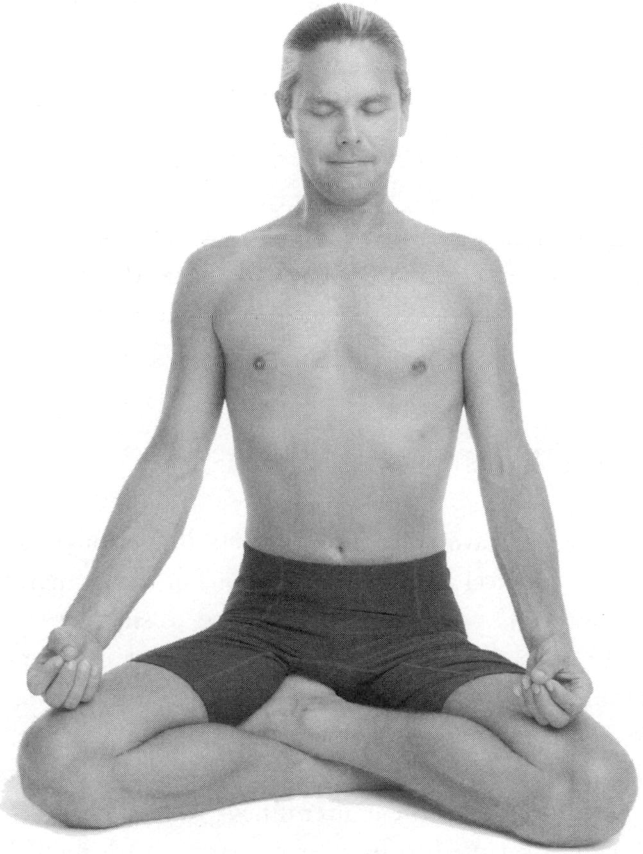

CHAPTER SIX

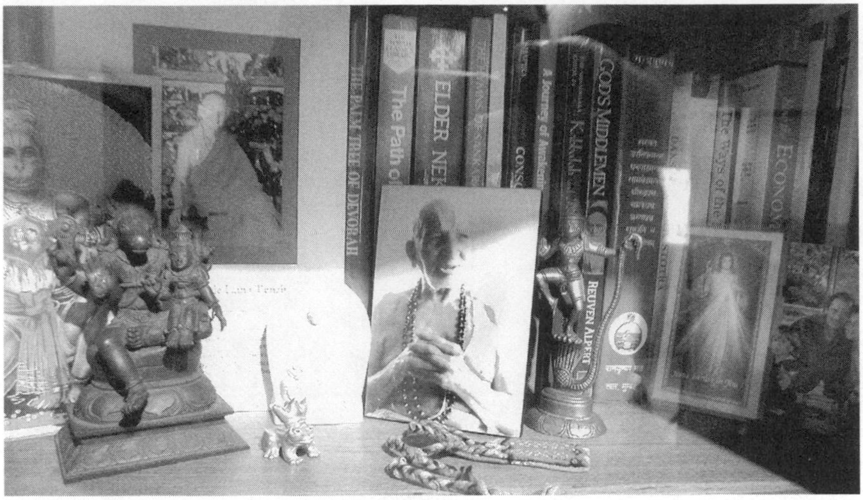

Educating the Intellect

THE *MANOMAYA* LEVEL

THE *MANOMAYA* DIMENSION is that part of us which takes in information from the outside via the senses. We may think of this as the dimension of our intellect, and, even more specifically, as our capacity to learn.

THE ROLE OF THE INTELLECT

Up to now we have considered aspects of personal practice that relate primarily to the physical and vital dimensions of the human system. We have considered how *āsana* practice can be adapted to support the balanced development of our physical body, to help preserve its integrity in the face of stress, and to rehabilitate it after injury. We have also seen how *āsana* practice can be adapted to serve as preparation for *prāṇāyāma*. And we have seen how *prāṇāyāma* practice can be adapted to nourish our vitality, to help maintain that vitality, and to help restore it after illness. In later chapters, we will see how *prāṇāyāma* can be adapted to serve as preparation for meditation and prayer.

Pivotal in all of these practices is the role of the intellect. In developing a personal practice relevant to our needs and intentions, it is obviously important to be educated about the different aspects of practice, and how and when to adapt and apply them.

As children, we have a tremendous unfulfilled potential. And the energy to fulfill this potential is fueled by curiosity. As we grow, we continue to accumulate knowledge through both school and life experiences. What we learn, and how we learn it, depends on many factors, both external and internal. What is clear, however, is that what we learn has a tremendous influence on who we become.

As adults, we often reach a point beyond which we stop learning. We are busy with work and family responsibilities. And what free time we have, after fulfilling our daily responsibilities, we use for entertainment. However, in order to stay as healthy and active as possible, it is important to continue to develop the mind; to continue to learn throughout our entire lives. I often ask students to consider areas of interest they have that they have not pursued. I encourage them to take up new fields of investigation, to stimulate their interest in learning.

Continued education is often an overlooked part of personal practice, and yet our intellects play an essential role in every aspect of our lives. As we have seen, personal practice is a tool to develop, refine, and integrate every dimension of our system.

We have seen how practices that serve the physical and vital dimensions of our system are mutually beneficial. For example, *āsana* practice can be adapted to serve our constitutional as well as our structural needs, and *prāṇāyāma* can be adapted to serve our structural as well as our constitutional needs.

As illustrated on the following page, developing our intellects will serve us at every level of our being. Consider how many structural problems are causally linked to daily physical activity. Learning about our structure and its needs will help us make intelligent choices in how we use our body. Many of the chronic diseases we suffer from as a society are linked to insufficient or inappropriate exercise, poor eating habits, misuse of substances, inadequate rest—in short, unhealthy lifestyles.

Learning about our constitution and its needs will also help us make intelligent choices in our lifestyle. It is true that many of us have a genetic

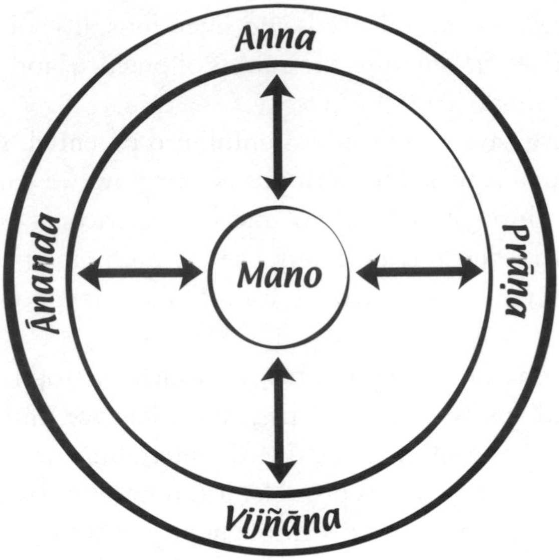

propensity for certain diseases. But if we learn about our family profile, what those propensities are, we can take steps to avoid certain conditions. For example, if there is heart disease in the family, we can modify our diet, increase exercise, and reduce stress. It takes education to recognize such needs and to adapt our behavior accordingly.

Thus, we have seen how the intellect can serve in refining the first two dimensions of our system—the physical and the vital. Later, we will see how the intellect can serve in the refinement of the personality and the heart as well. For now, however, we will concentrate on teachings related to the development of the intellect itself.

THE BREAKDOWN OF TRADITIONAL CULTURES

The rapid transformation of contemporary society, due to the mixing of cultures and advancements in science and technology, has resulted in a breakdown in traditional cultures—their institutions, customs, values, and forms of education. We have, to a large extent, lost confidence in the old ways.

Today we live in a new world—a world in which much of our education is public, secular, and oriented solely toward learning about the external world around us and how to function in it. Of course, we have made tremendous advancements in science, health care, and even human rights. But we are also witnesses to the degradation of our environment, the development of new diseases—which may, in fact, be linked directly with our genetic engineering experiments—and the breakdown of the family structure, with its related increase in unwanted pregnancy, divorce, depression, crime, and suicidal and even homicidal children. Clearly, with all our advancements, something is missing!

Personal practice, of course, does not address these larger collective issues directly. It is about helping us to become more integrated, healthy, happy, and productive in our personal lives. But one thing is certain: as we become more balanced and integrated, we will have a positive influence on those around us, especially our children. And, thus, it is a general benefit when we advance in our own personal practice, in relation to which the development of our intellect is vital.

TRAINING THE MIND THROUGH CHANT

Today most of our education is of a secular nature, and learning is intimately linked to reading rather than to chanting. However, in ancient times, before the printing press, books were handwritten and rare. Most knowledge, particularly sacred knowledge, was organized into compositions that could be preserved and transmitted through chants. Students would learn by listening and repeating scriptural and other texts, and by memorizing chants containing the knowledge to be transmitted. Thus, chanting and learning were intimately linked.

Compositions were "by-hearted" by young students, and, as the child matured, the teacher offered commentaries. This method of learning was very effective in both the preservation of knowledge and the development of intellect and memory. The advent of the printed and now digitized word has been a tremendous help in the accumulation, preservation, and dissemination of knowledge. And because we can have our reference texts close at hand, we no longer need to commit them to memory. But an unfortunate result is that we seem to have all but lost a time-honored and potent tool of mind training.

Learning to Listen

Learning to chant refines our capacity to listen, and listening requires an open mind. Chanting is therefore a potent method of mind training. The method of teaching chanting requires that the student repeat what the teacher chants exactly and without any mistakes; thus, the student has to be very attentive. As the student progresses, the chanting becomes more complex, the passages longer, and the pace quicker. This training makes the mind alert and able to shift focus quickly. It also strengthens memory. This use of chanting is, of course, only possible when we have a relationship with a teacher from whom we can learn.

The Energetics of Sound

There is a purely vibratory and energetic quality to chanting that can be modulated by several factors—including phonetics, pitch, volume, and pace—to produce either a more activating or soothing effect. Understanding these factors, we can use this subtle and complex science in our personal practice to enhance the effects of our *āsana* and *prāṇāyāma*.

PHONETICS

Different sounds are produced from different areas of the throat and mouth. Vowel sounds are different from consonant sounds. The ancients suggested that certain sounds such as *ra* or *śa* (pronounced *sha*) are more active and have a heating effect, while other sounds such as *ma* are more soothing and have a cooling effect.

PITCH

We can modulate the pitch in our chanting. As we raise or lower the pitch, we can feel the vibrations shifting in our body. Higher pitches generally create an increased sensation of vibration in the upper part of the torso and the head, while lower pitches create a sensation of vibration relatively lower in the torso.

VOLUME

We can vary the volume of our chanting. Softer chanting utilizes less air, and takes less energy to produce. Increased volume requires more air and takes more energy.

PACE

We can chant the same passages at different paces. Generally, faster-paced chanting is more energizing and stimulating to our systems, while slower-paced chanting is more calming and soothing.

Transmitting Information Through Chant

Chanting was, and in certain cultures still is, a primary means to transmit information. Chanting can be used as a powerful learning tool. For personal practice, once again, this necessitates a relationship with a teacher from whom we can learn. And it also requires that we have specific texts that are relevant to us. An example for a student of Yoga would be the Yoga Sūtra-s of Patañjali.

The Symbolism of Sound

The symbolism of sound is also a significant factor in the impact of chanting on the human system, as chanting is a powerful tool for evoking emotional response. Recognizing this, the ancients used chanting to cultivate and celebrate our relationship to ourselves, our society, our environment, and our source. The power of sound and chanting is its ability to penetrate to the core of our being—even if we don't know the meaning of what we are chanting. It takes us in the direction of its origin, and becomes a part of us (*saṃskāra*). And, if it gets too strong, it can take over. Therefore, if what we are chanting is not in harmony with what is already residing at this core, it can cause deep fragmentation. After all, if the mirror itself is cracked, so is the reflection that it mirrors back to us. It is for this reason that we are very careful about teaching our students chants, or giving them *mantra-s* to be used in their personal practice, which are of a sectarian nature and contain theological symbolism that comes from traditions other than their own and with which they have no deep inner resonance.

IN SUMMARY: While the primary method of nourishing and cultivating the intellectual dimension is through learning, the use of chant as a primary tool of mind training and learning is not a part of our contemporary culture. Nevertheless, it remains a powerful tool for use in personal practice. So, recognizing this fact, we will now consider how to utilize chanting in the service of mind training, education, and for the purpose of deepening self-understanding in preparation for self-transformation.

THE CAKRA MODEL

In personal practice, the process of receiving new teachings should be followed by the effort to understand, apply, and be transformed by them. The *cakra* model developed by the ancients offers a structure that contains teachings on the nature of the human system—teachings that, when understood and applied, have profound transformational value.

The first step is to learn the structure. Then we learn how *āsana, prāṇāyāma,* and chanting can be used together to enhance our ability to understand the *cakra-s*. Finally, we will apply this knowledge of the *cakra-s* in order to be transformed.

The Symbolism of Wheels and Lotuses

The ancients conceived of three main vertical channels (*nāḍī-s*) within our bodies: *suṣumnā* (central channel), *iḍā* (left channel), and *pingalā* (right channel). The *cakra* model describes seven reference points in the body, organized around the central channel (*suṣumnā*), which represent the meeting point of these three major channels. They are described variously as wheels and lotuses. Each of the *cakra-s* corresponds to specific natural elements, sensory functions, and vital organs. They also represent certain emotional characteristics and qualities. Each also has a corresponding *bīja mantra* (seed syllable) and *yantra* (geometric form) that the ancients revealed. The seed syllable and the geometric form represent, respectively, the revealed sound and shape that expresses each center.

The ancients taught that the *cakra-s* are vital and active. Their movement is linked to the movement of energy (*prāṇa*) in the channels (*nāḍī-s*), as discussed in the previous chapter, much like a water wheel is spun by the flow of water. For *prāṇa* to reach the *cakra-s,* the passages must be clear. The wheels can inappropriately spin too fast, too slow, and either discontinuously or intermittently. They can also be tilted on their axes, displaced to the right or left, pulled up too high, or dropped down too low. And the lotuses can inappropriately sag or fold, bend to one side or another, be lifted too high or dropped too low. These defects in the *cakra-s* can have a local effect on organ function as well as a detrimental influence on specific emotional characteristics.

Āsana, prāṇāyāma, and meditation can be used to correct these defects in the *cakra-s*—through appropriate practices, we can purify the passageways and correct and enhance the flow of *prāṇa* in the *cakra-s.*

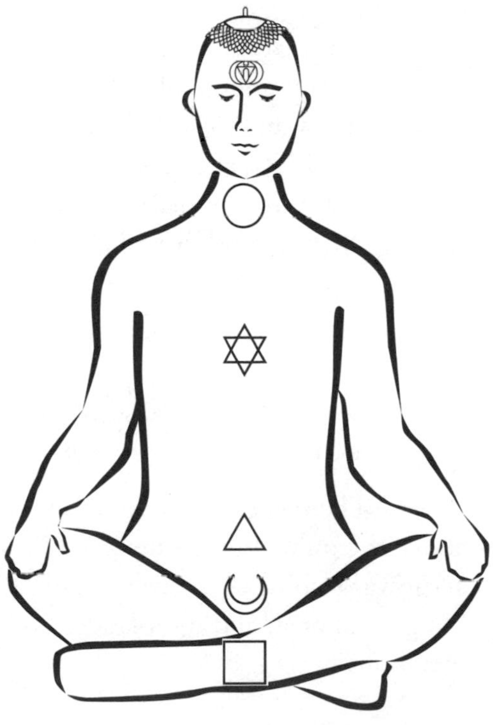

The Seven Major Cakra-s

Starting from the base of the human system and moving upward, the *cakra-s* are described in the following list in terms of their locations, corresponding elements, sensory function, and vital organs, corresponding sound (*bīja mantra*) and form (*yantra*). Finally, examples of some of the emotional characteristics and qualities that the *cakra-s* represent, and some of the emotional disturbances that may appear when they are defective will also be given. The details of this model are adapted from the *Ṣaṭ-cakranirūpana,* one of the authoritative texts on the *cakra* model.

FOUNDATION: *MŪLĀDHĀRA* 

The root *cakra,* known as the *mūlādhāra,* is located in the perineal floor. It relates to the feet, ankles, knees, hips, and anus. The *bīja mantra* for this *cakra* is **lam** and the *yantra* is a square.

The meaning of the term *mūlādhāra* is "root support." This center reflects basic survival issues, and, accordingly, it corresponds to the earth element and to the sense of smell. In evolutionary biology, smell has been the primary means by which animals of most species were able to identify food and danger, as well as reproductive potential. In our own experience, we often use the expression "I don't like the smell of this" to describe a situation in which we feel uncomfortable. We use our nose, as it were, to help us know the character of a situation.

As foundation, this *cakra* represents stability in the system—physically, mentally, and emotionally. Its corresponding emotional characteristic is the sense of safety and trust. When there is a defect in this *cakra,* the characteristics of fear, instability, and mistrust appear. We can say that if we are insecure, we lack a solid foundation. If the foundation of any structure is weak, tilted, or sinking, there is a risk it will collapse.

CREATION: *SVĀDHIṢṬHANA* (THAT WHICH SUSTAINS BY ITSELF—SELF-SUSTAINING) 

The *svādhiṣṭhana cakra* is located two inches above the *mūlādhāra,* just above the pubic bone. The *bīja mantra* for this *cakra* is **vam** and the *yantra* is an upward-pointing crescent moon. It is related to the sacrum and pubic bone, the genital area, and the bladder and kidneys, which are involved with water metabolism.

Accordingly, this *cakra* corresponds to the water element and to the sense of taste. The meaning of the term *svādiṣṭhana* is "self-sustaining." The water element represents creation. Taste, like smell, is a primary sense by which we judge whether or not we are attracted to something. Thus, taste represents the flavor of a relationship, which we may like or dislike, and, in this sense it is a measure of our appreciation of the essence of a relationship.

As creation, this center corresponds to our vitality, our capacity for play, and, in particular, our ability to have a healthy sexual relationship. When there is a defect in this *cakra,* it will manifest as feelings of inhibition, being stifled or repressed in our sexual energy, excessive sexual preoccupation, or the inability to have children.

TRANSFORMATION: *MAṆIPŪRAKA* △

The *maṇipūraka cakra* is located in the region of the navel. It is related to the lumbar spine, the large and small intestines, liver, pancreas, and adrenal glands. The *bīja mantra* for this *cakra* is **ram** and the *yantra* is an upward-pointing triangle (sometimes it is depicted as a downward-pointing triangle).

This *cakra* corresponds to the fire element and to the sense of sight. The meaning of the term *maṇipūraka* is "full of gems." Sight, which reveals form, is linked to light and color. This *cakra* corresponds to our self-esteem and our self-image. Thus, we often say that someone with high self-esteem looks "bright," whereas someone with low self-esteem looks "dull."

This center is the seat of *agni,* the digestive fire. It relates to digestion at every level. The fire that digests food the ancients called *jaṭhara agni*. The fire that digests experience the ancients called *jñānagni*. With good strong fire, we are able to digest not only physical food but also sensations and experiences. We can say that when a person has a strong fire, they can digest or "handle" more. As digestion is a process of transformation, this center is also responsible for change, and it reflects our ability to grow. When the digestive fire is strong, we can handle challenges and we are able to adapt.

When there is a defect in this *cakra,* however, characteristics such as low self-esteem, depression, a difficulty to accept change, and an inability to adapt may appear. We can think of the expression "I can't swallow that," which we may use in a situation which is too bitter, which we cannot absorb. In addition, when the fire is weak, impurities accumulate in our system.

RELATION: *ANĀHATA*

The *anāhata cakra* is located at the base of the sternum. It relates to the thoracic spine, the heart and lungs, and the spleen. Its *bīja mantra* is **yam** and its *yantra* is a hexagon.

This *cakra* corresponds to the air element and to the sense of touch, which represents the ability to make contact with others. *Anāhata* means "that which cannot be destroyed." It also corresponds to the qualities of openness, compassion, self-acceptance, and self-confidence, as well as to the ability to have deep relationships, to love, and to be devoted. The ancients taught that it is the place where *dharma* resides.

The *anāhata cakra* is often described as a lotus. The ancients said that when this *cakra* is closed, the lotus droops downward, but that when it opens it is like an open flower that is turned upward, receiving light from the sun. We can understand this image when we think of how we feel when we are in love.

This *cakra* reflects emotional issues. Sudden outbursts of emotion indicate some disturbance in it. When there is a defect in this *cakra,* characteristics such as insecurity, nervousness, anxiety, anger, impatience, fanaticism, and an overly critical nature may manifest. Other characteristics, such as a tendency to be withdrawn, an inability to have deep relationships, to express emotion, and to actualize dreams may also manifest.

COMMUNICATION: *VIŚUDDHI*

The *viśuddhi cakra* is located in the throat, at the level of the Adam's apple. It is related to the cervical spine, thymus and thyroid glands, throat, and voice. The *bīja mantra* for this *cakra* is **ham** and the *yantra* is a circle.

Viśuddhi means "extraordinarily pure." This center corresponds to the element of space, the quality of the voice, and the sense of hearing. It is involved with the production of sound, and reflects our ability to communicate. It also corresponds to our ability to speak clearly and appropriately, to say the right things at the right time. Space is required to communicate properly. When we feel a lack of space in a relationship, for example, our communication skills are often compromised. This may even manifest in the quality of our voice. In addition, fear or hesitation to communicate, repressed communication, incessant talking, hasty or inappropriate communication, and speaking too rapidly are characteristics that may appear when there is a defect in this *cakra*. Most of us have had the experience of feeling "all choked up."

EVALUATION: ĀJÑA

The *ājña cakra* is located in the region above the nose and between the eyes. It is related to the brain, the eyes, and the ears. The *bīja mantra* for this *cakra* is **am** and, although there is no specific geometric form given, it is often depicted as an upward-pointing crescent moon above a downward-pointing triangle with a phallic shape within it.

This *cakra* is beyond the gross elements. It corresponds to intelligence—the higher functions of the brain—including our ability to discern, evaluate, discriminate, decide, and set a direction for action, as well as our capacity for insight and intuition (*prātibhā*). *Ājña* means "command" or "all-knowing."

We know how much is revealed through our eyes. But our ability to perceive and understand through our eyes is influenced by our past conditioning. The ancients taught that when this *cakra*—often referred to as our "third eye"—prevails, we are able to see from a deeper place within us. The ancients suggested that deep insight and flashes of intuition themselves are the result of a link to something beyond our minds. Usually this is explained in the context of a higher force. In such moments it is as if the "normal" eyes of perception surrender to this "higher" eye.

This *cakra* is closely associated with the symbolism of the *nāḍī-s,* which we discussed in the last chapter. Defects in this *cakra* that relate to the lunar channel include doubt, lack of clarity, indecision, and confusion. Defects that relate to the solar channel include being stubborn, uncompromising, and of an adamant nature.

Until this center "opens," we experience bondage and suffering in life.

INSPIRATION: *SAHASRĀRA*

The last major *cakra,* known as the *sahasrāra,* is located at the crown of the head. The *bīja mantra* is **om** and, although there is no geometric form given, it is often represented as a full moon–like circle.

Sahasrāra means "thousand spokes." It corresponds to consciousness itself and to the Divine. The ancients taught that this center is what protects and sustains our life. It is symbolized as a downward-turning lotus. When it "opens," this center enables us to touch our higher consciousness and the Divine, and to realize freedom (*mokṣa*).

The ancients developed the *cakra* model to express their tremendous insights into the nature and function of our complex systems. The preceding information represents only a small part of the profound teaching about the human system that is coded into this ancient model.

Of course, ours is a living and dynamic system. It is difficult to understand much about our lumbar spine without understanding its functional relation to our thoracic spine. It is difficult to understand much about our cardiovascular system without understanding its functional relationship to our respiratory system. In the same way, it is difficult to truly understand any one of these *cakra-s* without understanding their functional relationship with each other. Defects in one center "spill over" and impact another.

Using this model, it was the intention of the ancient *yogī-s* to resolve the constituent elements of the body and mind back into their respective sources; and, ultimately, to resolve consciousness back into the Divine. In other words, it was their intention to use it as a means to realize with their conscious awareness what they understood to be the process that occurs at death and to codify that understanding for others. Mapping the death process as they understood it to occur in relation to the *cakra* system, the ancient *yogī-s* strove to dissolve the earth element into water; water into fire; fire into air; air into space; space into consciousness; and consciousness into the Divine.

From a contemporary perspective, but still in relation to the *cakra* system, we can use our personal practice to help us to become more stable, vital, empowered, loving, expressive, discriminating, and awakened.

As our awareness of the *cakra-s* deepens through practice, we can utilize the symbolism of this ancient model to help us identify dysfunctional patterns in our system; and as our understanding of the tools of practice deepens through application, we can refine our ability to use them in the transformational process. In order to facilitate this, we introduce chanting in *āsana* practice—and, specifically, vocal chanting while repeating as well as staying in postures as well as silent, mental chanting during the retention of the breath after inhalation and suspension of the breath after exhalation. In the practice below, we will also continue the use of ratio development, introducing the techniques of *śītalī,* in which we inhale through a curled tongue and exhale through alternate nostrils, and *nāḍī śodhana,* in which we inhale and exhale through alternate nostrils, as well.

We recommend that you begin by chanting softly during practice. As you gain experience, you may want to modulate the volume for different effects. We also recommend that you begin with a comfortable pitch and that, as you gain experience, you vary the pitch to explore different effects.

The practice presented below is both complex and long. It can be simplified and shortened by focusing on only one *cakra,* rather than all seven, throughout each practice. In this way, the sequence below can be divided into seven practices that can be explored cyclically: choose the particular *cakra* you want to focus on; skip postures #3A, #3B, #9, #11A, #11B, #13, #15A, #15B, #17A, and #17B; practice only one *prāṇāyāma,* either #14 or #16; and chant only the *mantra* associated with the *cakra* of your choice, mentally or vocally, wherever chanting is indicated throughout the rest of the practice.

MANOMAYA PRACTICE

1.

POSTURE: *Uttānāsana/Ardha Utkaṭāsana* combination.

EMPHASIS: To introduce chanting **lam** on exhalation, and to bring awareness to Foundation center (*mūlādhāra*).

TECHNIQUE: Stand with feet slightly apart, arms over head.

On exhale: Bend forward, bending knees slightly, bringing chest to thighs, and palms to sides of feet.

Repeat **lam** one time more with each successive repetition, from one to eight times.

On inhale: Return to starting position.

On exhale: Bend forward, bending knees until thighs are parallel to ground, hips are at knee level, chest to thighs, and palms to sides of feet.

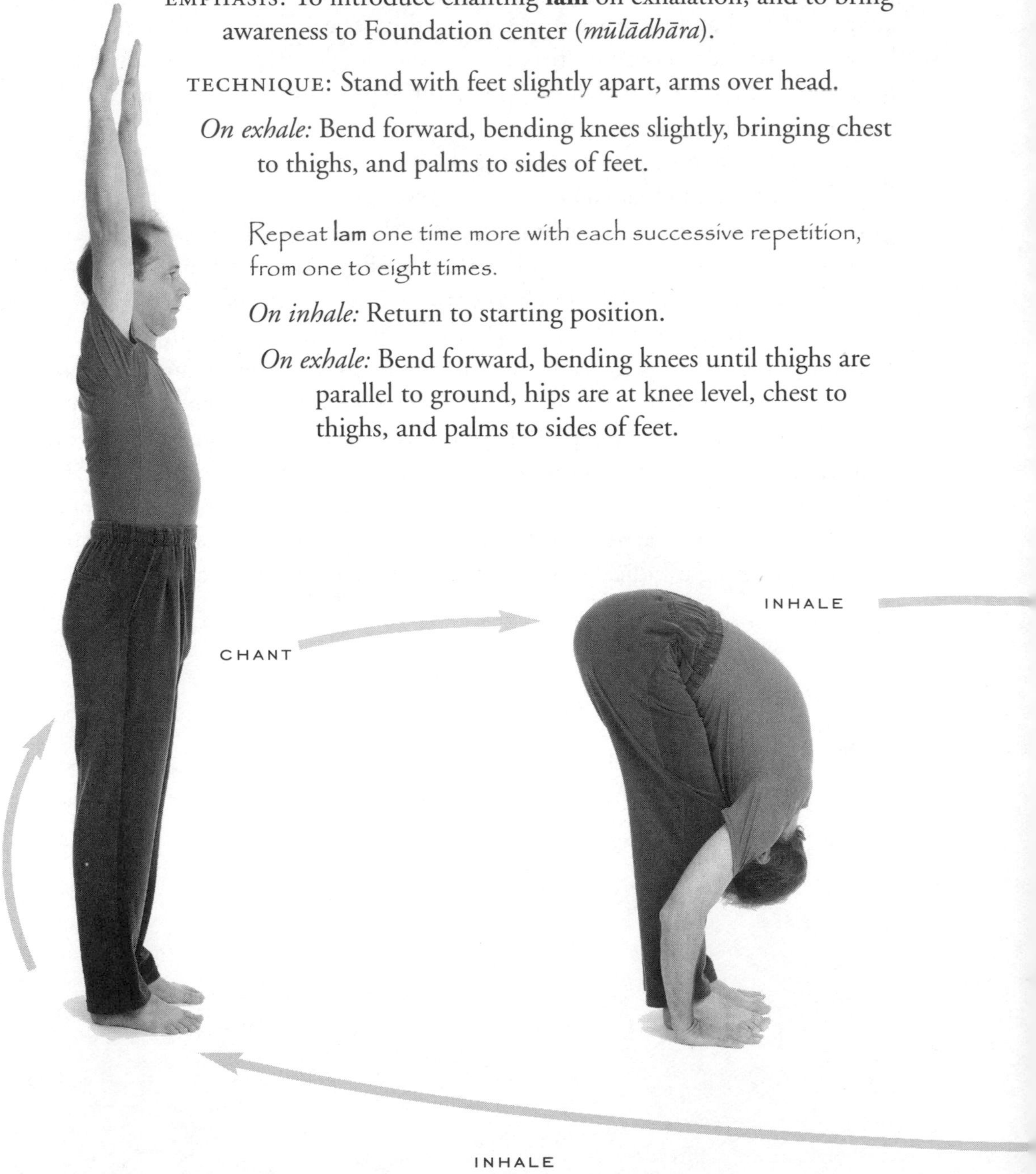

Repeat **lam** one time more with each successive repetition, from one to eight times.

On inhale: Return to starting position.

Number: Eight times.

DETAILS:

On exhale: Make exhalation progressively longer with each repetition. Chant **lam** softly and at a lower pitch. Bend knees to facilitate stretching in lower back. Push heels firmly, and reach arms forward.

On inhale: Lift chest up and away from thighs, flattening upper back, without exaggerating lumbar curve. Keep knees bent until last part of movement.

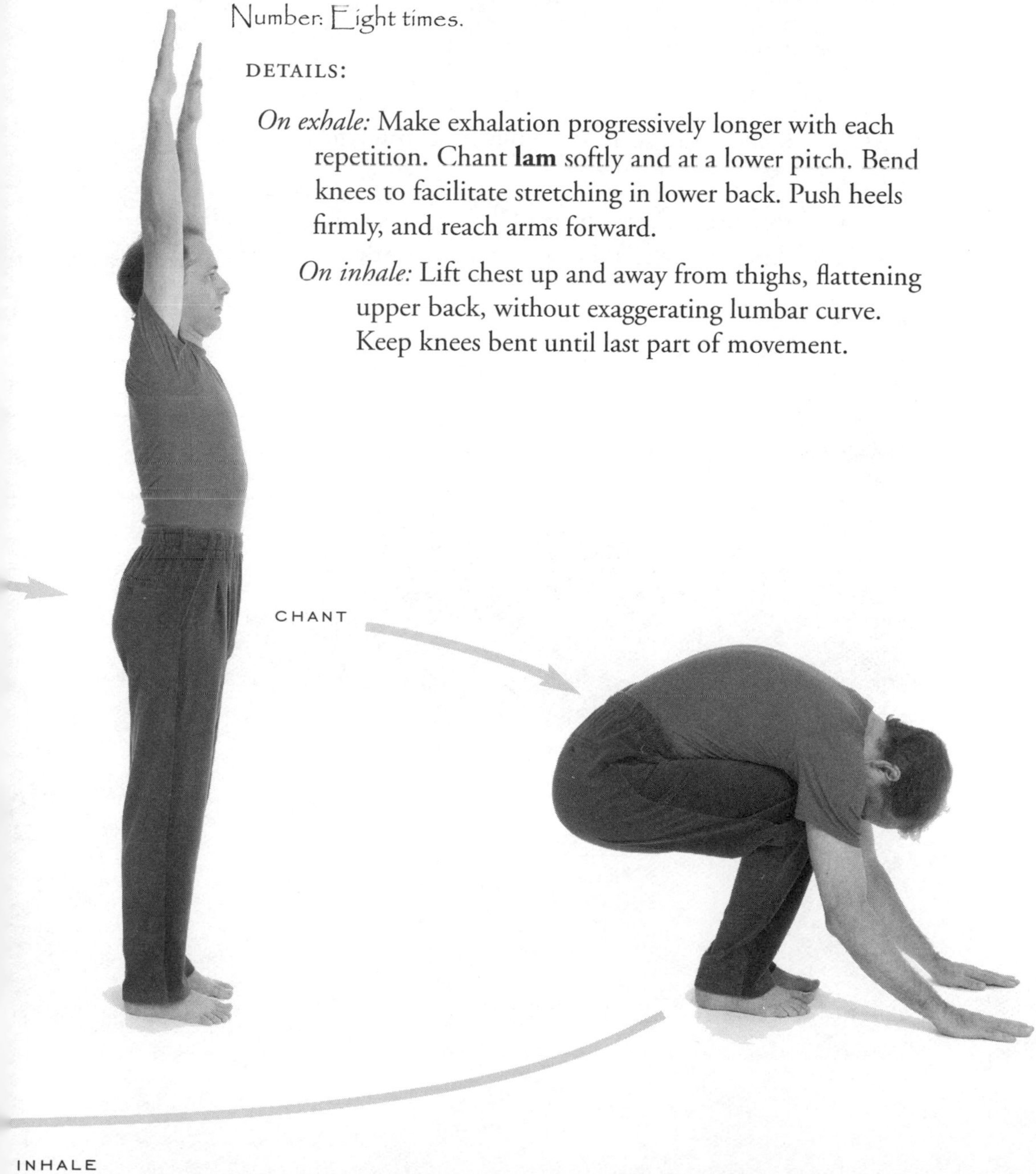

2.

POSTURE: *Vajrāsana/Cakravākāsana/Adho Mukha Śvānāsana/Ūrdhva Mukha Śvānāsana*

EMPHASIS: To chant **lam** mentally on each exhalation, keeping focused on the Foundation center (*mūlādhāra*).

TECHNIQUE: Stand on knees with arms over head.

On exhale: Bend forward, bringing arms to floor in front of you.

On inhale: Lift chest up and away from belly, coming forward onto hands.

On exhale: Push buttocks upward, lifting knees off ground and pushing chest toward feet. Stay one breath.

On inhale: Stretch body forward and arch back. Stay one breath.

On exhale: Return to previous position.

Repeat six times.

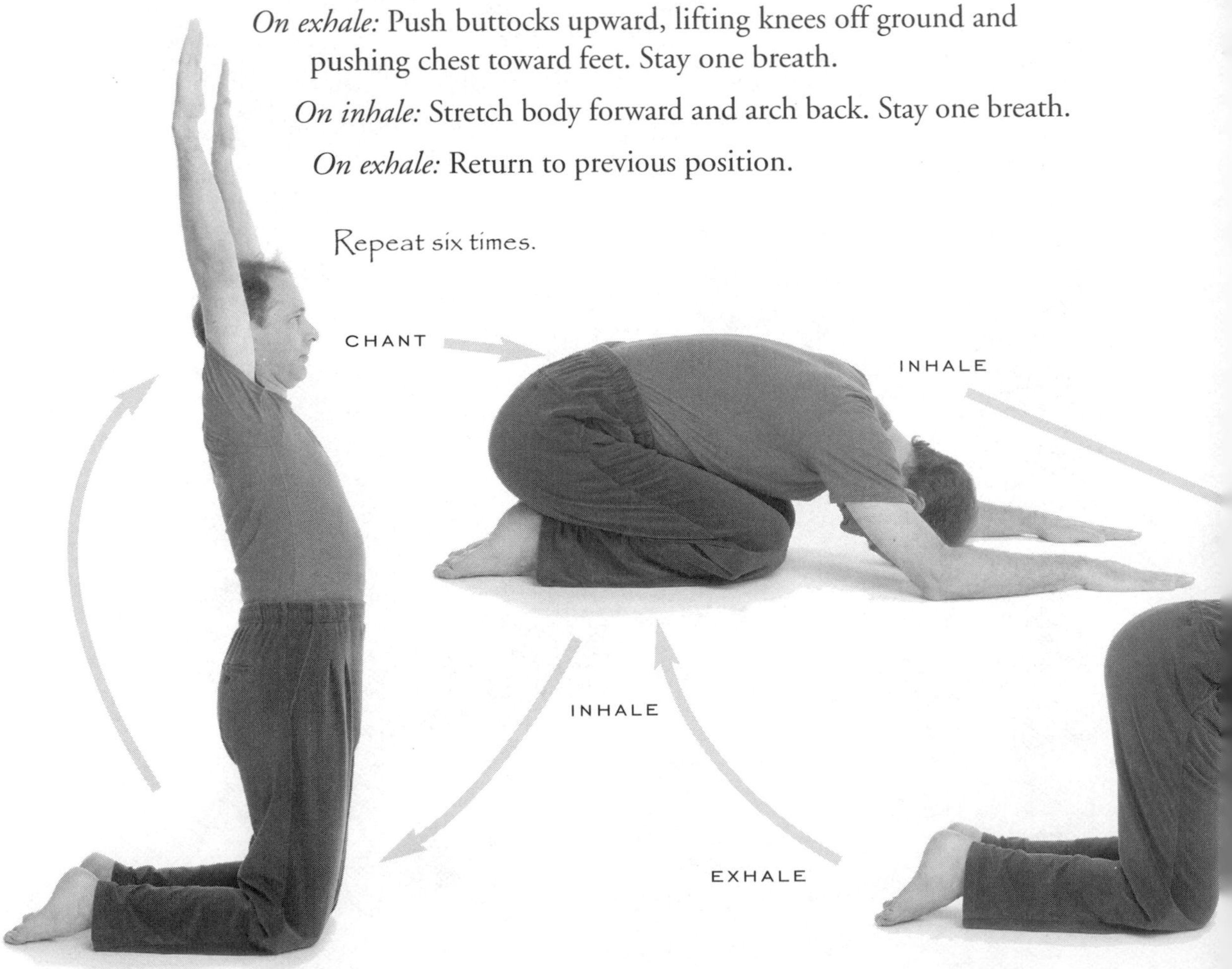

On inhale: Return to knees, lifting chest up and away from belly, coming forward onto hands.

On exhale: Tighten belly, round lower back, and bring chest toward thighs.

On inhale: Return to starting position.

Number: Eight times.

DETAILS:

On exhale: Repeat **lam** mentally one time more with each successive repetition, from one to eight times. End in kneeling forward bend and rest.

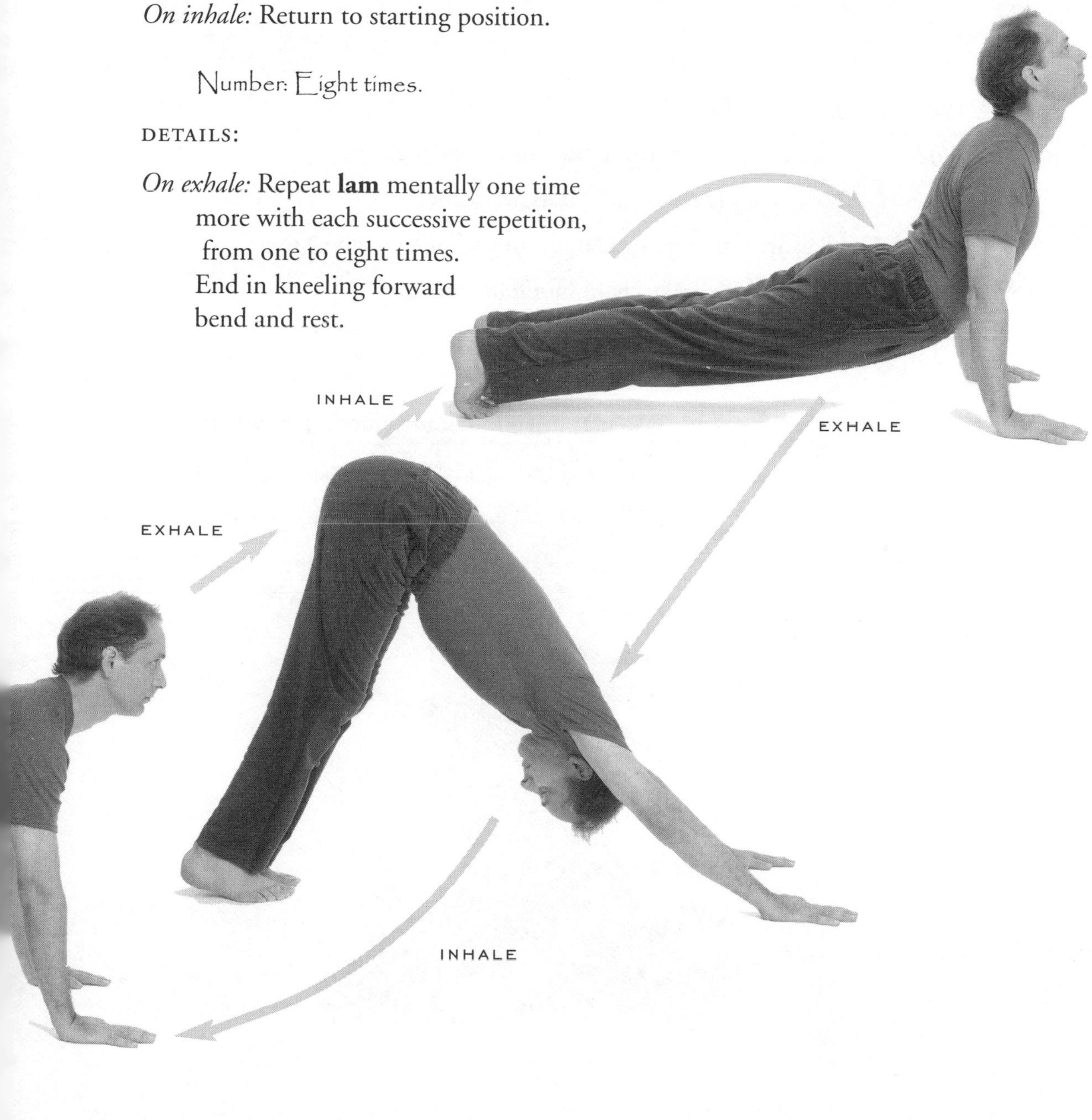

3.

POSTURE: *Siddhāsana*

A: EMPHASIS: *Ujjāyī Prāṇāyāma* to bring awareness to Foundation center (*mūlādhāra*). To repeat **lam** mentally on hold after inhale and exhale.

Ratio: 8-4-8-4

TECHNIQUE: Sit comfortably.

Inhale: Move awareness to perineal floor as inhale deepens.

On hold after inhale: Mentally chant **lam** four times.

Exhale: Hold awareness at perineal floor throughout exhale.

On hold after exhale: Mentally chant **lam** four times.

Number: Twelve times.

B: EMPHASIS: Rest with awareness in Foundation center for some time.

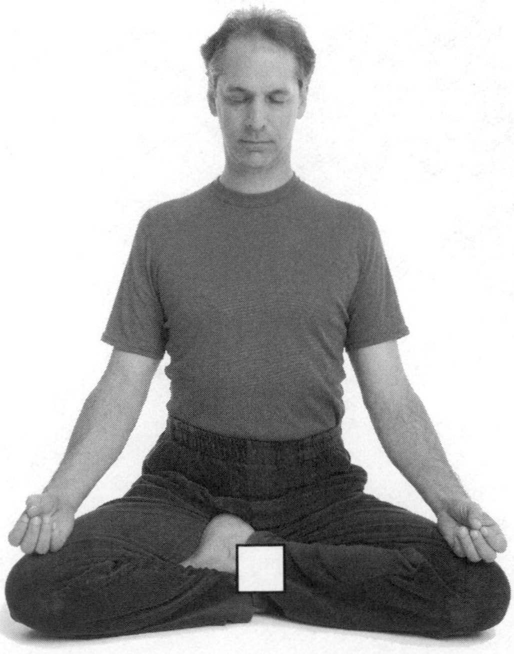

4.

POSTURE: *Dvipāda Pīṭham*

EMPHASIS: To relax neck and upper and lower back, and to gently stretch between belly and thighs.

TECHNIQUE: Lie on back with arms down at sides, knees bent, feet slightly apart on floor and comfortably close to buttocks.

On inhale: Press down on feet, raising pelvis, keeping chin down until neck is gently flattened on floor, while raising arms over head to floor behind.

On exhale: Return to starting position.

Number: Repeat eight times.

DETAILS: *On inhale:* Lift spine, vertebra by vertebra, from bottom up.

On exhale: Unwind spine, coming down vertebra by vertebra.

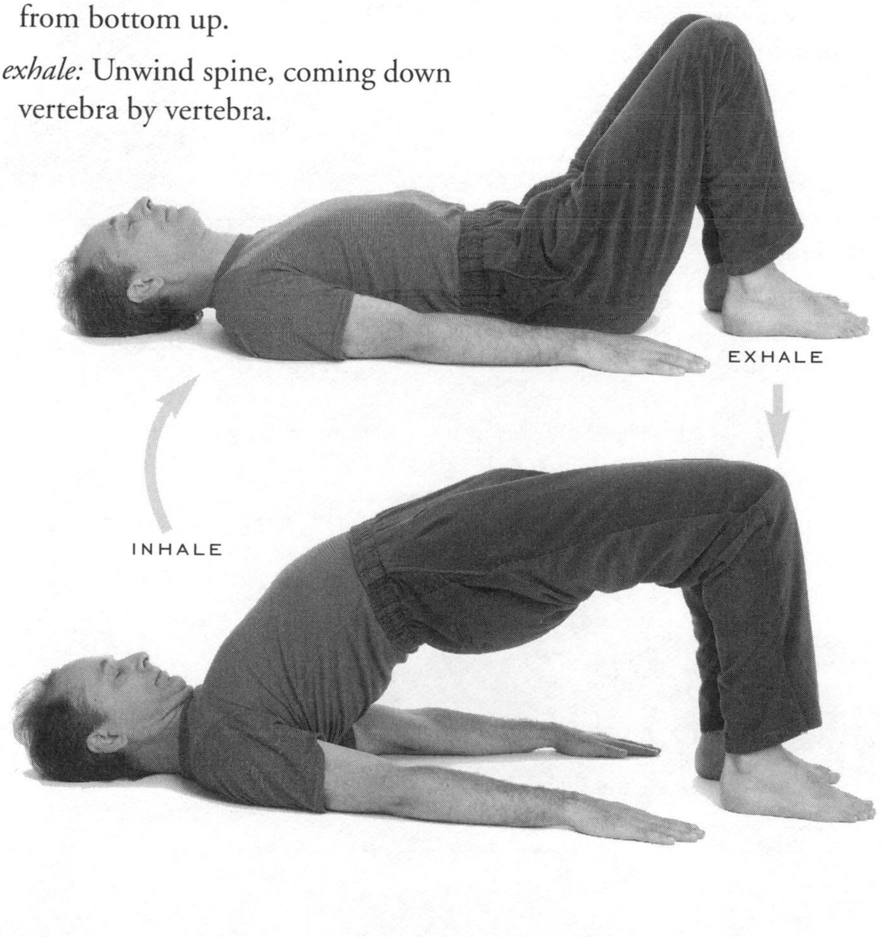

5.

POSTURE: *Apānāsana*

EMPHASIS: To gently stretch and relax lower back.

TECHNIQUE: Lie on back with both knees bent toward chest and feet off floor. Place each hand on its respective knee.

On exhale: Pull thighs gently but progressively toward chest.

On inhale: Return to starting position.

Number: Eight times.

DETAILS:

On exhale: Pull gently with arms, keeping shoulders relaxed and on floor. Press lower back down into floor and drop chin slightly toward throat.

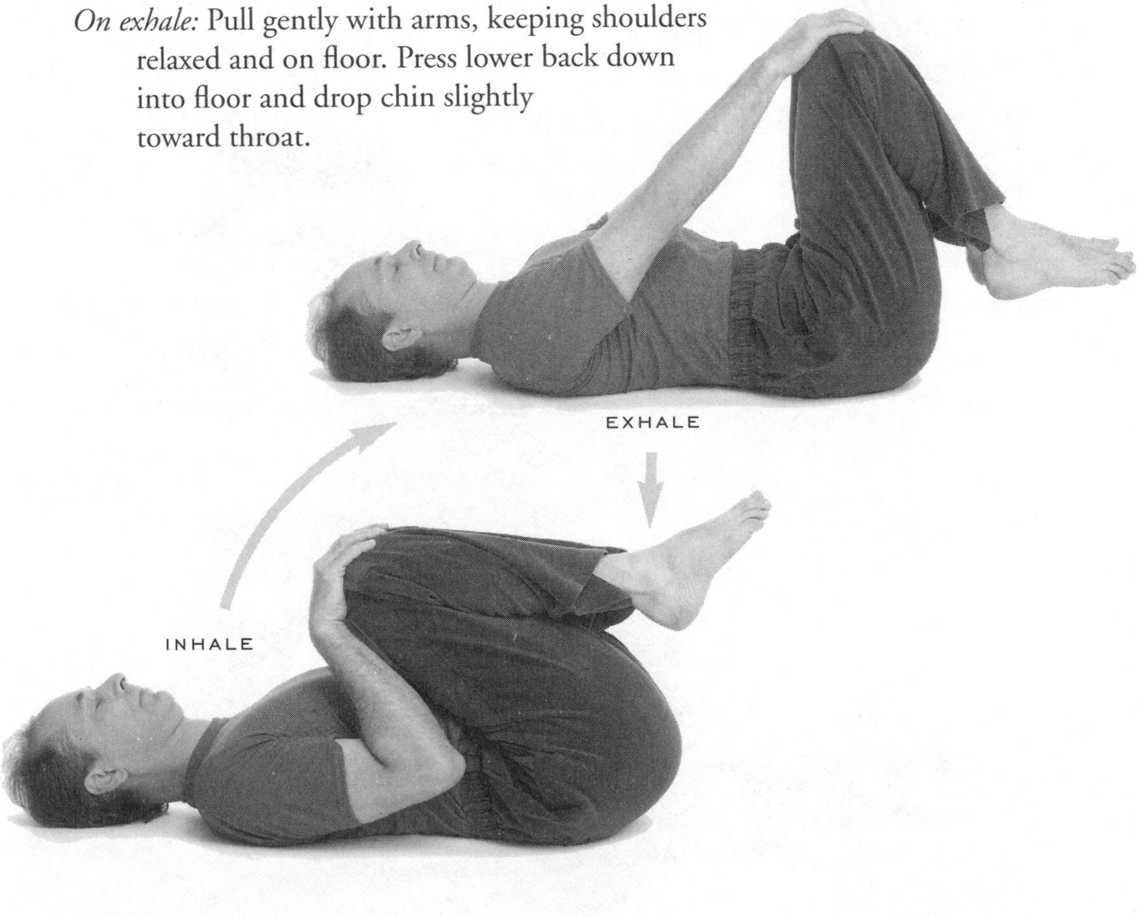

6.

POSTURE: *Jaṭhara Parivṛtti*

EMPHASIS: To gently twist and compress belly. To chant **vam** mentally on each exhalation, and to bring awareness to the Creation center (*svādhiṣṭhana*).

TECHNIQUE: Lie on back with both knees bent, thighs lifted toward chest, and both feet off the ground. Arms out to sides, slightly less than right angles to torso.

On exhale: Bring both knees toward floor on left side of body, twisting abdomen while simultaneously turning head to right.

Repeat **vam** mentally one time more with each successive exhalation, from one to eight times.

On inhale: Return to starting position.

Number: Eight times, alternating sides.

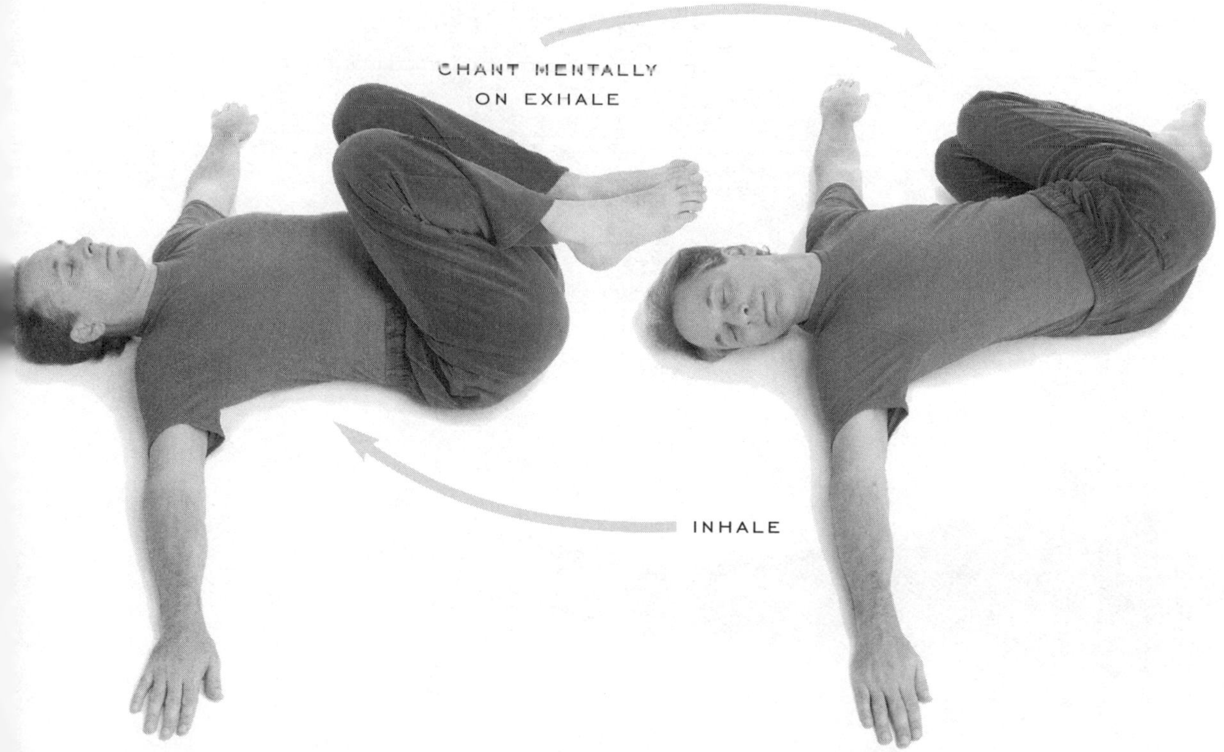

7.

POSTURE: *Jānu Śirṣāsana*

EMPHASIS: To introduce chanting **vam** on exhalation, and to bring awareness to Creation center (*svādhiṣṭhana*).

TECHNIQUE: Sit with right leg folded in, heel to groin, left leg extended forward, and arms over head.

On exhale: Bend forward, bringing belly and chest toward left leg and bringing hands to left foot.

Repeat **vam** one time more with each successive repetition, from one to eight times.

On inhale: Return to starting position.

Number: Repeat eight times each side.

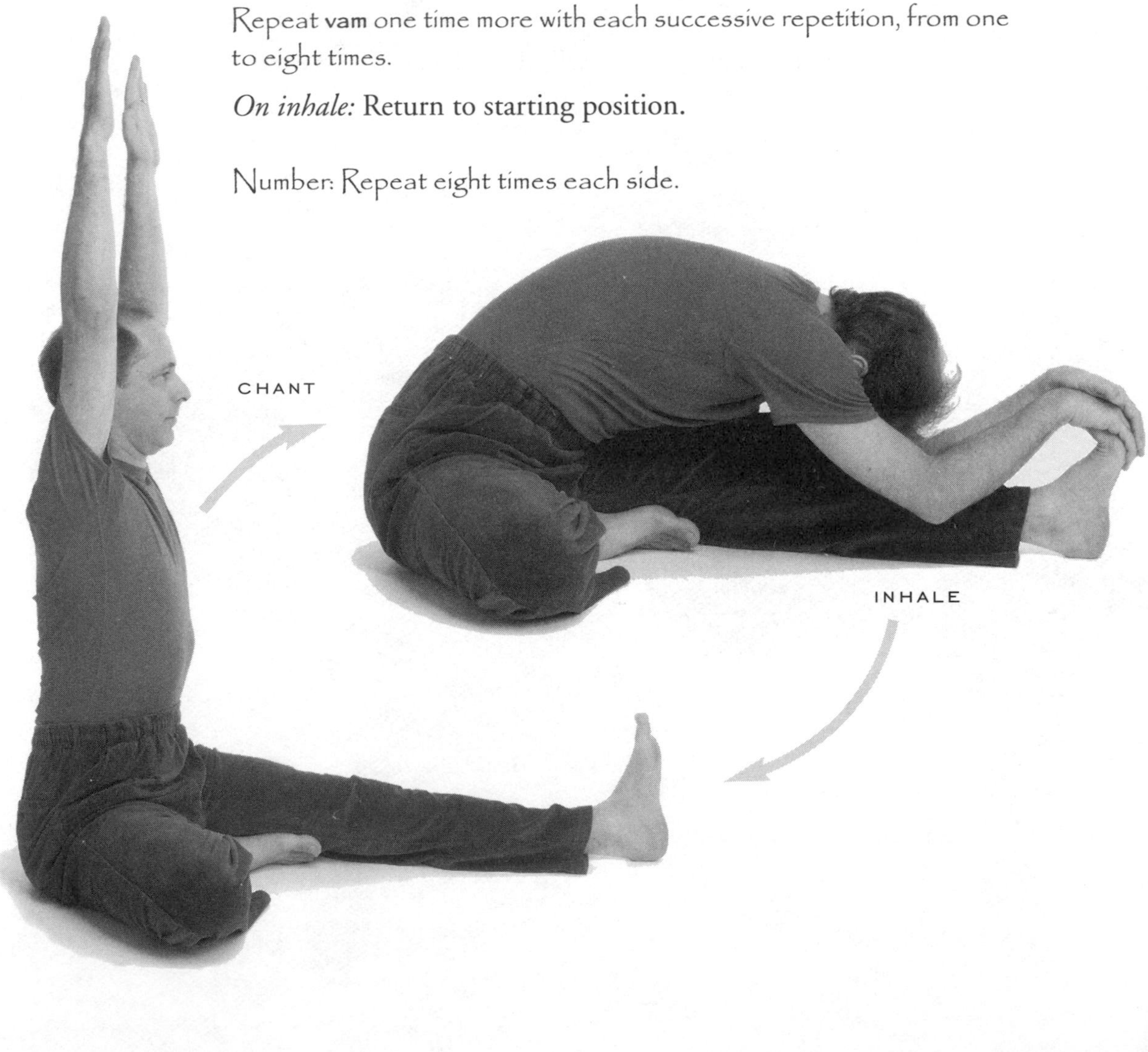

8.

POSTURE: *Bhāradvājāsana*

EMPHASIS: To deepen awareness of Creation center (*svādhiṣṭhana*). To chant **vam** mentally on suspension of the breath after exhalation.

TECHNIQUE: Sit with the right leg folded back, right foot on the floor to the right of right hip, and the left leg folded with left foot on upper right thigh. Wrap left arm behind back and grasp left foot, and place right palm down on floor on outside of left knee with fingers pointing toward right knee.

On inhale: Extend spine upward.

On exhale: Twist shoulders left and turn head right.

On hold after exhale: Repeat **vam** mentally one time more with each successive repetition, from one to eight times.

Number: Stay eight breaths each side.
Then rest for a few moments.

DETAILS: Lean firmly on right palm, allowing right sitz bone to lift off floor.

On exhale: Twist shoulders left and turn head right. Focus on Creation center.

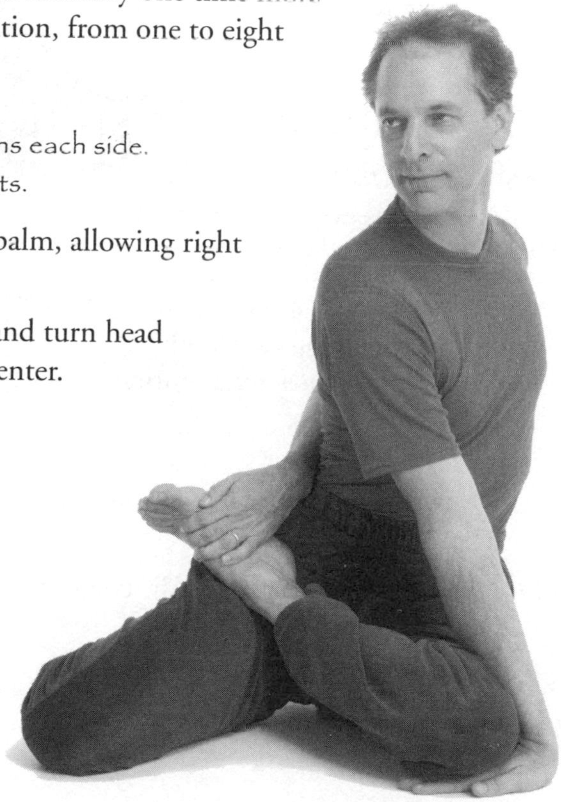

9.

POSTURE: *Siddhāsana*

EMPHASIS: Rest with awareness in Creation center (*svādhiṣṭhana*) for some time.

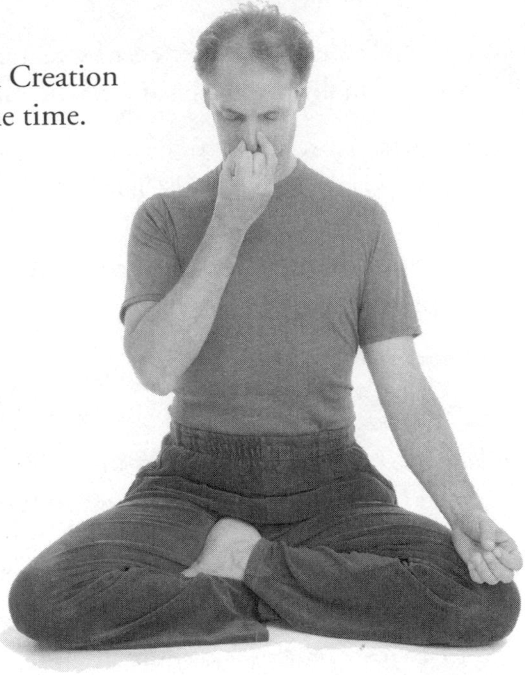

10.

POSTURE: *Paścimatānāsana*

EMPHASIS: To bring awareness to Transformation center (*maṇipūraka*).
To chant **ram** on exhalation.
To introduce movement during suspension of the breath after exhalation.

TECHNIQUE:

A: Sit with legs forward, back straight, and arms raised over head, palms forward.

On exhale: Bending knees slightly, bend forward, bringing chest to thighs, and palms to balls of feet.

On inhale: Return to starting position.

Repeat four times

B: Sit with legs forward, back straight, and arms raised over head.

On exhale: Stay in position. Pull belly inward while chanting **ram**.

Repeat **ram** one time more with each successive repetition, from one to eight times.

On hold after exhalation: Bending knees slightly, bend forward, bringing chest to thighs, and palms to balls of feet.

On inhale: Return to starting position.

Number: Repeat four times.

DETAILS:

On exhale: Bend knees to facilitate stretching lower back and bring belly and chest to thighs. Move chin down toward throat.

On inhale: Lift chest up and away from thighs, flattening upper back.

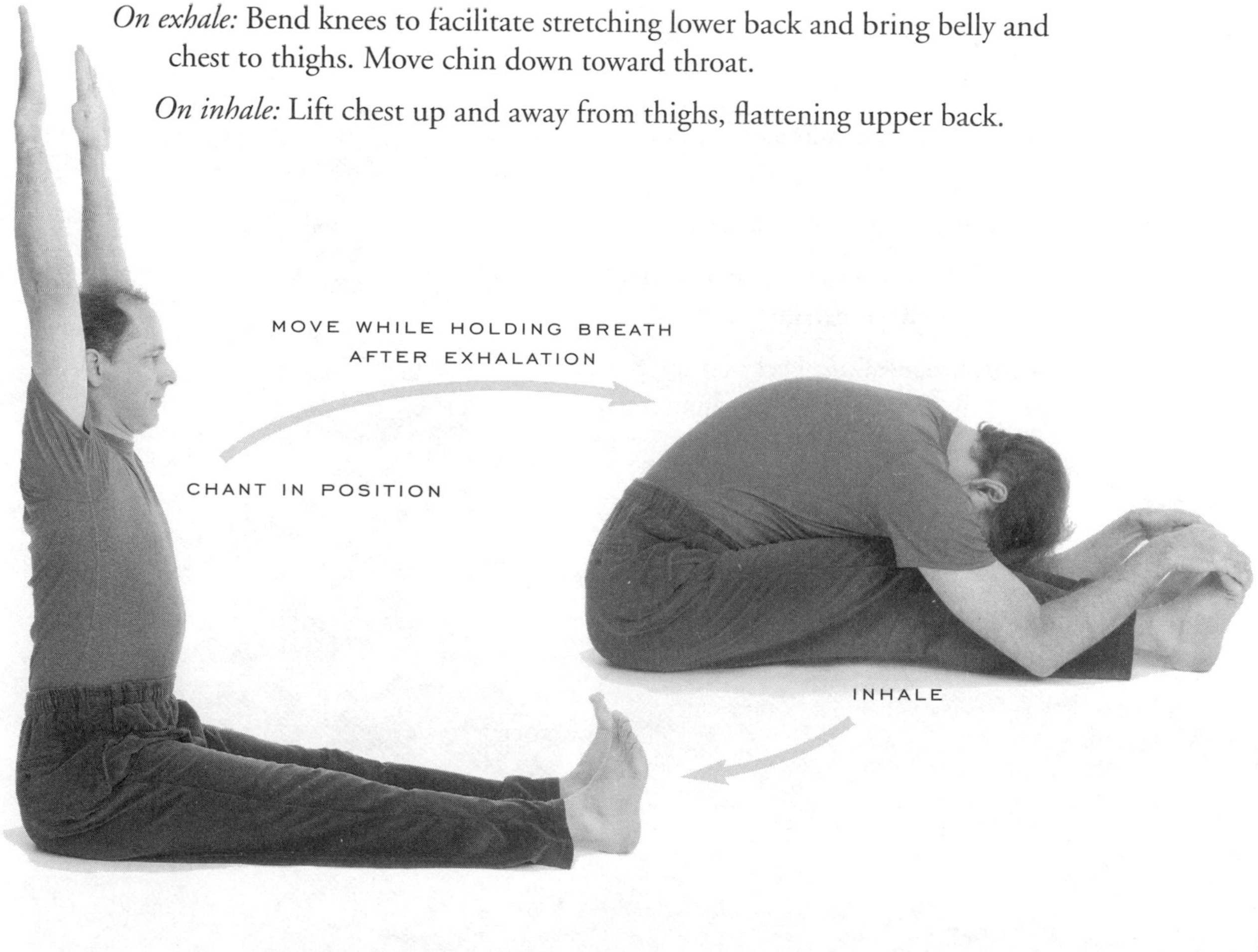

11.

POSTURE: *Siddhāsana*

A: EMPHASIS: *Prāṇāyāma* with *uddīyāna bandha*–like focus, during which the lower abdomen is pushed deeply inward and upward toward the rib cage. To deepen awareness of Transformation center (*maṇipūraka*).

Ratio: To build to 8-8-8-8

TECHNIQUE: *Ujjāyī*

Inhale	*Hold*	*Exhale*	*Hold*	*Number*
8	4	8	4	4
8	8	8	4	4
8	8	8	8	8
8	0	8	0	4

DETAILS:

On inhale: Move awareness to navel area as inhale deepens.

On hold after inhale: Hold awareness at navel.

On exhale: Continue holding awareness at navel throughout exhale.

On hold after exhale: Feel as if navel area is still pulling in and pushing up.

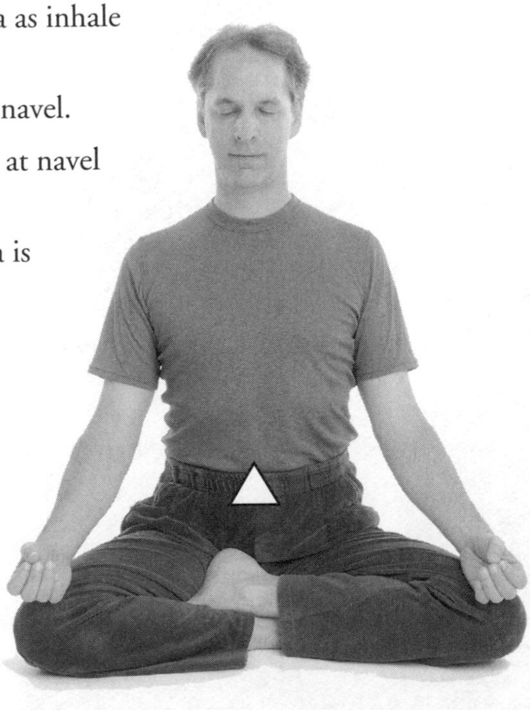

B: EMPHASIS: Rest with awareness in Transformation center (*maṇipūraka*) for some time.

12.

POSTURE: *Vajrāsana* with gesture and chant

EMPHASIS: To bring awareness to Relation center (*anāhata*).
To chant **yam**, at a slightly higher pitch, while bringing hands to heart.

TECHNIQUE: Kneeling on the floor with belly and chest on thighs, forehead on floor, and palms on floor near knees.

On inhale: Expand chest and raise arms up and out to sides, palms up, while standing on knees.

On exhale: Bring palms to heart while chanting **yam**.

Repeat **yam** one time more with each successive repetition, from one to eight times.

On inhale: Raise arms up and out to sides again, palms up, and slightly arch back.

On exhale: Return to starting position.

Number: Eight times.

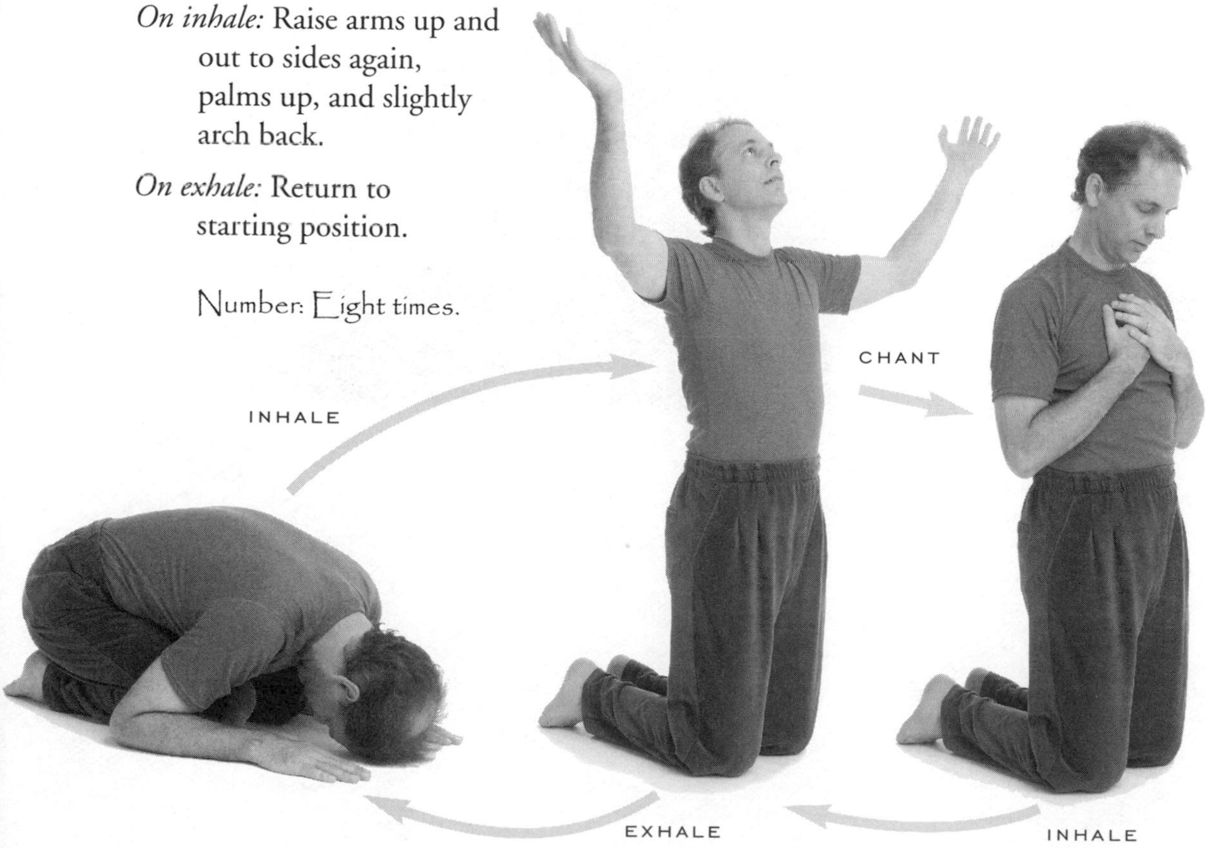

13.

POSTURE: *Siddhāsana*

EMPHASIS: Rest with awareness in Relation center (*anāhata*) for some time.

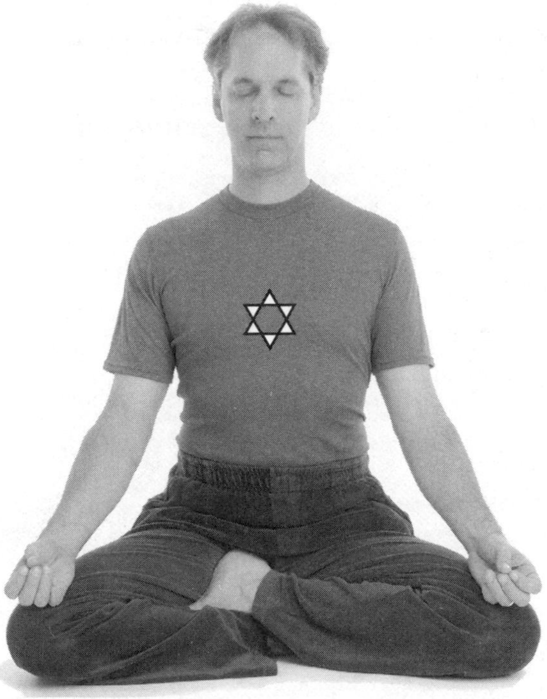

14.

POSTURE: *Siddhāsana*

EMPHASIS: *Śītalī prāṇāyāma* with alternate nostril exhalation.
To bring awareness to Communication center (*viśuddhi*).

Ratio: 8-4-12-4

TECHNIQUE: Sit comfortably.

Inhale through an extended curled tongue—like a straw—while raising chin slightly. Close mouth, curl tongue backward, drop chin, raise right arm, and seal right nostril.

Exhale through left nostril.

Inhale through curled tongue.

Then, following same procedure, *exhale* through right nostril.

Number: Six times each side, alternately.

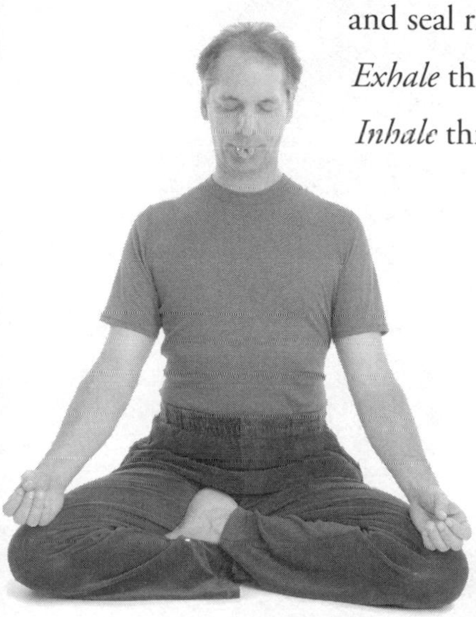

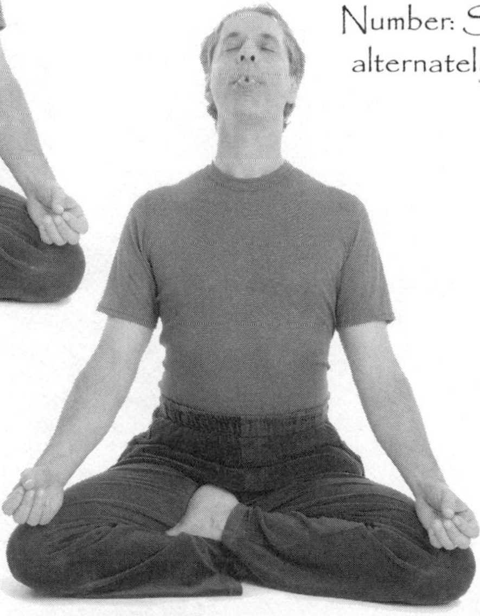

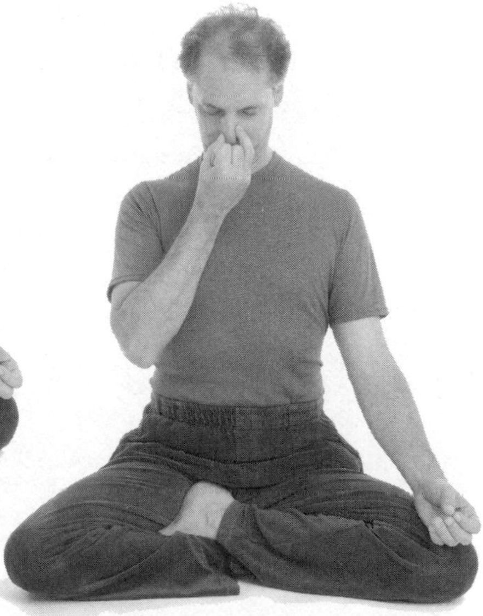

15.

POSTURE: *Siddhāsana*

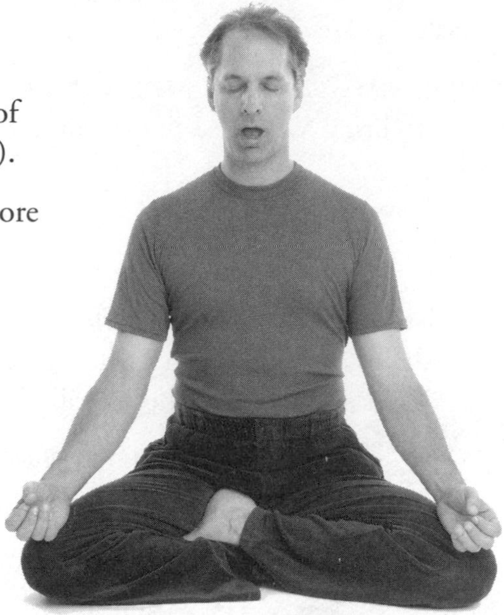

A: EMPHASIS: To deepen awareness of Communication center (*viśuddhi*).

TECHNIQUE: Chant **ham** one time more with each successive exhalation, from one to eight times.

Number: Eight times.

B: EMPHASIS: Rest with awareness in Communication center (*viśuddhi*) for some time.

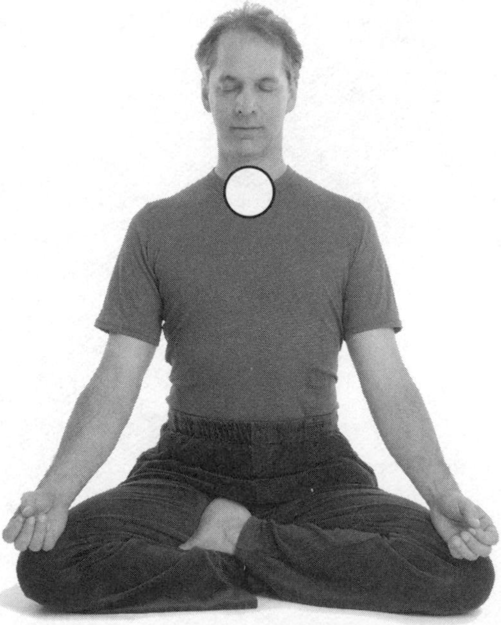

16.

POSTURE: *Siddhāsana*

EMPHASIS: To deepen awareness of Evaluation center (*ājña*).

Ratio: To build to 8-8-12-8

TECHNIQUE: *Nāḍī Śodhana* (alternate nostril inahalation and exhalation)

Inhale	*Hold*	*Exhale*	*Hold*	*Number*
8	4	12	4	4
8	8	12	4	4
8	8	12	8	8
8	0	12	0	4

DETAILS: One round equals two breaths:

Inhale left nostril.
Exhale right nostril.
Inhale right nostril.
Exhale left nostril.

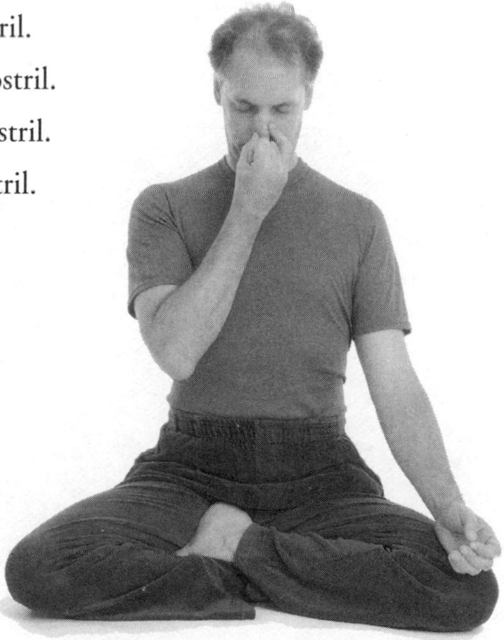

17.

POSTURE: *Siddhāsana*

A: EMPHASIS: To deepen awareness of Evaluation center (*ājña*).

TECHNIQUE: Chant **am** softly one time more with each successive exhalation, from one to eight times.

Number: Eight times.

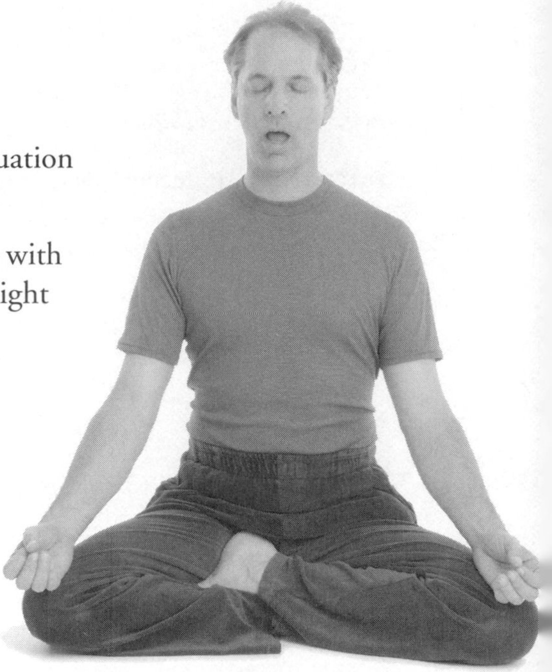

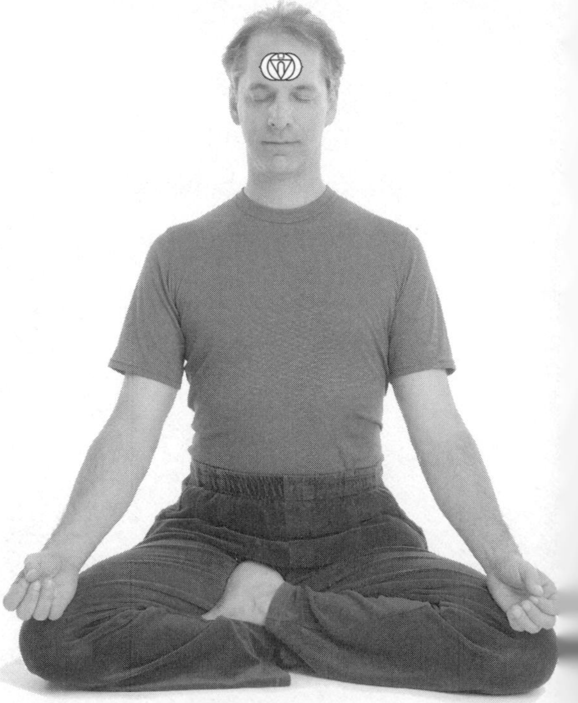

B: EMPHASIS: Rest with awareness in Evaluation center (*ājña*) for some time.

18.

POSTURE: *Siddhāsana*

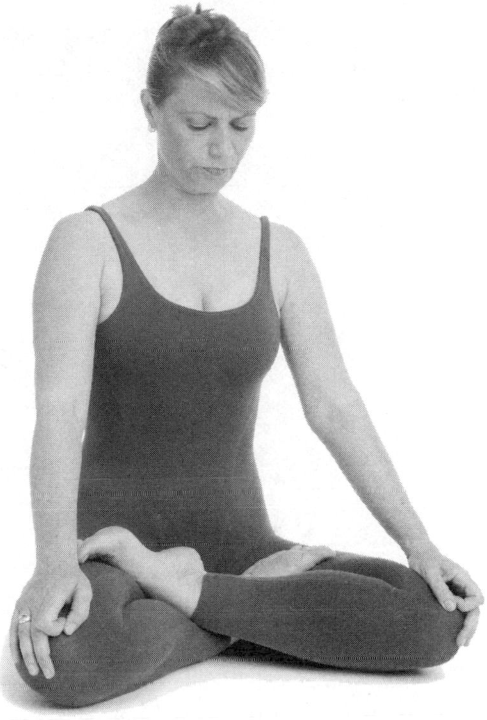

A: EMPHASIS: To bring awareness to the Inspiration center (*sahasrāra*).

TECHNIQUE: Chant **om** softly one time more with each successive exhalation, from one to eight times, at a slightly higher pitch.

Number: Eight times.

B: EMPHASIS: Rest with awareness in Inspiration center (*sahasrāra*) for some time.

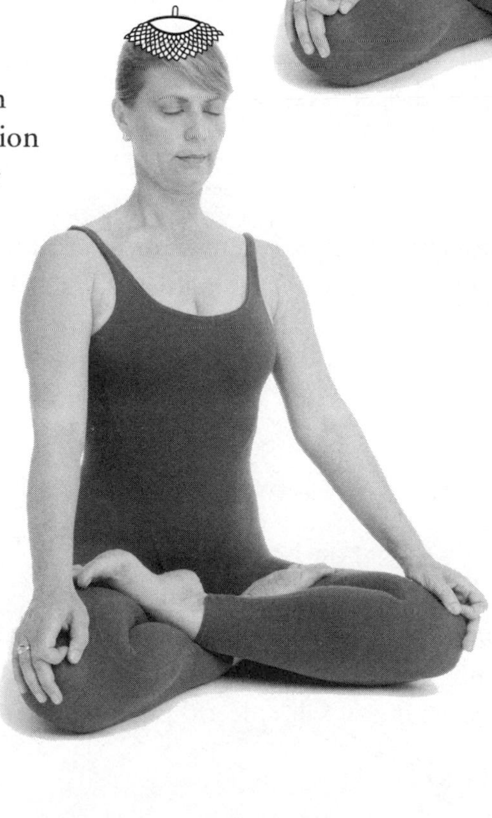

CHAPTER SEVEN

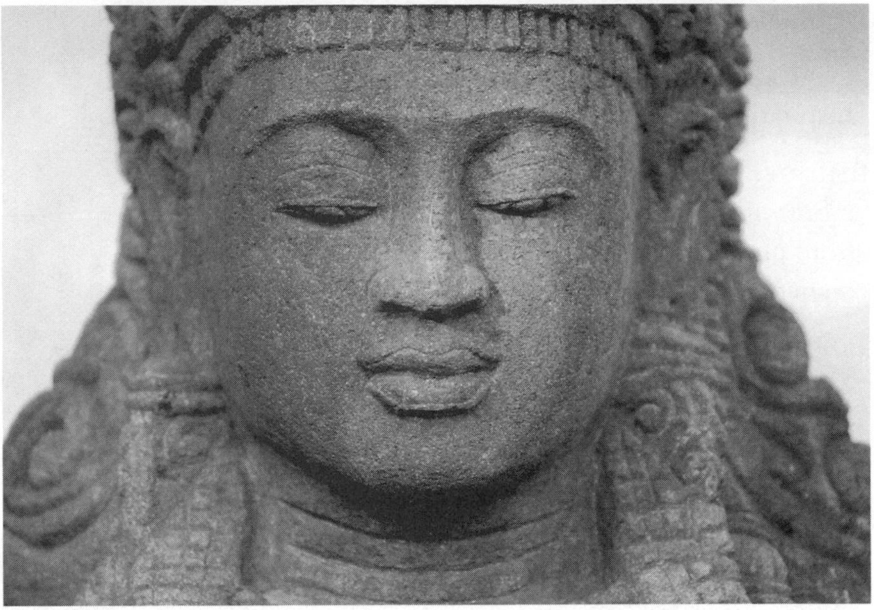

Refining the Personality

THE *VIJÑĀNAMAYA* LEVEL

THIS *VIJÑĀNAMAYA* DIMENSION represents the level of the personality. The personality, as we have seen earlier, is strongly influenced by our past. And this influence conditions our attitudes and perceptions, our priorities and goals, our values, and the content and style of our communication.

THE NATURE OF PERSONALITY

The ancients used the image of a crystal to symbolize the relationship between the role of the mind, as an instrument of perception, and the character of the personality, which conditions and, in that sense, distorts our perception.

A pure quartz crystal will absorb and reflect accurately the qualities of any object it is placed on; it will reflect things as they are. A pure quartz crystal is rare. We are much more likely to find a quartz that is smoky or rosy. And the inclusions and imperfections in these ordinary crystals will distort and obscure the qualities of any object it is placed upon. Our attitudes and beliefs distort our perceptions in much the same way. So, for example, pessimism—represented by a smoky quartz crystal—represents a mental quality that tends to view things negatively, while optimism—represented by a rosy quartz crystal—represents one that views things positively. There are many who go through life with the attitude that the "glass is half empty," focusing their attention on what they don't have and what is not right, while others go through life with the attitude that the "glass is half full," focusing instead on what they have received, with a feeling of appreciation for their good fortune. Thus, our attitude, or our personality, largely determines how we experience the world around us.

As we can influence our physical structures through the intelligent practice of *āsana* and our energy through the intelligent practice of *āsana* and *prāṇāyāma,* so too we can influence our personality through the practice of meditation.

THE FUNCTION OF MEDITATION

The normal state of mind fluctuates between distraction and attention, fueled by internally conditioned patterns and external stimulations. Like the crystal, the mind takes on the character of the objects toward which it is directed. And, in the normal course of perception, the flow of energy is toward the external: that is, we use our minds to perceive our environment, so that we can function in the world.

Meditation is a means of developing progressively subtler, more deeply internalized levels of perception until, at its deepest level, it breaks the external connection altogether—and the mind takes on the character of "that which we are." Discriminative insight arises as we are established in our true nature. This represents the highest goal of Yoga, which, according to the ancient Seers, we can only understand through experience. As the great Chinese mystic Lao-Tzu said, "He who knows does not speak. He who speaks does not know."

Between that deepest level and our normal waking consciousness there are many steps. Meditation practice therefore involves reducing mental agitation, shifting attention away from distractions, and progressively linking our attention to something of a deeper and deeper character. In fact, establishing this link is the basic meaning and purpose of meditation practice.

Thus, as we meditate, our primary intention is to develop a one-pointed flow of energy toward progressively subtler objects of perception—from the external to the internal, from the gross to the subtle. And, it is toward this end that the various techniques of meditation were developed and can be usefully applied.

One-Pointed and Self-Reflective Meditation

Popular methods of meditation usually use a variety of techniques that can all be categorized under the heading of one-pointedness. These might include gazing at an external object, such as a candle, a *yantra,* a part of the body, or some representation of a form of the Divine. They may include gazing internally at an image developed in the imagination, resting the attention on an inner part of the body, or resting the attention on the breath. And they may also include vocally or mentally repeating a *mantra* or a phrase from a song or sacred text, listening to music, singing, and reciting poems or prayers. All of which come under the general category of "directed" meditation.

And still another popular technique is what might be called "nondirected" meditation, in which attention rests on attention itself.

These types of meditation have different effects, depending on the object of focus, but they all reflect the process of mind training in which we develop our ability to sustain focused attention in one direction, without distraction, over a period of time. And yet, as potent as these mind-training techniques may be, they may not help us to see ourselves more clearly. In order to rise above our conditioning, free ourselves from suffering, improve our relationships, or find a deeper meaning and purpose in life, we must "go within ourselves." For it is only when we return to our core that we can overcome our reactive tendencies and free ourselves from the attitudes and behaviors that are born from them. Self-reflective meditation may be the most potent aid in our journey toward transformation.

As we have seen, the teachings and practices of meditation are fundamentally about the phenomenon of attention. The normal pattern of attention, according to the Yoga Sūtra of Patañjali, is characterized as the fluctuation between distraction and attention. In fact, Patañjali uses the word *vyutthāna,* loosely translated as "rising up, scattering," which suggests that thoughts arise and move in different directions habitually and haphazardly through successive moments.

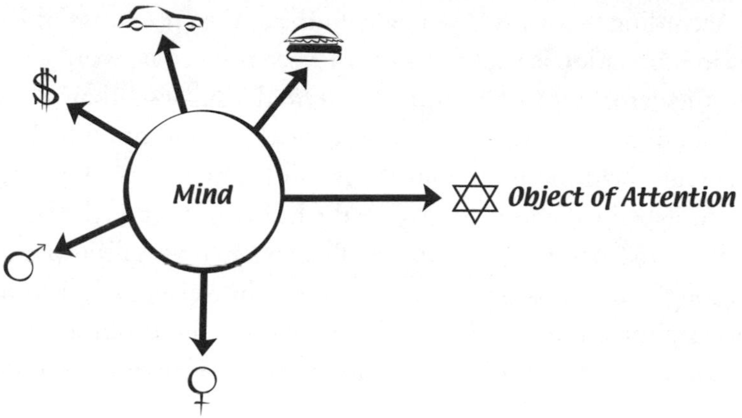

The teachings of Yoga suggest that the mind is fundamentally an instrument of perception and cognition. Normal perception, as we have seen, is mediated through the conditioned mind.

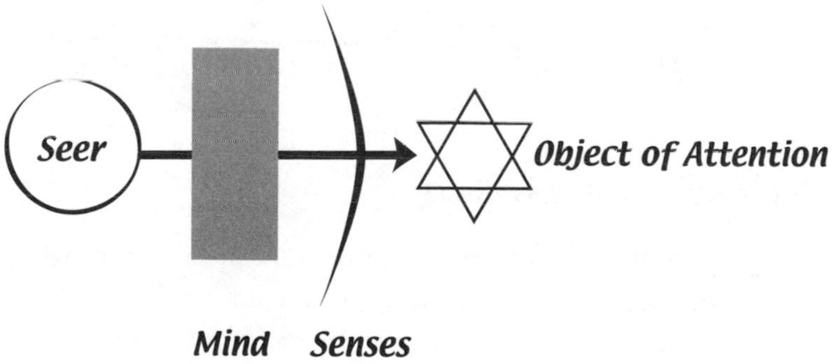

Initial Goals of Meditation Practice

Two initial goals relate to the mind-training methods suggested by these teachings. One, as mentioned above, is to develop the capacity for the attention to stay linked to an object of choice without distraction over a period of time. The other is to progressively reduce the degree to which past conditioning distorts our perception.

Basic Steps in the Meditation Process

THE FIRST STEP: *DHĀRAṆĀ*

According to the *aṣṭāṅga* (eight-limbed) Yoga teachings of Patañjali, the first step in meditation is the state known as *dhāraṇā*. The word *dhāraṇā*, coming from the verbal root *dhā* (or *dhṛ*), "to hold," suggests that in this state the object of meditation serves as a support for the attention, which is linked to one object and held there without distraction. The object of attention can be variable. As explained above, it may be the breath, a part of the body, a *mantra* or sound, an external image, an internally generated visualization, a feeling, or even a thought or an idea. From experience, however, we all know that the things we are most interested in are most likely to hold our attention. Therefore it is important that the object of attention be something that captures our interest.

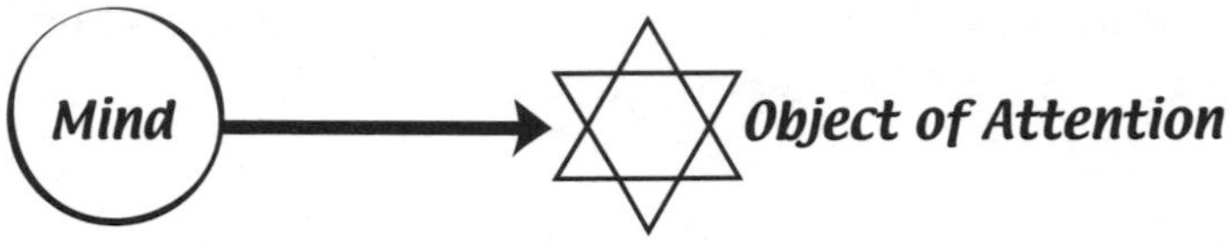

Dhāraṇā

THE SECOND STEP: *DHYĀNAM*

The next step in meditation, the state of *dhyānam*, occurs when the oriented state of attention (*dhāraṇā*) has been prolonged until there begins to be a relationship between the mind and the object of attention. The word *dhyāna*, coming from the verbal root *dhī*, "to reflect," suggests that some intelligence or knowledge is derived from this relationship. As symbolized by the following drawing, the mind is, as it were, closer to the object and the arrows move in both directions. That is, something returns to the mind from the object, at which point the significance of the choice of object can be seen. Knowledge derived from this state of meditation is of the object and, as we have seen, that object can be either gross or subtle, secular or spiritual.

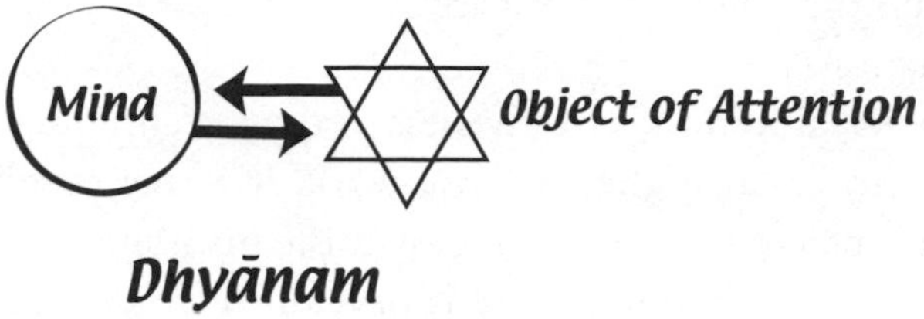

THE THIRD STEP: *SAMĀDHI*

The final step in meditation is the state known as *samādhi,* wherein the relationship between the object and the mind becomes so close that it is as if they have merged. There are many levels of *samādhi* described. The basic idea here, however, is that it is as if the mind becomes progressively freed from its conditioning until all that remains is the object itself. The mind has absorbed the true nature of the object as it is.

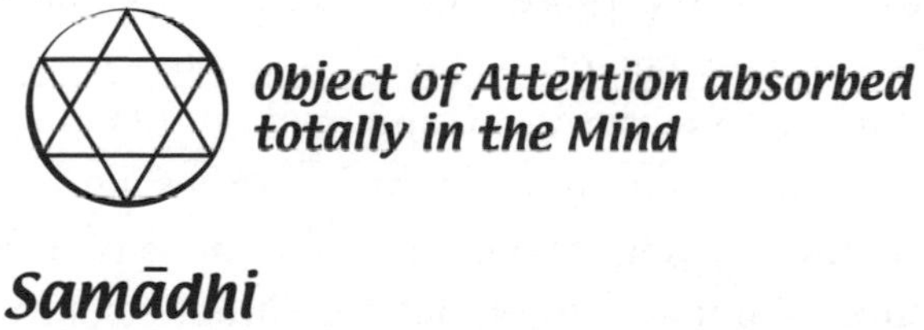

At the root of the personality are drives and motivations that guide our actions and behavior. To be transformed at the root, we need meditative processes that will impact our deepest drives and motivations. It is clear that we can use meditation techniques in the process of mind training to develop our concentration skills, deepen our focus, and achieve one-pointedness. Beyond simply developing one-pointedness, however, we can use the meditative process as a means of transforming our character, reassessing our priorities, improving our relationships, and setting a new direction for our future.

Many and varied methods of meditation have evolved toward this end. They utilize the body, through movement and breathing; the emotions, through music and prayer; and the intellect—both abstractly and personally—through study and contemplation.

However, without faith in the effectiveness of these techniques and without the commitment to practice, they will not work. It is therefore important to consider what will inspire faith. For some, it is the inspiration of the spiritual masters who have come before us and is developed by meeting spiritual friends who can give instruction, or by reading the life story of a great being. For others, it is the eagerness to be free from suffering, to enjoy happiness, to engage in positive actions, and to avoid negative actions. For still others, it is faith in the sources of refuge that have been offered through the spiritual lineages of their ancestors or through other lineages that they have encountered along their journey through life.

Whatever the method, it will be most effective when the motivation to practice arises from the depths of our hearts. Faith is like a seed from which the commitment to practice will grow, and from which that practice will bear fruit. Thus, faith is perhaps the most precious of all our resources, for it carries us along on our path.

In the practice that follows, we will demonstrate how to use deep self-reflective meditations to initiate the process of "returning to oneself"—the place from which, as the ancients taught, our faith is awakened. In the next chapter we will turn our attention to the means and methods of cultivating, refining, and celebrating our relationship to that which inspires our faith.

A common theme in the teachings of the spiritual traditions of the East as well as the West is the effect of our actions on our condition. There appears to be an almost universal agreement that action can lead to suffering. And that those actions occur at the level of the body, at the level of speech, and at the level of the mind. According to these nearly universal teachings, actions are influenced by past conditioning, and influence future conditions. Therefore, it is important to become progressively more conscious of our actions, so that we can set a positive direction for our future.

The following practice demonstrates how we can use *āsana* and *prāṇāyāma* as a preparation for meditative self-reflection. These preparatory steps enable the reflections to penetrate to a deeper level within us and, therefore, they facilitate the transformational potential of the meditations. These particular reflections can be used in the context of personal practice again and again. We encourage you to take them to your heart, and use them often.

VIJÑĀNAMAYA PRACTICE

1.

POSTURE: *Padmāsana*

A: EMPHASIS: *Bhāvana* (absorption/contemplation) of consciousness as clear as a blue sky.

TECHNIQUE: While sitting, bend right knee and place right foot on top of left thigh, close to groin. Then bend left knee and place left foot on top of right thigh, close to groin. Rest in *bhāvana* for some time.

B: EMPHASIS: Deepen inhalation and exhalation while sustaining *bhāvana.*

TECHNIQUE:

A: Progressively deepen inhalation and exhalation to a comfortable maximum length of inhalation. Let exhalation pace inhalation.

B: Sustain this breathing.

C: Progressively reduce length of inhalation and exhalation to normal breathing.

Number: Repeat A, B, and C six times each.

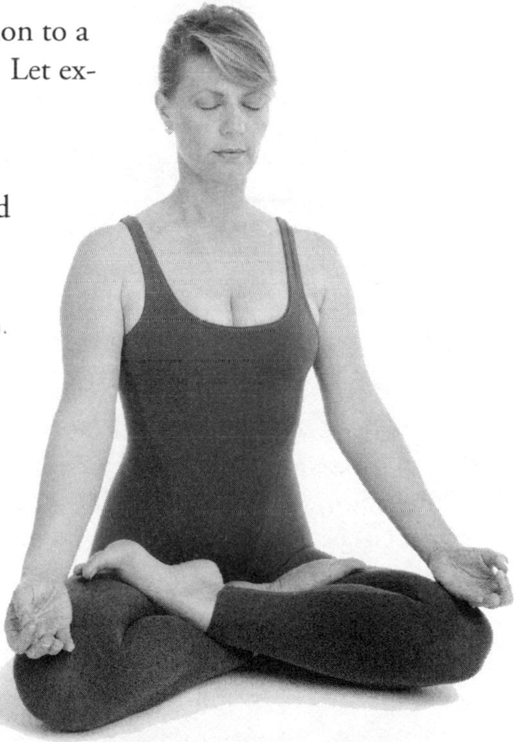

DETAILS:

On inhale: Follow the downward flow of inhalation, expanding progressively from chest to belly.

On exhale: Follow the upward flow of exhalation, contracting progressively from pubic bone to navel.

C: EMPHASIS: Reflect on the questions: What is my highest value? What is most important to me? What are my highest priorities?

TECHNIQUE: Personally consider these questions for some time.

2.

POSTURE: *Vajrāsana*

EMPHASIS: To stretch back gently and symmetrically.
To open chest and mobilize shoulders.

TECHNIQUE: Stand on knees with arms over head.

On exhale: Bend forward, sweeping arms behind back, and bringing hands to sacrum, keeping palms up, forehead to the floor.

On inhale: Return to starting position.

Number: Six times.

DETAILS:

On exhale: Bring chest to thighs before bringing buttocks to heels. Rotate arms so palms are up and hands are resting on sacrum.

On inhale: Expand chest and lift it up off of knees as arms sweep wide.

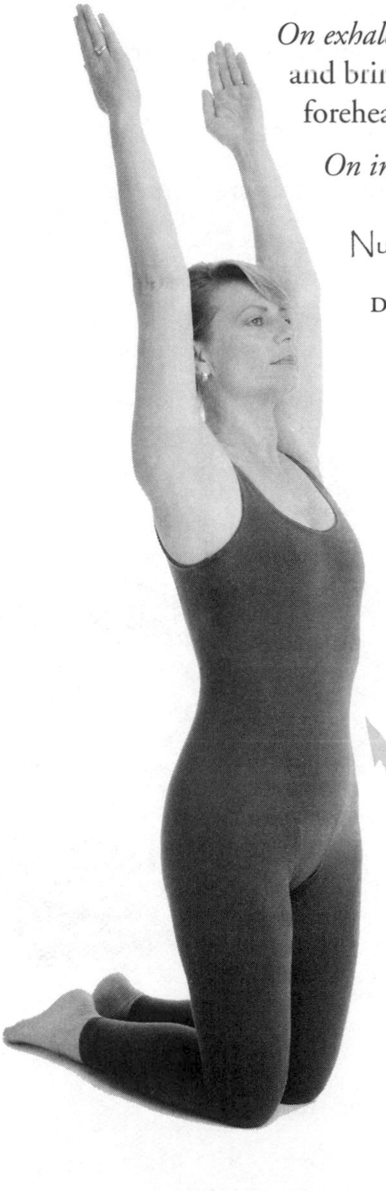

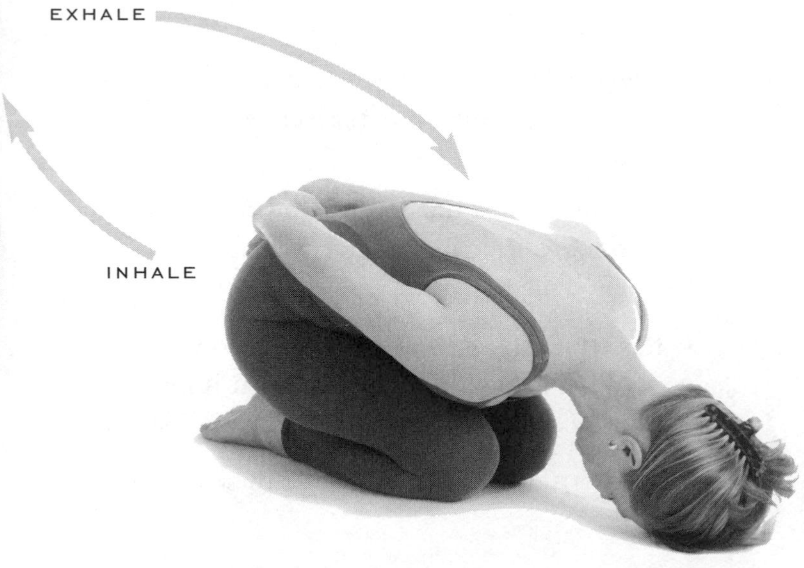

3.

POSTURE: *Bhujaṅgāsana*

EMPHASIS: To arch upper back while mobilizing arms. To warm up and stabilize lower back.

TECHNIQUE: Lie on belly, forehead on floor, with elbows bent and palms on floor in line with diaphragm, fingers facing forward.

On inhale: Lift chest, arching back.

On exhale: Return to starting position.

Number: Six times.

DETAILS:

On inhale: Lift chest using back muscles, engaging arms toward the end of inhale. Lead with chest, lifting chin slightly at end of inhale.

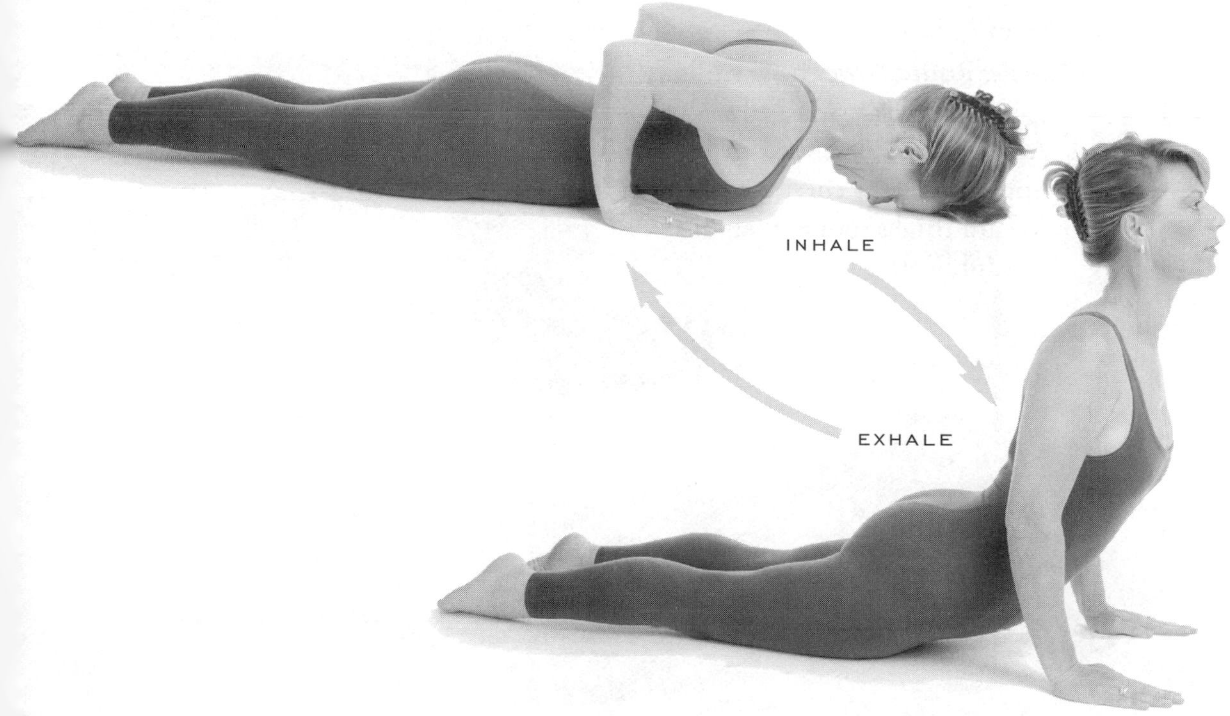

4.

POSTURE: *Cakravākāsana*

EMPHASIS: To stretch lower back after back bend. To prepare for seated meditation posture.

TECHNIQUE: Get down on hands and knees, with shoulders vertically above wrists, and with hips above knees.

On inhale: Lift chest up and away from belly.

On exhale: Gently contract belly, round lower back, and bring chest toward thighs.

Number: Six times.

DETAILS:

On inhale: Lead with chest, keeping chin slightly down. Avoid compressing lower back; rather, feel chest expanding.

On exhale: Round lower back without collapsing chest over belly. Avoid increasing curvature of upper back. Let chest lower toward thighs sooner than hips toward heels.

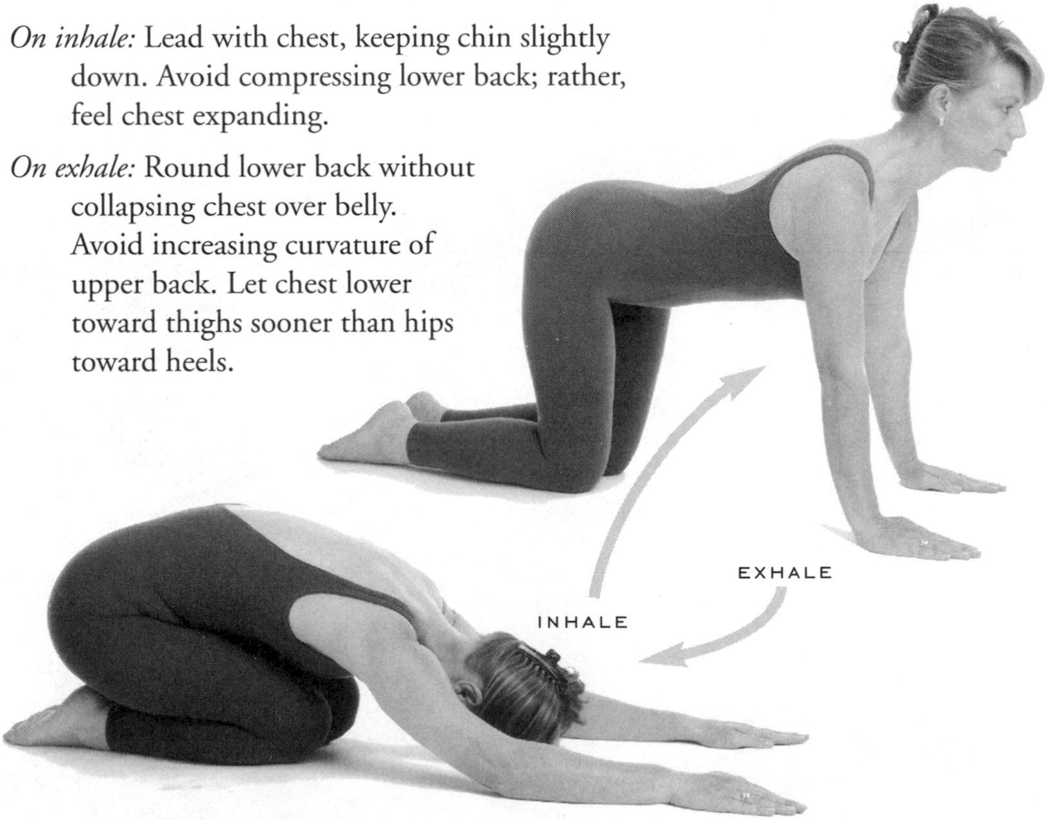

5.

POSTURE: *Padmāsana*

A: EMPHASIS: To deepen inhalation. To energize system.

TECHNIQUE: While sitting, bend right knee and place right foot on top of left thigh, close to groin. Then bend left knee and place left foot on top of right thigh, close to groin.

Prāṇāyāma: Anuloma Krama—segment inhalation in stages

TECHNIQUE:

A: Two-stage inhalation

Exhale deeply and fully.

Inhale first half of breath in five seconds.

Pause five seconds.

Inhale remainder of breath in five seconds.

Pause five seconds.

Exhale slowly and fully.

Number: Six times.

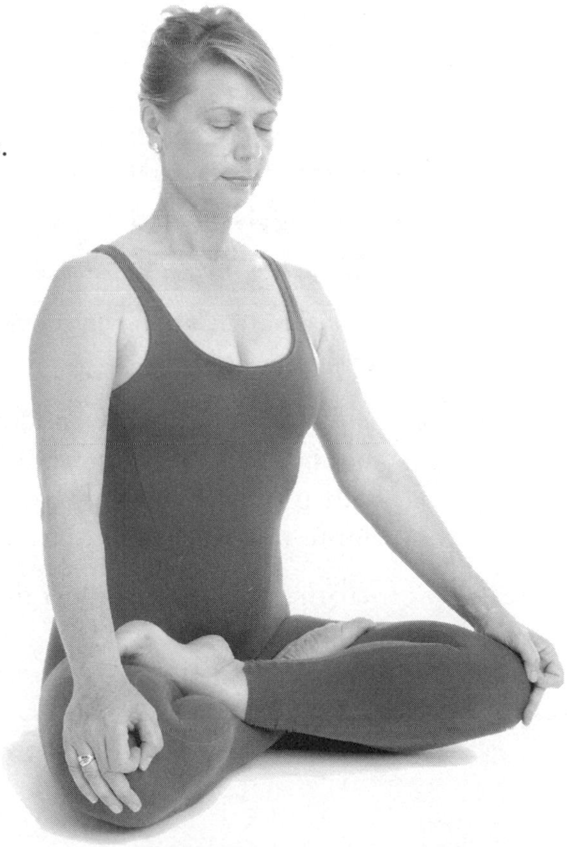

DETAILS:

On first stage of inhale: Expand chest from pit of throat to sternum.

On second stage of inhale: Expand abdomen from sternum to pubic bone.

On exhale: Contract abdomen progressively from pubic bone to navel to sternum.

TECHNIQUE:

B: Three-stage inhalation.

Exhale deeply and fully.

Inhale first third of breath in four seconds.

Pause four seconds.

Inhale second third of breath in four seconds.

Pause four seconds.

Inhale last third of breath in four seconds.

Pause four seconds.

Exhale slowly and fully.

Number: Six times. Then rest for a few moments.

DETAILS:

On first stage of inhale: Expand chest from pit of throat to sternum.

On second stage of inhale: Expand abdomen from sternum to navel.

On third stage of inhale: Expand abdomen from navel to pubic bone.

On exhale: Contract abdomen progressively from pubic bone to navel to sternum.

B: EMPHASIS: To reflect: Consider your usual daily activity and the level of your **body**. What percentage of your daily activity at the level of your **body** is truly oriented toward your highest value? What is most important to you, your highest priorities?

TECHNIQUE: Personally consider this question for some time.

6.

POSTURE: *Tāḍāsana*

EMPHASIS: To encourage balance. To extend the spine. To strengthen calves and feet. To equalize length of inhalation and exhalation.

TECHNIQUE: Stand with arms at side, feet parallel.

On inhale: Raise up on toes while simultaneously raising arms up over head, bringing palms together.

On exhale: Return to starting point.

Number: Six times.

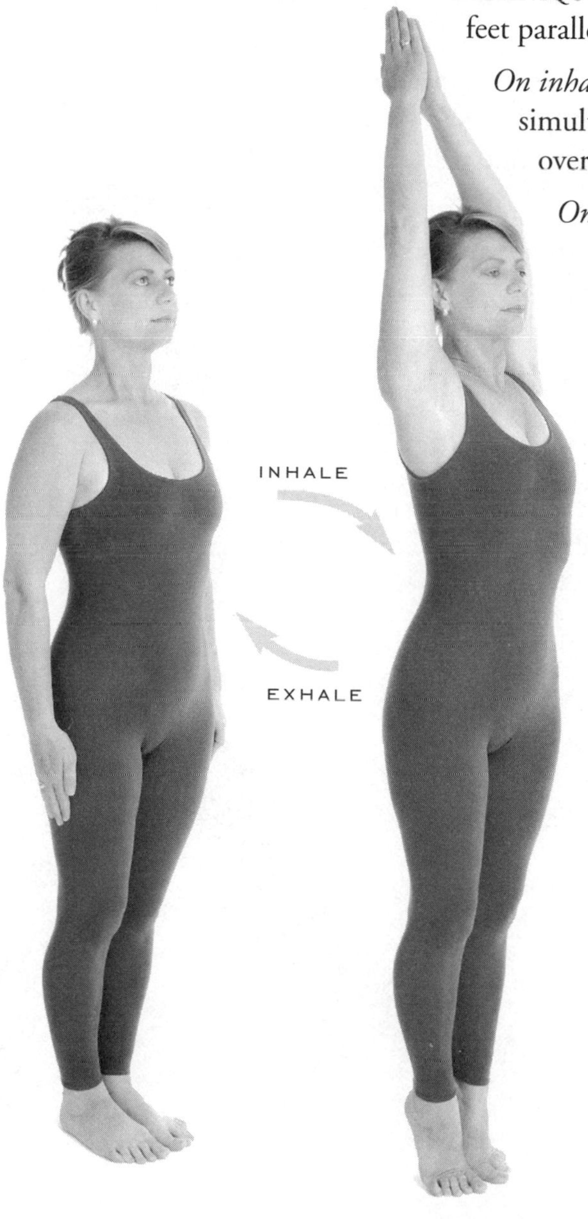

DETAILS: Equalize inhalation and exhalation at approximately eight seconds.

On inhale: Slightly arch back and lift head.

On exhale: Slightly flatten lower back, chin down.

7.

POSTURE: *Vīrabhadrāsana*

EMPHASIS: To strengthen muscles of back and legs, expand chest, and flatten upper back. To equalize length of inhalation and exhalation.

TECHNIQUE: Stand with left foot forward, feet as wide as hips, and arms at sides.

On inhale: Simultaneously bend left knee, displace chest slightly forward and hips slightly backward, and bring arms forward and up over head, palms together. Arch upper back.

On exhale: Return to starting position.

Number: Six times each side.

DETAILS: Equalize inhalation and exhalation at approximately eight seconds.

On inhale: Feel expansion of chest. Avoid compressing lower back.

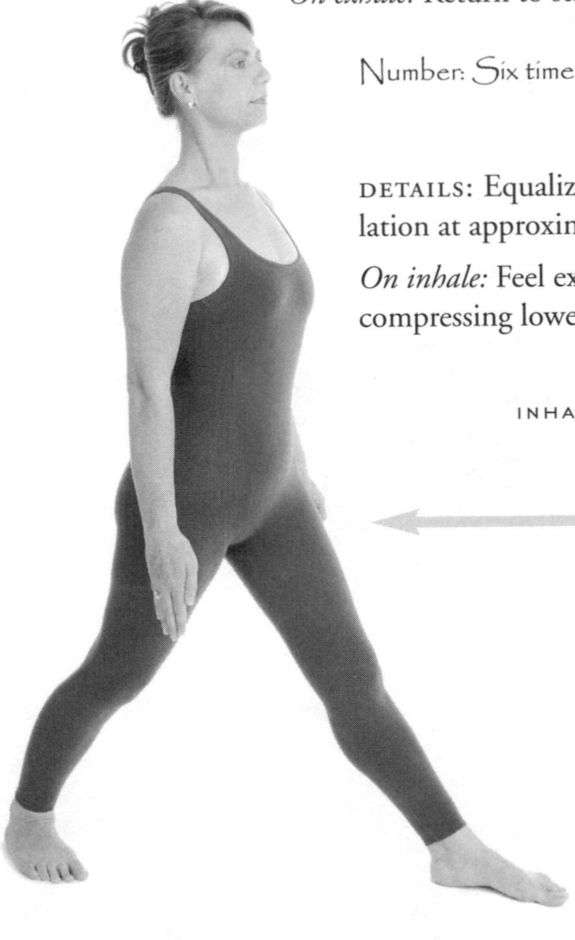

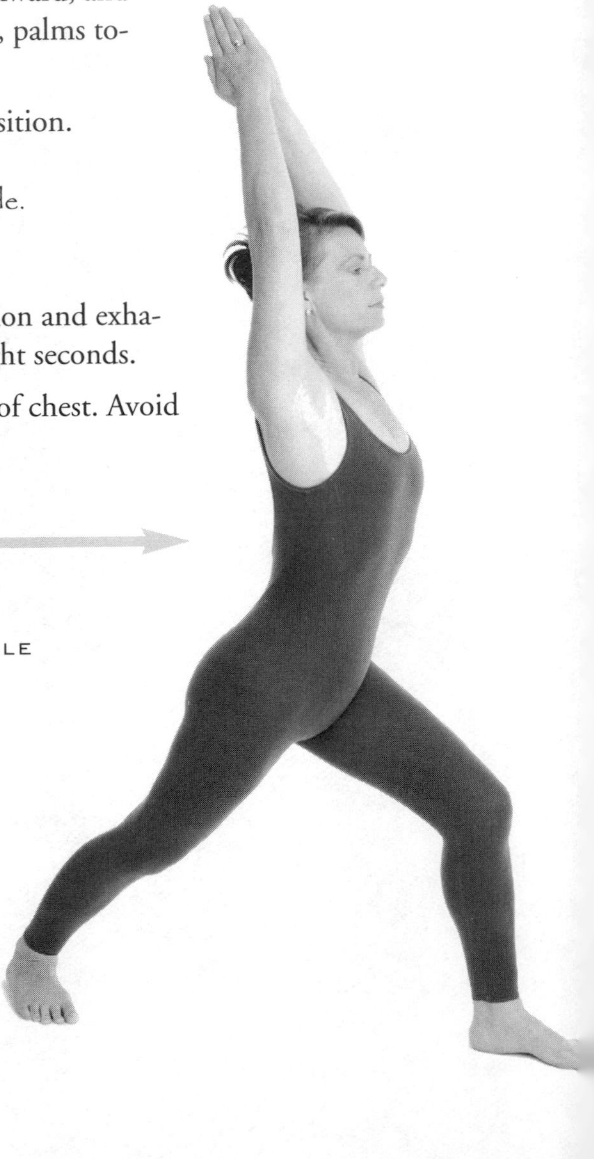

8.

POSTURE: *Uttānāsana*

EMPHASIS: To equalize length of inhalation and exhalation.
To warm up back and legs.

TECHNIQUE: Stand with arms over head.

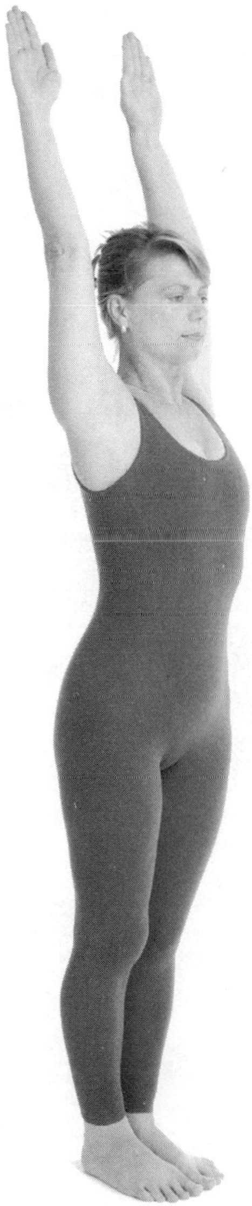

On exhale: Forward bend, bringing belly and chest toward thighs, and bringing hands to feet.

On exhale: Return to starting position.

Number: Six times.

DETAILS: Equalize inhalation and exhalation at approximately eight seconds.

On exhale: Bend knees to facilitate stretching of lower back. Move chin down toward throat.

On inhale: Lift chest up and away from thighs, flattening upper back. Keep knees bent until end of movement.

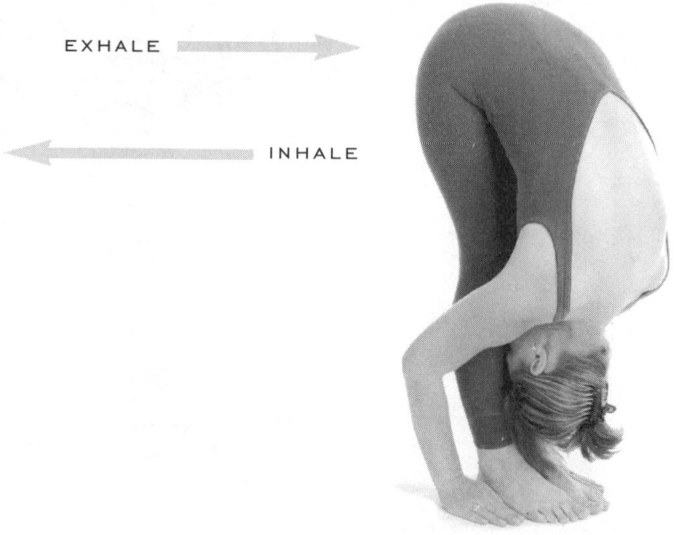

9.

POSTURE: *Vīrabhadrāsana* variation

EMPHASIS: To strengthen legs, hips, and back. To focus attention and increase balance. To experience a standing balance posture. To equalize length of inhalation and exhalation.

TECHNIQUE: Stand with arms over head, palms together.

On exhale: Bend forward, extending arms forward and lifting straight right leg behind, until torso and right leg are parallel to floor. Left leg knee can be slightly flexed.

On inhale: Return to starting point.

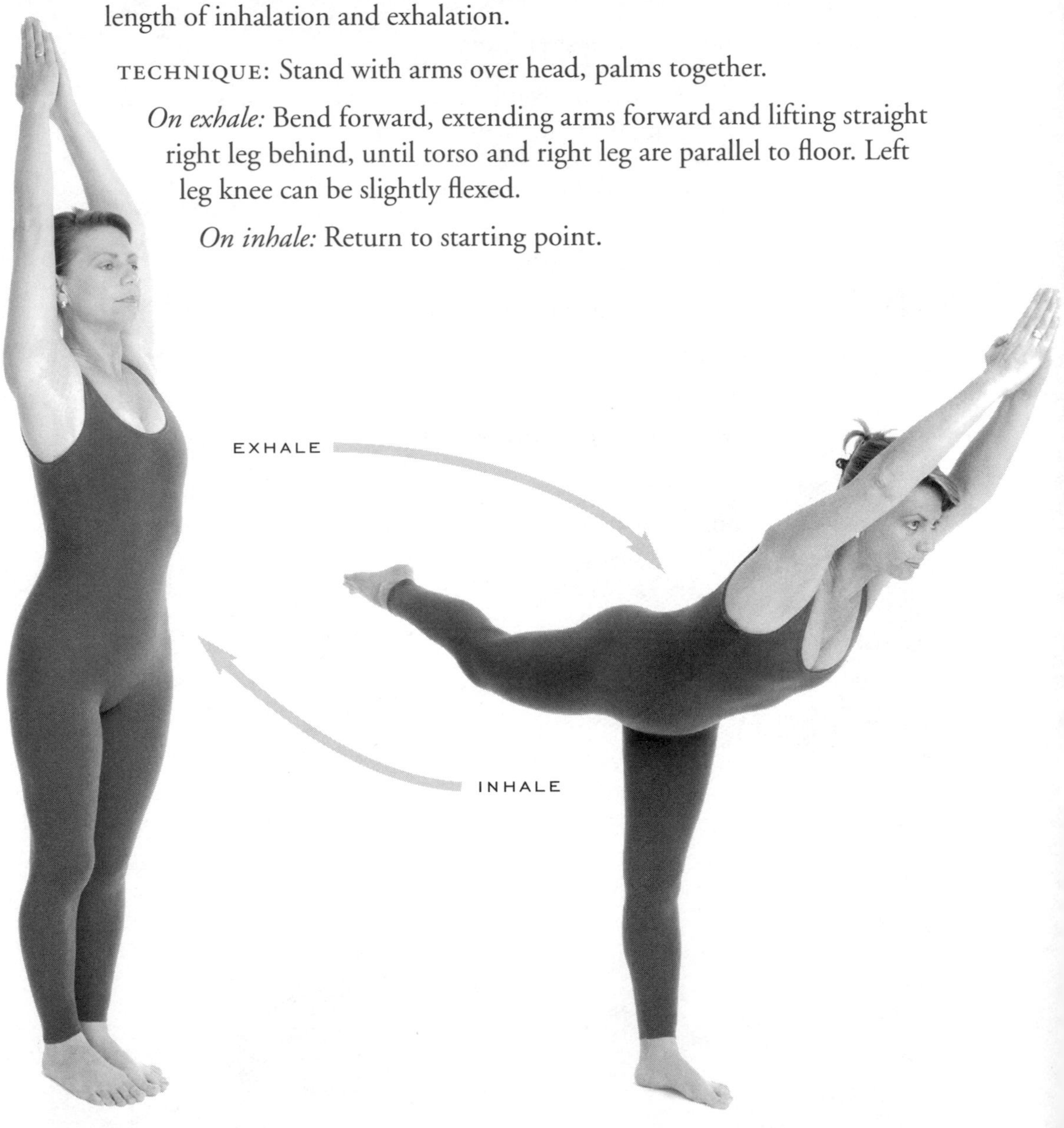

Repeat three times.

Then stay in balance position six breaths.

Repeat on other side.

DETAILS: Equalize inhalation and exhalation at approximately eight seconds.

On inhale: Arch back and lift right leg. Keep arms level with ears.

10.

POSTURE: *Vajrāsana/Cakravākāsana/Adho Mukha Śvānāsana/Ūrdhva Mukha Śvānāsana*

EMPHASIS: To energize system by engaging musculature of upper body, expanding chest, and stretching belly. To equalize length of inhalation and exhalation.

TECHNIQUE: Stand on knees with arms over head.

On exhale: Bend forward, bringing arms to floor in front of you.

On inhale: Lift chest up and away from belly, coming forward onto hands.

On exhale: Push buttocks upward, lifting knees off ground, and pushing chest toward feet.

On inhale: Stretch body forward and arch back.

On exhale: Return to previous position.

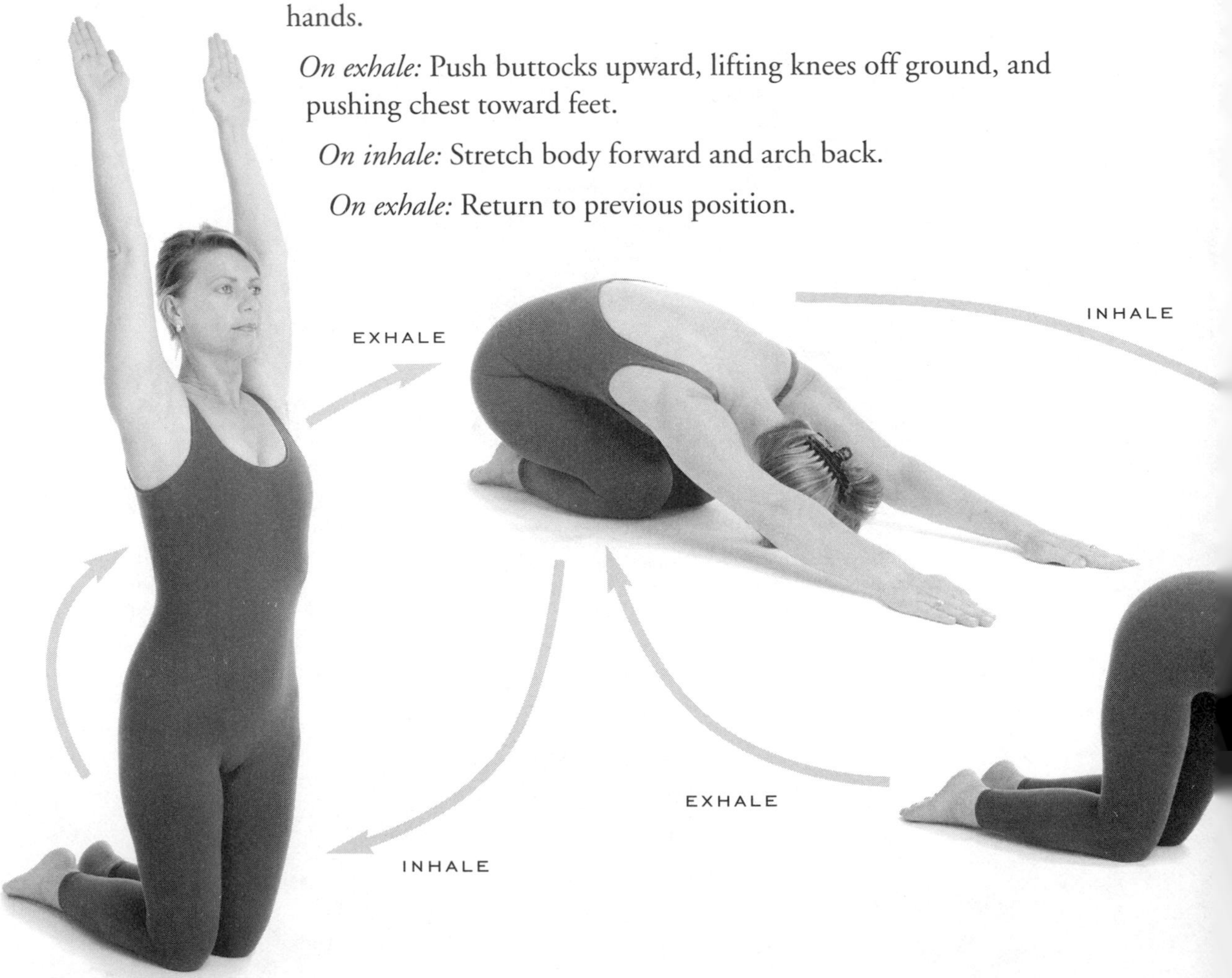

On inhale: Return to knees, lifting chest up and away from belly, coming forward onto hands.

On exhale: Tighten belly, round lower back, and bring chest toward thighs.

On inhale: Return to starting position.

Number: Six times.

DETAILS: Equalize inhalation and exhalation at approximately eight seconds.

On inhale: Expand chest, stretch belly, and avoid compressing lower back.

On exhale: End in forward bend position.

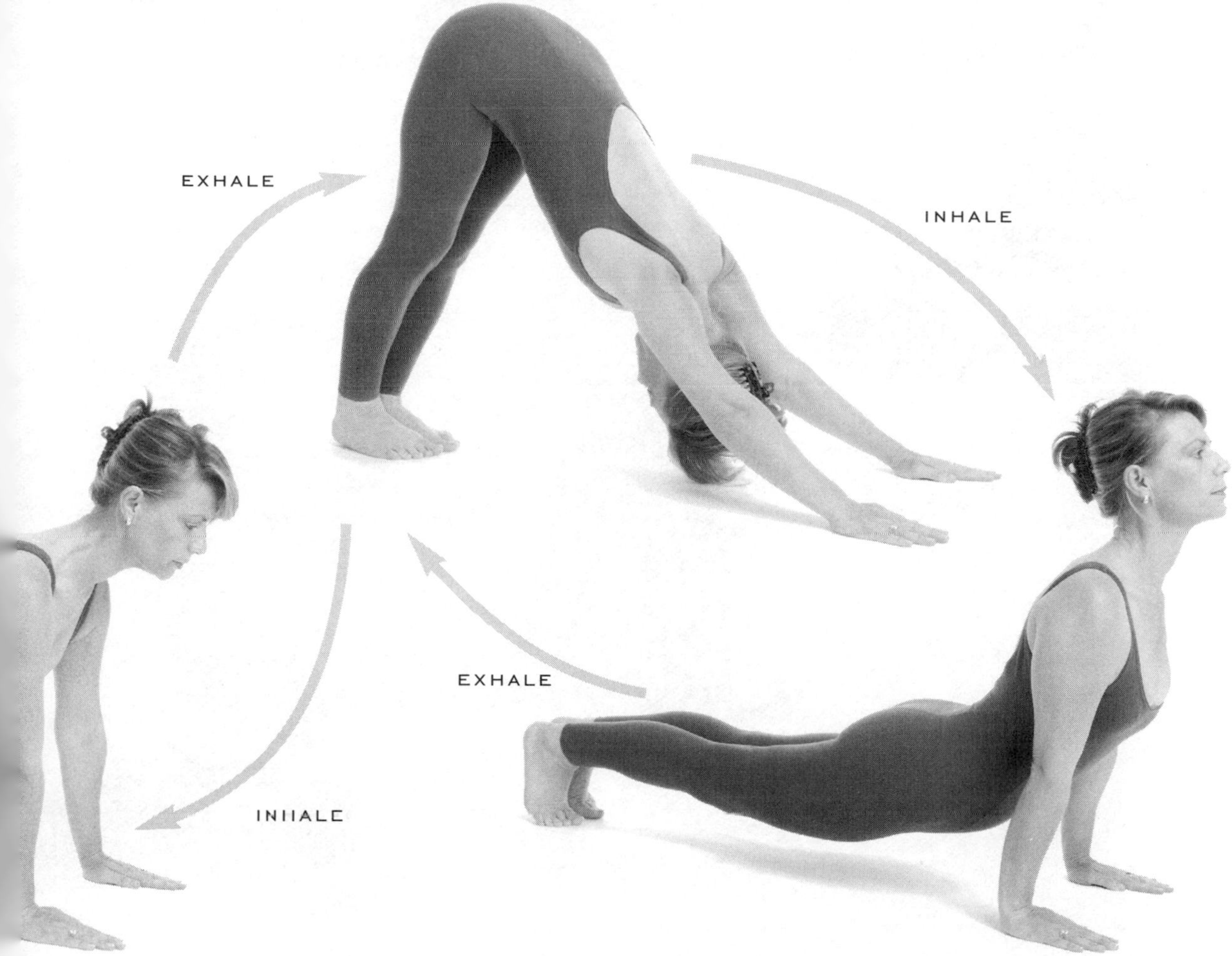

11.

POSTURE: *Padmāsana*

A: EMPHASIS: To open throat and bring awareness to the Communication center.

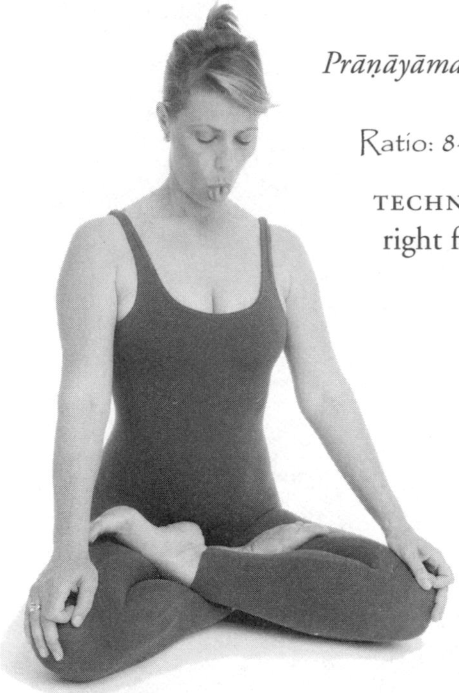

Prāṇāyāma: Śītalī prāṇāyāma with alternate nostril exhalation

Ratio: 8-4-12-4

TECHNIQUE: While sitting, bend right knee and place right foot on top of left thigh, close to groin. Then bend left knee and place left foot on top of right thigh, close to groin. Place hands on knees.

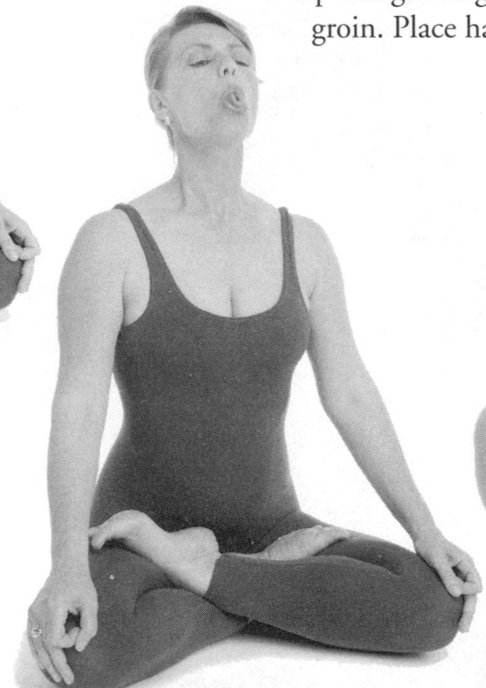

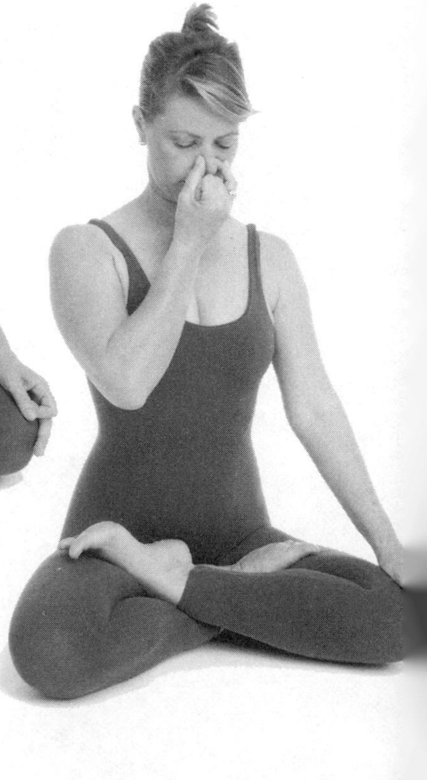

Inhale through an extended curled tongue—like a straw—while raising chin slightly. Close mouth, curl tongue backward, drop chin, raise right arm, and seal right nostril.

Exhale through left nostril.

Inhale through curled tongue.

Then, following same procedure, *exhale* through right nostril.

Number: Six times each side, alternately. Then rest for a few moments.

B: EMPHASIS: To reflect: Personally consider your usual daily activity and the level of your **communication**. What percentage of your daily activity at the level of your **speech** is truly oriented toward your highest value? What is most important to you, your highest priorities?

TECHNIQUE: Personally consider this question for some time.

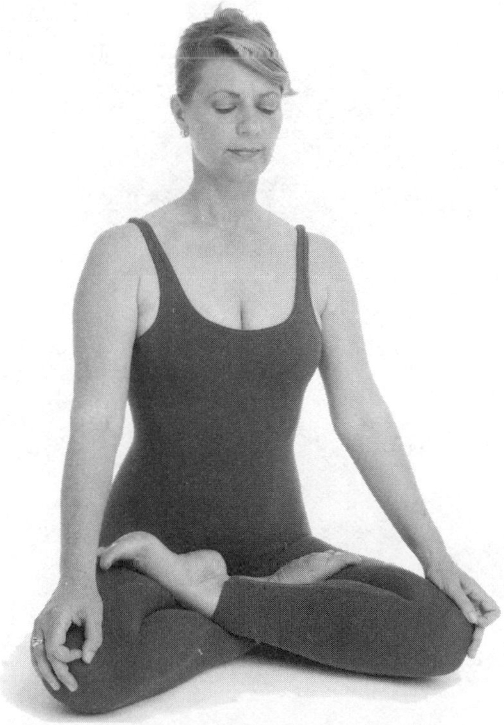

12.

POSTURE: *Dvipāda Pīṭham*

EMPHASIS: To relax upper back and neck, and to mobilize lower back after sitting.

TECHNIQUE: Lie on back with arms down at sides, knees bent, and feet slightly apart on floor and comfortably close to buttocks.

On inhale: Pressing down on feet and keeping chin down, raise pelvis until neck is gently flattened on floor, while raising arms up over head to floor behind.

On exhale: Return to starting position.

Number: Six times.

DETAILS: *On inhale:* Lift spine, vertebra by vertebra, from bottom up.

On exhale: Unwind spine, coming down vertebra by vertebra.

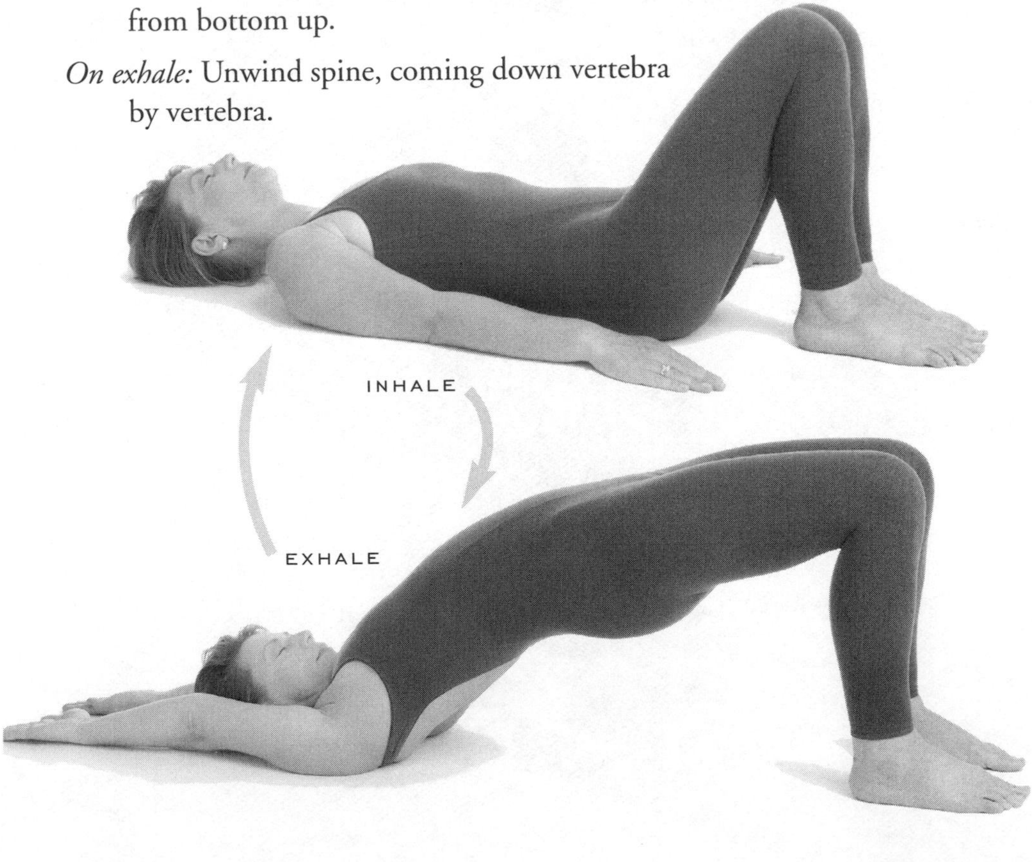

13.

POSTURE: *Ūrdhva Prasṛta Pādāsana*

EMPHASIS: To extend spine and flatten it onto floor. To stretch legs.

TECHNIQUE: Lie on back with arms down at sides, legs bent, and knees lifted toward chest.

On inhale: Raise arms upward all the way to floor behind head, and raise legs upward toward ceiling.

On exhale: Return to starting position.

Number: Six times.

DETAILS: *On inhale:* Flex feet as legs are raised upward. Keep knees slightly bent, and keep angle between legs and torso less than ninety degrees. Push lower back and sacrum downward. Bring chin down.

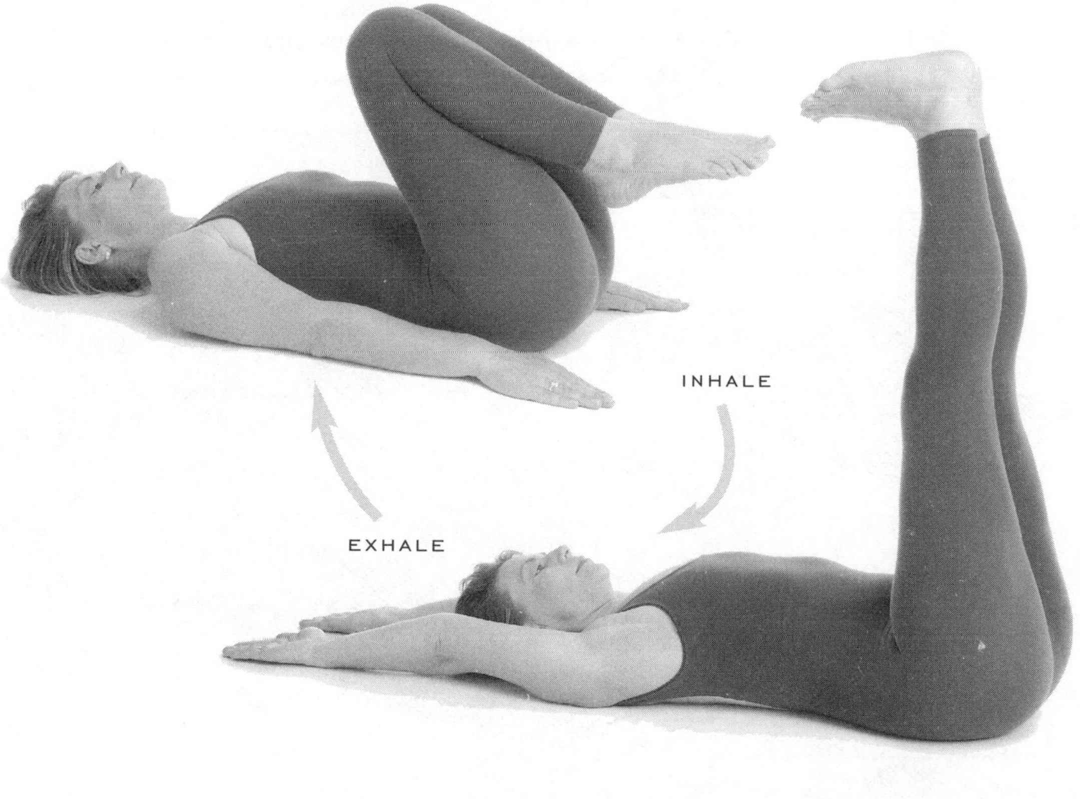

14.

POSTURE: *Jaṭhara Parivṛtti*

EMPHASIS: To gently twist and compress belly, and stretch hips. To prepare for seated twist.

TECHNIQUE: Lie on back with both legs straight, at right angles to torso, feet flexed and facing upward. Arms out to sides, slightly less than right angles to torso.

On exhale: Bring both legs toward floor on right side of body, bringing feet to right hand, twisting abdomen while simultaneously turning head to left.

On inhale: Return to starting position.

Number: Six times each side, alternating sides.

DETAILS:

On inhale: Bend knees slightly while raising legs, if necessary.

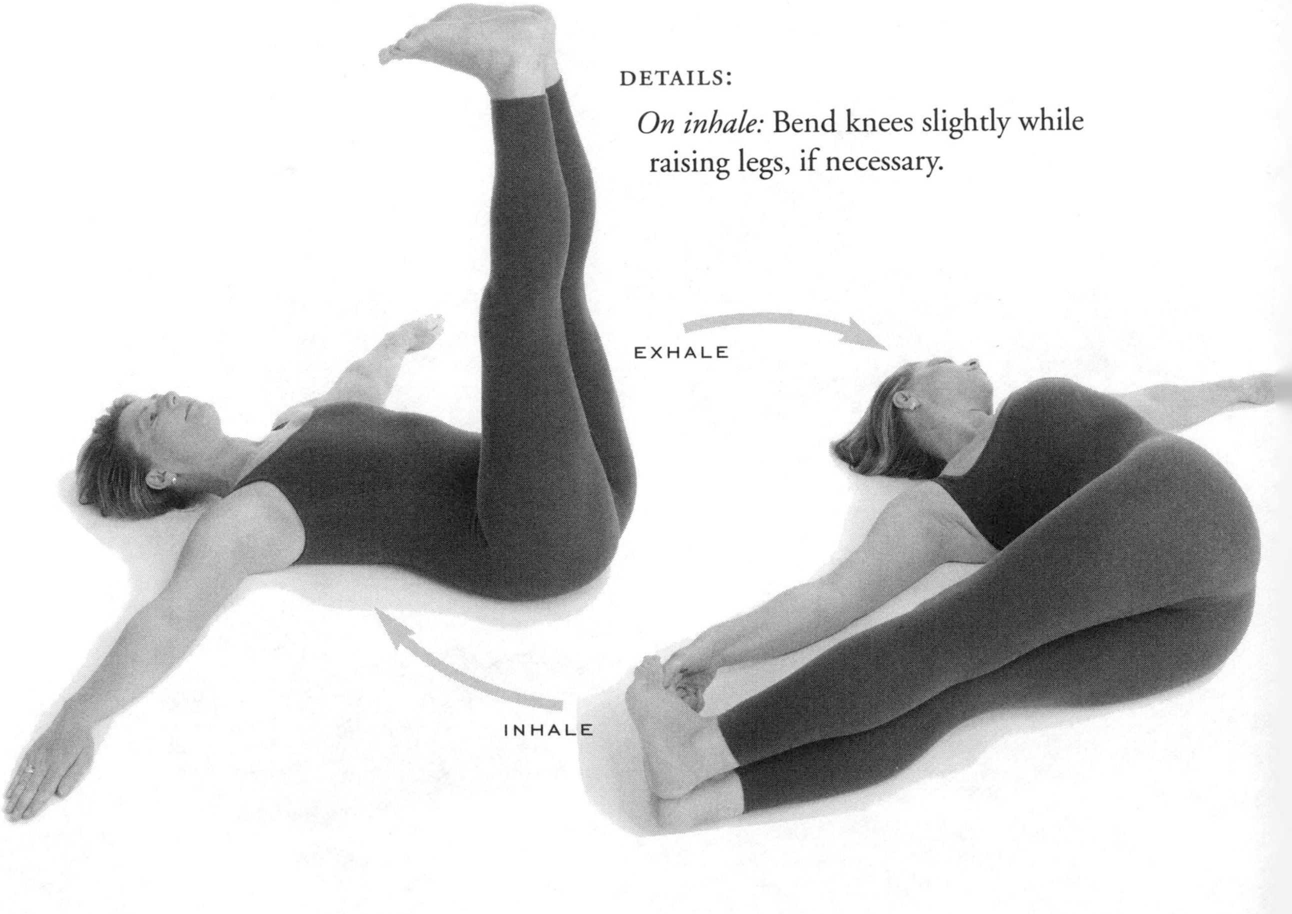

15.

posture: *Ardha Matsyendrāsana*

emphasis: To twist spine.

technique: Sit with left leg bent beneath right leg, left foot by right hip, and right leg bent, right knee straight up, right foot crossing over on outside of left knee, right arm behind back with palm down on floor by sacrum, and left arm cradling outside of right thigh, left elbow on right knee, left hand on right hip.

On inhale: Extend spine upward.

On exhale: Twist torso and look over right shoulder.

Number: Six breaths each side.

details: *On exhale:* Control torsion from deep in belly, using arm leverage only to augment twist.

On inhale: Subtly untwist body to facilitate extension of spine.

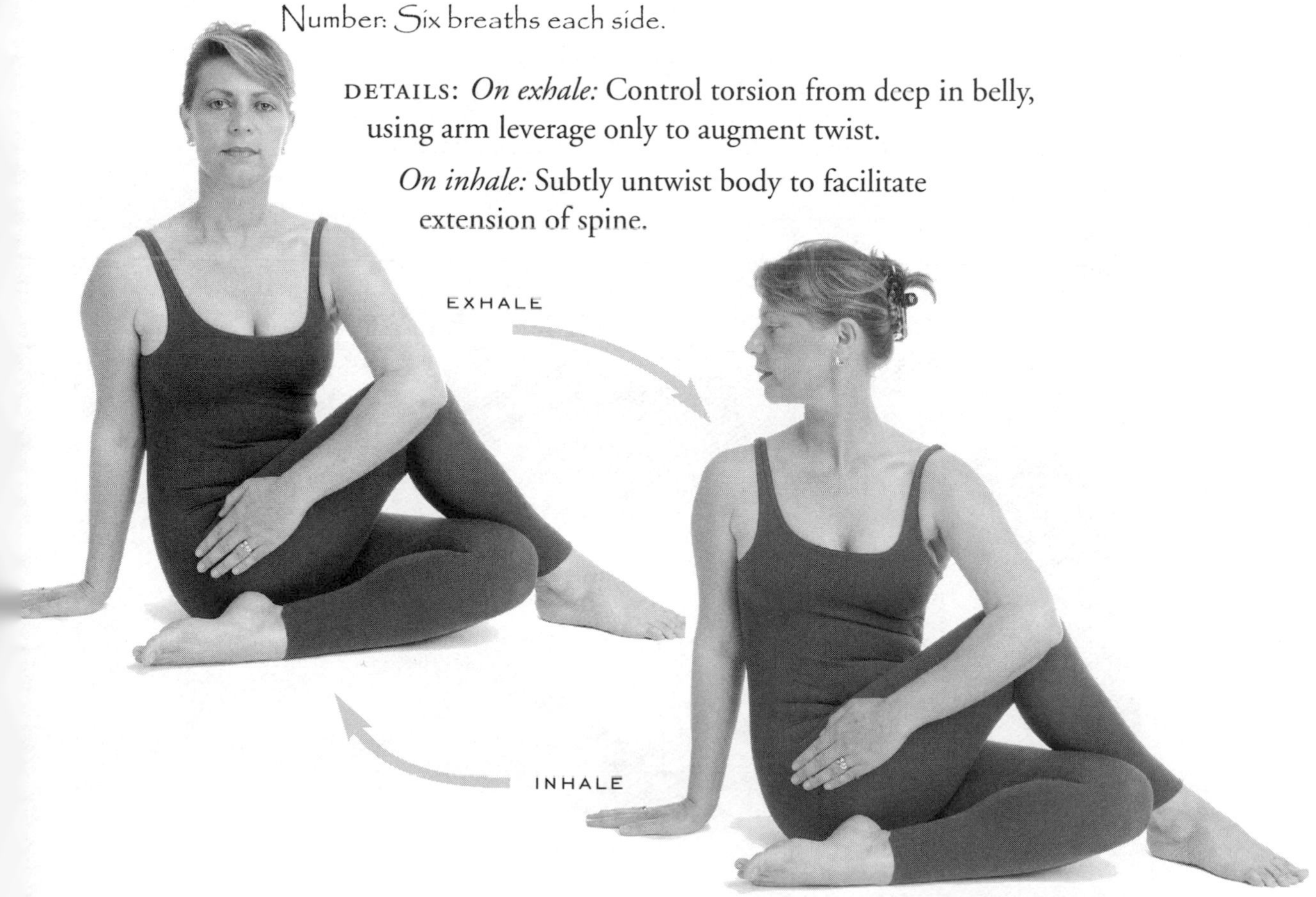

16.

POSTURE: *Paścimatānāsana*

EMPHASIS: To stretch back symmetrically after twist.

TECHNIQUE: Sit with legs forward, back straight, and arms raised over head, palms facing forward.

On exhale: Bending knees slightly, bend forward, bringing chest to thighs, and palms to floor beyond feet.

On inhale: Return to starting position.

Number: Six times.

DETAILS:

On exhale: Bend knees to facilitate stretching lower back, and bring belly and chest to thighs. Move chin down toward throat.

On inhale: Lift chest up and away from thighs, flattening upper back.

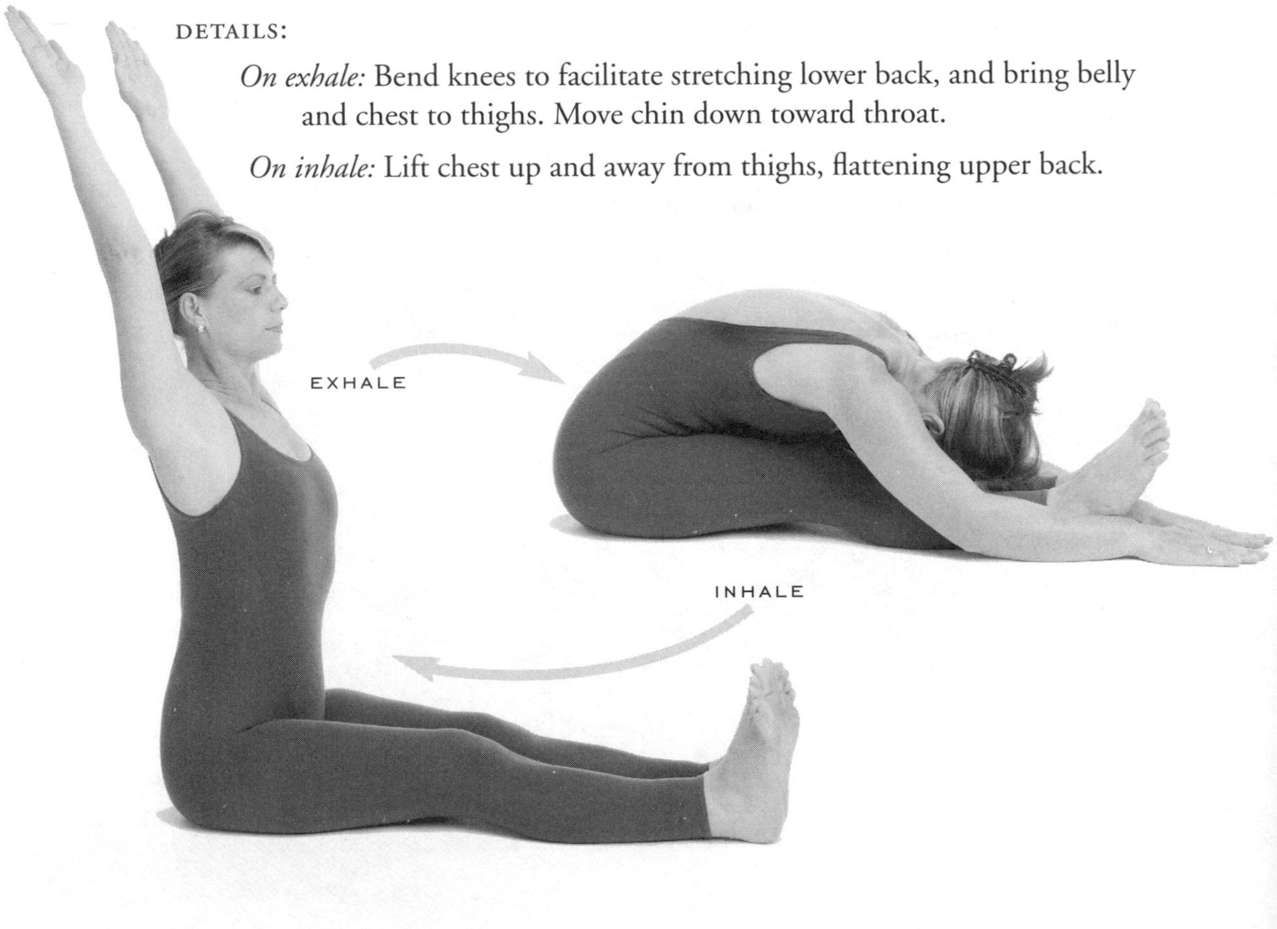

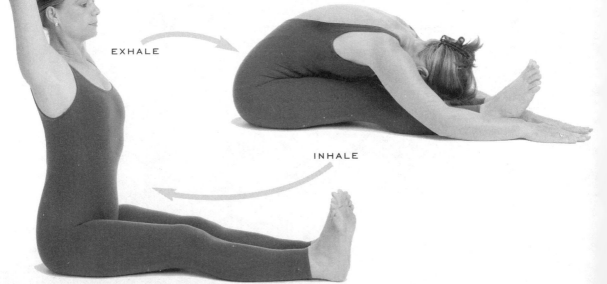

17.

POSTURE: *Padmāsana*

TECHNIQUE: While sitting, bend right knee and place right foot on top of left thigh, close to groin. Then bend left knee and place left foot on top of right thigh, close to groin.

A: EMPHASIS: To clear the mind and bring awareness to the Evaluation center.

Prāṇāyāma: Kapālabhāti followed by deep, slow breathing.

TECHNIQUE: Establish a moderate rhythm of rapid exhalation by contracting the abdomen below the navel forcefully, and quick spontaneous inhalation by relaxing the abdomen immediately after each contraction. Follow each round of rapid breathing by deep, slow breathing.

Number:

Eighteen fast breaths; three deep and slow breaths.

Thirty-six fast breaths; six deep and slow breaths.

Fifty-four fast breaths; nine deep and slow breaths.

Then rest for a few moments.

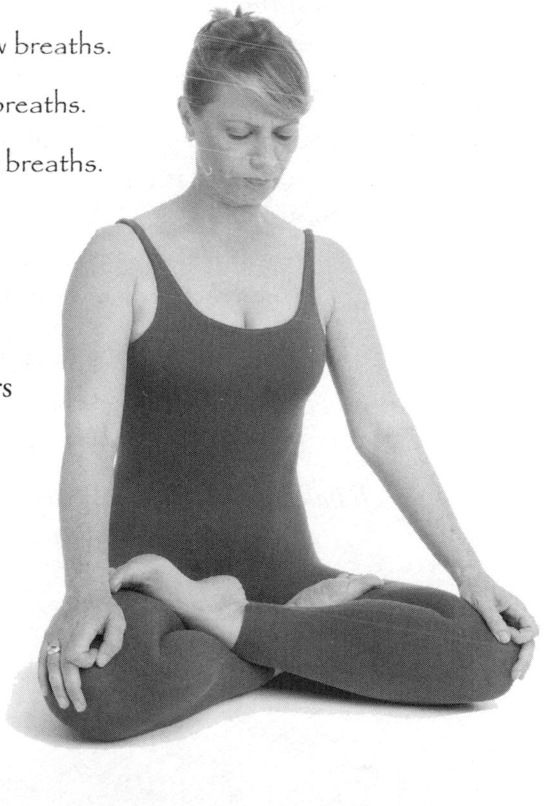

DETAILS:

During the fast breaths: Keep the shoulders and head still. Keep a steady rhythm, avoiding the tendency to speed up.

During the slow breaths: Use *ujjāyī* (inhale through the nose with a partial contraction of the glottis). Make the breaths long and subtle. Be patient.

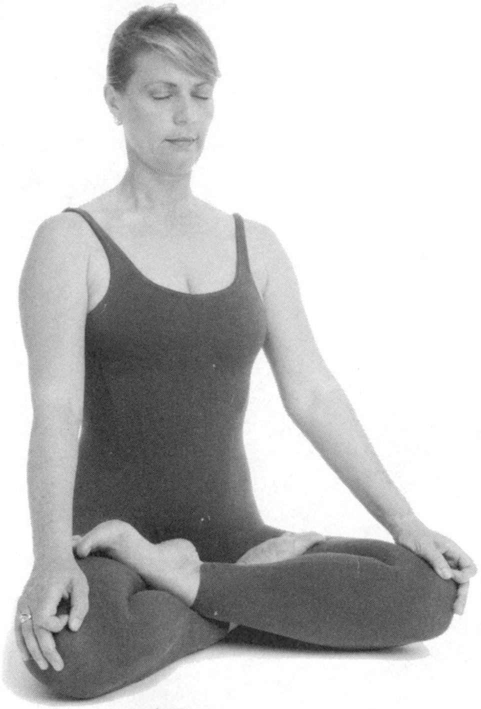

B: EMPHASIS: To reflect: Personally consider your usual daily activity and the level of your **thought**. What percentage of your daily activity at the level of your **mind** is truly oriented toward your highest value? What is most important to you, your highest priorities?

TECHNIQUE: Personally consider this question for some time.

C: EMPHASIS: To balance and integrate.

Prāṇāyāma: Pratiloma Ujjāyī

Ratio: 12-4-12-4.

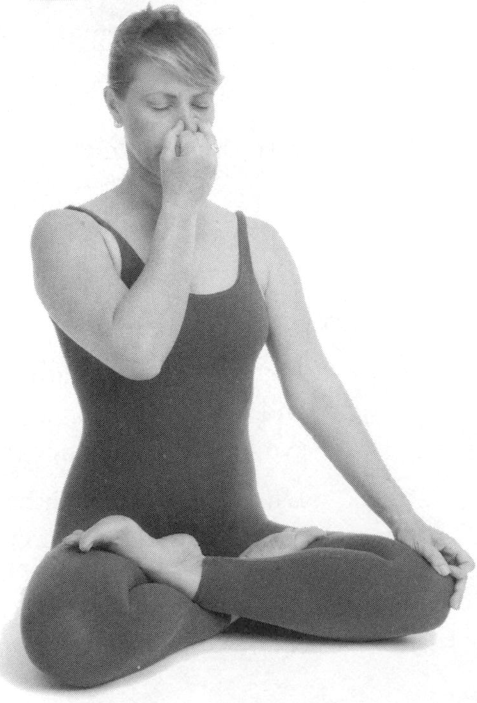

TECHNIQUE: Establish a deep, slow inhalation and exhalation.

Number: Twenty-four breaths.
Then rest for a few moments.

DETAILS: One round equals four breaths:

Inhale ujjāyī, exhale left nostril; *inhale* left nostril, *exhale ujjāyī*.

Inhale ujjāyī, exhale right nostril; *inhale* right nostril, *exhale ujjāyī*.

D: EMPHASIS: To reflect: Personally consider your daily action at the level of body, speech, and mind. From the perspective of your highest value, what is most important to you, your highest priorities? Are your actual daily actions in harmony with your highest values? If not, what does that mean?

TECHNIQUE: Personally consider this question for some time.

E: EMPHASIS: Return to the *bhāvana* of consciousness as clear as a blue sky.

TECHNIQUE: Rest in *bhāvana* for some time.

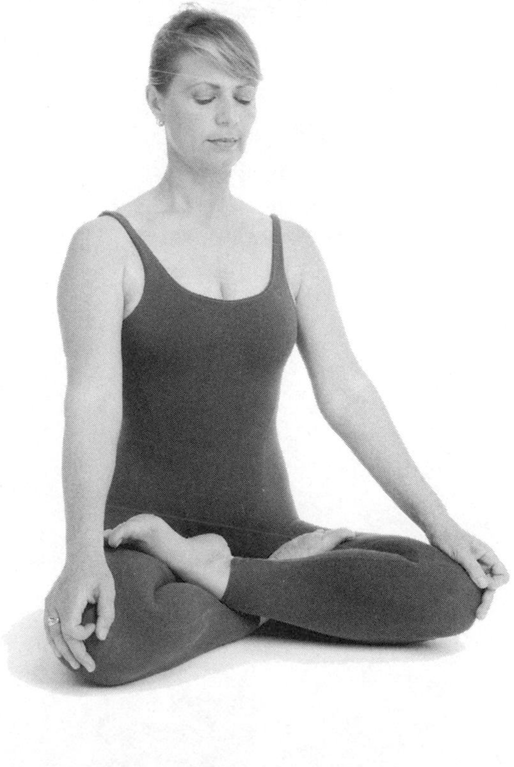

18.

POSTURE: *Śavāsana*

EMPHASIS: To rest.

TECHNIQUE: Lie flat on back, arms at side, palms up, and legs slightly apart. Close eyes. Relax body fully, keeping mind relaxed and alert to sensations in body.

Duration: Minimum ten minutes.

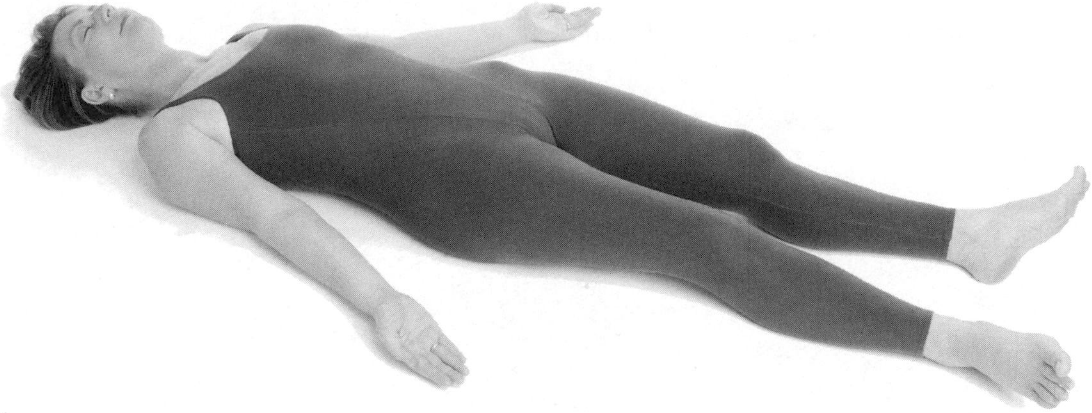

CHAPTER EIGHT

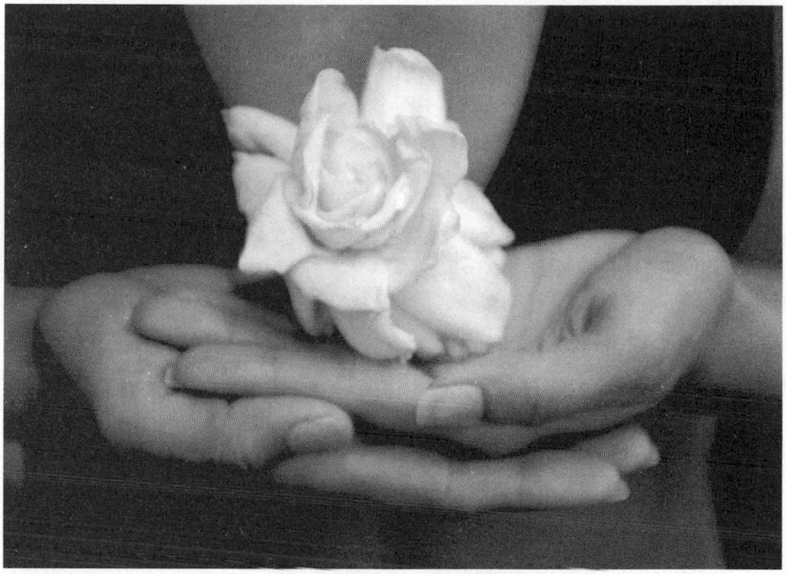

Fulfilling the Heart

PRAYER AND ABSORPTION: WORKING THROUGH THE HEART AND VOICE THE *ĀNANDAMAYA* LEVEL

THIS LEVEL IS KNOWN AS *ĀNANDAMAYA*. It represents the dimension of our emotional structure—and, in particular, of our "hearts"—in the sense of what we are seeking. According to the model of this tradition, derived from the *Taittirīya Upaniṣad,* it represents the part of us which informs and guides our attitudes and behavior, prompts our actions, and gives our lives a sense of meaning and purpose. This is the dimension of ourselves where our passions, longings, and potential for happiness and joy reside. And it is this dimension of our being that the mystics have named our spiritual center.

THE ULTIMATE GOAL OF OUR PRACTICE

Developing *Ānanda* Through Relationship

This *ānanda* level is refined and cultivated through relationships. There may be people in our lives who inspire us, who bring out the best in us, who share our deepest aspirations and orientations. These people can include our teachers, therapists, ministers, priests, rabbis, parents, mentors, spouses, friends, and others as well. Remember, too, that a relationship at this level does not necessarily imply living people. It can also include people from the past who were great sources of inspiration to us.

Perhaps there is such a person who has inspired you in your own life—a spiritual leader, a social activist, a visionary, a great scientist, or a doctor. Or maybe you have been touched and inspired by something in nature—the majesty of a mountain, the vastness of the sky, the expanse of the ocean, the mystery of the forest, the flight of the eagle, the glory of the sun. Or the source of your inspiration may have been a sublime concept, insight, or idea—the infinite reaches of space, the luminosity of the stars, the mysterious perfection of the DNA code, for example. Or it may even have been an emotional quality, such as love, kindness, courage, compassion, or wisdom; a value, such as honesty or integrity; or a form of the Divine, which resonates most deeply in your heart—the name of God or an image of the Divine, for example.

At the level of personal practice, it is important to become progressively more aware of what can help to remind us of our highest values, to orient our lives toward achieving our goals, and ultimately to facilitate the "descent into the heart" that enables us to awaken to spiritual awareness. Therefore, the purpose of practice at this level is to strengthen our connection to that source of inspiration that takes us beyond our own self-importance and that reminds us of our higher aspirations, goals, and values.

This connection is cultivated and celebrated through various methods that may include *āsana, prāṇāyāma,* chanting, and meditation. It may also include other practices such as prayer, the ritual use of objects, bodily gestures, silence, or writing. These various means and methods can be collectively understood as personal ritual.

Developing Relationship Through Ritual

There are many examples of ritual in contemporary life, some religious and some sectarian, some personal and some social. Rituals most of us are familiar with include graduation, marriage, saying grace before meals, and saying prayers before going to sleep. These serve as potent reminders of who we are, why we are here, what we are doing, and where we are going.

Communal rituals are part of the glue that keeps a society together. In some segments of society, it is the ritual of church and prayer. In others, it's the ritual of football or soccer. These rituals create and support community and give each member some sense of belonging to a larger whole. Personal ritual is equally important, for it helps us to recognize and celebrate a meaningful life. Just as communal rituals are essential for a healthy society, personal rituals are essential for a healthy individual.

Ritual is a form of structured activity that has symbolic meaning. For rituals to be living symbols, they cannot be mechanical. If they remain at the level of the mindless repetition of words and actions, they will have no meaning for us. Perhaps that is why so many of us have rejected the rituals from our childhoods.

A living ritual is an active process, which engages our full attention. Although there are rituals of passage that happen only once, rarely, or seasonally, there are other rituals that can be performed daily. It is the daily repetition, with full attention, that empowers the ritual, and that enables the ritual process to empower us. Thus, ritual is a way of sanctifying our daily activity and making it holy.

Ritual and the Fulfillment of Our Highest Potential

The idea behind developing a personal ritual is that we establish a regular process by which we can recognize, remember, cultivate, refine, and celebrate our relationship to that which inspires us toward our highest potential. It is a way to find meaning, to be fulfilled, and to link to our source.

Rituals generally consist of the integration of several elements into a cohesive whole. Some of these elements include the use of a special or sacred space, ceremonial clothing, gestures of the body, vows, prayers, images and other objects, or special foods. These various tools of ritual practice are used to focus our intention and to facilitate inner transformation. They are ways of bringing the sacred into the profane, and of elevating the profane to the level of the sacred.

The Ingredients of Personal Ritual

To create personal rituals, we must find the symbols that resonate most deeply in us, the objects that have the most meaning to us, and the language that speaks most directly to our hearts. We can then integrate these elements with the dimensions of personal practice presented in the previous chapters—on *āsana, prāṇāyāma,* chanting, study, and meditation—to create a truly multidimensional practice that is adapted to our unique needs and interests.

Taking Root in the Heart

At this level, it is very important that we become rooted in who we truly are, that we are authentic, that we are rooted in the heart.

We have seen what happens when our root *cakra* is weak: we become full of doubt and confusion and, as a result, are very vulnerable. The more firmly rooted we are, the stronger and more confident we become. So the key to a really deep transformation is to have a strong root, to be rooted in a place where we won't be plagued by doubt and confusion as we undergo the demanding process of transformation. And that is why, at this level, we are talking about taking root in the heart and about using ritual to help us toward this goal. With this as a motivation, we can go deeper into our practice, and as we go deeper, our practice will enrich and nourish our lives. We will discover ourselves, and will find what is most precious to us. The ancients suggested that there is a natural progression through which we come to recognize the deeper meaning in our lives and from which we can derive a practice to help us remember and celebrate this meaning. But we must do the inner work, our work to become a better person.

The Natural Progression Toward Deeper Meaning

According to the ancients, the first wisdom is the recognition of **suffering**. Suffering is a wake-up call. And if we pay attention, and listen to our suffering, there is a tremendous opportunity to learn. So suffering can lead to **knowledge**. The recognition of suffering and the knowledge of the causes of that suffering, however, are not enough to end suffering. There must arise in us a strong **wish** to come out of suffering, and that wish must lead to **action**. Through this process of action, we begin to understand ourselves and our **values**. This leads us to a refocusing of our **direction,** and a progressive **letting go** of things that have no bearing on that direction. The ancients say that as this letting go occurs, the heart of **devotion** emerges. And ultimately this devotion leads to the state of total **dedication** of one's life to God.

THE ELEMENTS OF COMMUNAL WORSHIP

Communal worship, prayer, and ritual are present at the heart of all traditions. If we take a close look at the structure of sanctioned prayer, we will see that there are certain common elements that can be identified, regardless of the particular tradition. There are at least eight components to prayer that are developed in some form in nearly all sectarian faiths, and that are woven throughout traditional worship services. These provide a model from which we can develop our own meaningful personal rituals.

The First Step: Turning Within to the Source

The first step is a progressive shift from the outward orientation of attention as we engage in our normal day-to-day activities to an inward orientation, within the mind and heart, toward the source. This shift is facilitated by transitional activities. In a traditional religious context this is achieved, for example, by leaving the place where we live and work, and entering the sacred space of the church or temple. It is also accomplished by going on a pilgrimage.

The Second Step: Confessing Our Faith or Taking Refuge

When a community of the faithful is gathered in their house of worship, the prayer service is usually initiated through some formal confession of faith, what the Buddhists call "taking refuge." In essence, it is a collective affirmation of shared belief and commitment. Just as entering the church or temple is symbolic of entering the house of God, the confession of faith is symbolic of asking God to enter our hearts. These prayers form the foundation for communal worship, as well as for the personal practice of the faithful.

Examples of this confession of faith include:

The Nicene Creed of the Orthodox Church (the first two sentences):

I believe in one God, Father Almighty,
Maker of heaven and earth
and of all things visible and invisible.
And in one Lord Jesus Christ, the Son of God,
The only begotten, begotten of the Father
before all ages, Light of Light, true God of true God;
begotten, not made; of one essence of the Father,
by whom all things were made.

The Triple Refuge of Buddhism:

To the Buddha, Supreme *Dharma,* and Noble *Saṅga*
I go for refuge until Enlightenment. May I, through merit gained by gifts and so on, accomplish Buddhahood for the sake of all beings.

The *Shema* of Judaism:

Hear O Israel, the Lord is our God, the Lord is One.
Praised be His glorious kingdom, forever and ever.

The *Shahada* of Islam:

There is no God but God, and Mohammed is His Prophet.

Even the Yoga teachings of Patañjali begin with this idea. The first word in his classic Yoga Sūtra is ***atha***. The ancients taught that this word represents the proclamation of commitment on the part of the student, which is the necessary starting point to begin the Yoga journey.

A couple of years ago, my wife, son, and I went to a *dharma* dance that was a fund-raiser for the Tibetan Buddhist society on Maui in a big public community center. When we got there a little early to help set up, the room was almost empty. My son was about three at the time, and you know how little kids are when they are in a big space—they go crazy, they run all around . . . and I had my eye on him.

But over the next little while, the room was getting fuller and fuller. And after a while there were many people in the room, and all of a sudden he couldn't see me or his mom. And he just started to freak, and tremble. And then he saw me, and he ran, and he jumped into my arms. And he was so tense his breathing was agitated, but it wasn't long before he let out a deep sigh . . . and melted into my arms.

Refuge. Faith.

The Third Step: Joyous Expression of Praise

The joyous expression of praise most often follows the confession of faith. At this stage, the community of the faithful collectively affirm the greatness and glory of God or that toward which their faith is directed. In the great theistic religions of the world, God is praised as the source of creation, from whom the gifts of light, life, and love continually emanates.

The Fourth Step: Petitionary Prayer

A very important element in traditional prayer is asking for help. This kind of petitionary prayer may be for oneself—asking for healing, forgiveness, guidance, courage, wisdom, prosperity, or other personal supplications. It may also involve supplications for the sake of others such as members of one's family or community or for all peoples that are striving to improve their condition. It may even include asking for blessing for the environment.

The Fifth Step: Communion

Perhaps the pinnacle of prayer is the letting go of one's fixation on personal identity, and merging, in silent communion, with the source. An example of this would be the Communion rituals of the Orthodox and Catholic faiths, discussed in the *Kriyā Yoga* section above.

The Sixth Step: Return to Ordinary Life and Thanksgiving

After this stage, there is some formalized return to ordinary life, followed by expressions of thanksgiving.

The Seventh Step: Expression of Commitment

We may at this point include in our prayers some kind of affirmation, expression of intention, taking a commitment, or even taking a vow in regard to our future attitudes, behavior, or direction.

The Eighth Step: Dedication of Merit

The final step in prayer is usually some formal dedication of merit. Having returned to the ordinary mind with gratitude, we formally express our well wishes to all beings.

The above components of this generic model of worship, in which the community of the faithful pray together, are simple and at the same time complete. They represent the time-honored steps, found all over the world, that the ancients understood as essential in binding a community together in love and faith and in turning their hearts collectively toward their source.

In traditional paths, this corporate prayer is said to complement and enhance, but not replace, private prayer. In fact, the often unheard message of most spiritual lineages is that the faithful are called to "pray unceasingly." In other words, the ultimate goal of personal practice is the yoking of our hearts to that from which we came. For, as we have seen, it is only through this link that we will realize unceasing joy.

These steps can be adapted in a way that is applicable to practitioners from any faith or tradition, as well as to those who are nonsectarian, atheistic, or nontheistic. As we have seen, prayer and ritual are designed to help us link to and commune with whatever it is that is most important to us, that represents our highest value, and that we are most attracted to.

We may have discovered, for example, through the last practice, that there is a gap between our highest values and our daily action at the level of body, speech, and mind. Of course, it is important to reflect on that gap and what it means. Are we setting our values too high, or are we addicted to a cycle of habitual behavior that blocks our ability to act in harmony with our heart's desire? It would be particularly interesting to observe what, in fact, we are doing on a daily basis, for that will reveal where our attractions lie. And then we can work to refine our orientation.

THE SCIENCE OF PERSONAL RITUAL

The science of personal ritual and prayer gives us practical tools to use in healing our lives and achieving our highest potential. These tools include preparation (*pūrvaṅga*), establishing intention (*bhāvana*), achieving meditative absorption, petition, proclamation (*saṅkalpa*), gesture (*nyāsa*), and dedication (*maṅgala*).

Preparation (*pūrvaṅga*)

Preparation involves both setting up the outer surroundings and readying the inner environment.

In a personal and nonsectarian context we can facilitate this shift by creating a space within our home that is reserved for practice only. The physical act of entering this space reminds us to leave our worldly concerns at the threshold. Of course, it is easier to physically shift our body to a different location than to shift the direction of our thoughts. The conscious use of ceremonial objects like candles, bells, incense, water bowls, or flowers will facilitate the transition from ordinary to ritual activity.

The ancients considered the practice of *āsana* and *prāṇāyāma* to be a part of the preparatory steps for meditation and prayer; they help us to realign our attention away from its external and worldly preoccupations, and to progressively interiorize and attune our attention.

Establishing Intention (*bhāvana*)

With the above preparation, we are ready to direct our attention toward the object of our choice: to develop an appropriate attitude toward it. There are many possibilities at this point. We will offer two examples here, which take their inspiration from traditional paths, but are adapted to a more nonsectarian orientation.

USING SYMBOL TO DIRECT OUR ATTENTION

We begin with an image of a cross. This is a simple cross, based on the principle of self-sacrifice in which the individual ego is put in right relationship to the sacred so that the sacred may be manifested in the material world.

Using this cross as a device to focus our attention on the goals of our personal practice, let us determine:

- that the vertical line represents the connection between heaven and earth, the sacred and the profane, the Divine and the worldly, the spiritual and the material;
- that the horizontal line represents our connection to our community and the world around us; and
- that our intention, through practice, is to bring the spiritual to the plane of the material, or to lift the material to the plane of the spiritual.

Then, superimposing a body over the vertical and horizontal lines, visualize these lines intersecting at the heart. And, from our own hearts, state the intention to share this connection between the sacred and profane with our community and to live in the world with the intention to manifest the values that this represents.

- At the beginning of this practice, we set our intention: in this case, the intention to strive to live a meaningful life. The symbolism of the cross reminds us of that intention. And we gaze at it while holding its symbolism in our hearts.
- We contemplate the vertical line for a little while, and we close our eyes and feel the intention to grow spiritually. Then we open our eyes and contemplate the horizontal line for a little while.
- Then we close our eyes and contemplate sharing these values with our community.
- And, finally, we, as it were, become the cross. This is the communion stage. We become one with what is symbolized by the living cross. If we get distracted, we open our eyes and reconnect with the cross. Then we close our eyes again.

USING *MANTRA* TO DIRECT OUR ATTENTION

In this example, we will use the *mantra "namo namaḥ"* (pronounced nah-**mo** nah-**ma**-ha) as a device to focus our attention on our goals in personal practice as we did with the example of the cross.

The word *namaḥ,* as I once heard from my teacher, may translate as "not me." *Namo* is a different grammatical form of *namaḥ,* usually understood in either form as a reverential greeting. In an expanded way, we can understand this *mantra* to mean "not by me," "not for me," and "not through me"—implicit in these sentiments is "but by You," "but for You," and "but through You," respectively, where "You" represents the Divine, the Spirit, or whatever represents the Highest for us.

At the beginning of our practice, again we set an intention. In this case, that we will work to reduce our self-importance and to see the Divine working through us more and more. The symbolism of the chant reminds us of this intention. We chant the *mantra* **loudly**, then more **softly**, and then **silently**. The progressive softening of our chanting symbolizes and facilitates the progressive interiorization of our attention. And then we contemplate its symbolic meaning. If we get distracted we begin again, chanting the *mantra* loudly, then softly, then silently. And then we return to our contemplation.

Countless symbols and *mantra-s* have evolved over the centuries to help us bring our attention again and again to the object of our contemplation.

Meditative Absorption

This is the stage in which we rest in silence, communing, as it were, with the spirit of our reflection. This stage can last a few moments or a very long time.

Petition

This is the stage in which we ask for what we need or want. In the context of personal practice, we might ask for help for problems we are having at a particular level in our system. As an example, consider the following prayer that I composed as I reflected on the essence of what I want to convey to you through this book:

> May my physical body have strength, stability, and structural integrity,
> May my vital body have health, vitality, stamina, and immunity.

May my intellect be clear, capable, curious, eager, and open.
May my character have faith, wisdom, compassion, humility, integrity and patience.
May my emotions be stable and joyful.
May my heart be open.
May I be totally integrated structurally, physiologically, intellectually, psychologically, emotionally, and spiritually.

Proclamation (*saṅkalpa*)

This is the stage where we might make a personal affirmation or commitment to ourselves regarding the road ahead. For example, we might formally say, "May I remain on the path, not break my commitment to practice, and accomplish my intention," or, less formally, we might say, "I commit to creating more time in my life to go deeper into my own practice."

Gesture (*nyāsa*)

Physical gestures are a way to "anchor"—that is, to reinforce our intention or commitments. It is a way of bringing the meaning and intention of our meditations into our systems. There are many kinds of gestures that we can use. A familiar gesture from the Orthodox and Roman Catholic Church is the touching of the forehead, heart, left shoulder, and then right shoulder. In fact, there are many of these kinds of gesture that have evolved in different traditions, each with a slightly different symbolic meaning.

A beautiful gesture that can be used in a nonsectarian and/or secular way is as follows:

From standing with arms extended outward, we bring our hands toward our face and then down toward our heart. In this gesture, we are invoking some force to enter our hearts. We can then leave hands folded at our heart, feeling and connecting deeply to that toward which we are directing our prayers.

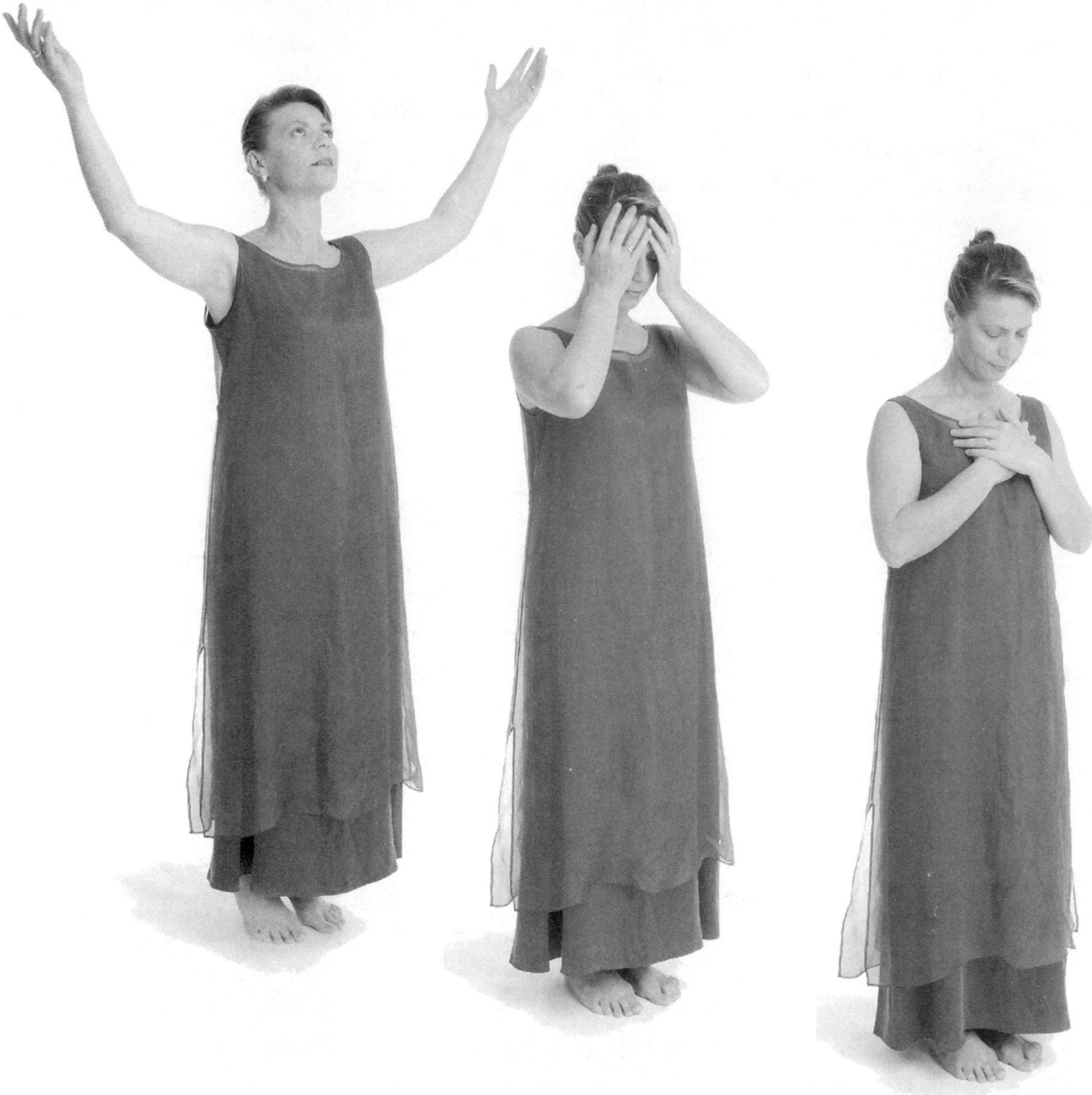

Other examples include bringing our palms to our eyes, ears, and mouth, or systematically touching the area of each *cakra*.

Dedication (*maṅgala*)

In this last stage, we are summing up our practice, with thoughts of thanks and appreciation, and sending out our well wishes to those around, those who are in our hearts, and to all others. This can be formalized in a beautiful gesture: while standing with hands folded on the heart, we extend our arms and spread our hands in a gesture of offering. This can be done in one direction, or offered in each direction. It can be done in silence or with a prayer of blessing or benediction. For example, we might say formally, "I dedicate the merit of my practice to all beings, that they swiftly find release from suffering, achieve their desires, fulfill their potential, and accomplish their goals." Less formally, we may say something like, "May all beings have happiness" or "May there be peace on Earth."

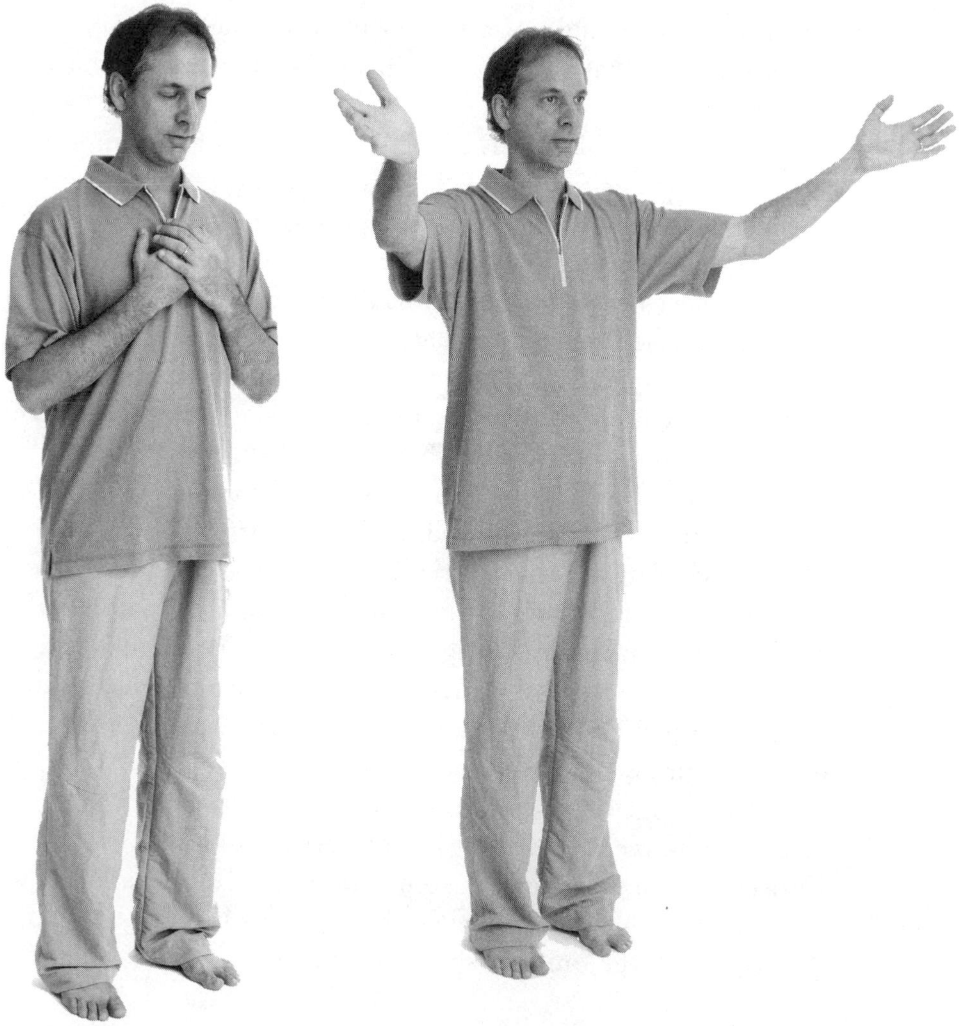

The crisis of faith in our contemporary society is that many of us are no longer able to believe in the images and concepts that gave expression to the faith of our ancestors. Nonetheless, we are impelled from within to find answers to life's ultimate questions. Without belief, our challenge is to discover the core of faith. We must, as it were, rediscover a deeper core that exists in each one of us—that same core from which the ancients drew their inspiration. It is with this in mind that we offer the practice that follows.

We begin with a reflection on an ancient Chinese proverb: "Nothing that enters through the front gate can be a family treasure." In the symbolism of the ancients, the "front gate" refers to our senses of perception. The image suggests that what is ultimately most precious to us, our "family treasure," is already within our homes and, in fact, hidden within the depths of our hearts. The message here is that we stop continually looking outside ourselves for satisfaction.

The effect of taking this expression as a seed for contemplation, following appropriate preparation, is much more profound than when it is simply considered intellectually. And this is the purpose of the practice that follows—a practice that shows how to integrate into a cohesive whole many of the elements we have been discussing throughout this book.

The practice includes *āsana, prāṇāyāma* (in which the lengths of the breath are measured by the mental repetition of a verse), vocal chanting, reflection, invocation, meditation, and ritualized gestures. The intention of this practice is to help us awaken to that "truth which constantly calls from within" and to recognize that the path to connect to the unending source of joy, which is the promise of all spiritual traditions, is the path of the heart.

The challenge of this practice is the use of *Vedic* Sanskrit, the language of the Seers of ancient India. This chant, however, is of a **nonsectarian** nature. There are **no theological images** at all. The ancient symbolism of this chant suggests that our essential self resides in the "cave of our hearts" and that, if we bring our attention into this "cave of the heart," we will discover that the true nature of our essential self is eternal bliss.

This image is present, in different forms, in many traditions. The Chinese, for example, regarded the heart as the seat of intelligence. In the Gospels, Christ speaks of the heart as the center of spiritual awareness. The writers of the *Philokalia,* the great testament of the Eastern Orthodox Church, considered the heart to be the "inner chamber" of the spirit.

The chant appears below with an adapted English translation. We encourage you to read through the practice until you understand its various elements and are able to associate the Sanskrit words with their respective meanings. The verse can be taken as a kind of prayer. Prayers from the heart are more effective, the ancients suggested, than prayers from the head. So take the time you need to understand these words until you feel them arise from your own heart. Please feel free to put any melody to the chant that you are comfortable with. Or, if the Sanskrit is too foreign or complicated for you, please also feel free to substitute this verse with any verse that inspires similar feelings in you. The trick is to have short phrases that can be integrated into both the *āsana* and the *prāṇāyāma* practices. We hope you enjoy the practice.

ĀNANDAMAYA PRACTICE

Ātmā Hṛdaye	Let my life force be linked to my Heart.
Hṛdayam Mayi	Let my Heart be linked to the Truth within me.
Aham Amṛte	Let this Truth be linked to the Eternal.
Amṛtam Ānandam	That Eternal which is Unending Bliss.

1.

POSTURE: *Siddhāsana*

A:

EMPHASIS:

Deepen inhalation and exhalation.

TECHNIQUE:

A: Progressively deepen inhalation and exhalation to a comfortable maximum length of inhalation. Let exhalation pace inhalation.

B: Sustain this breathing.

C: Progressively reduce length of inhalation and exhalation to normal breathing.

Number: Repeat A, B, and C eight times each.

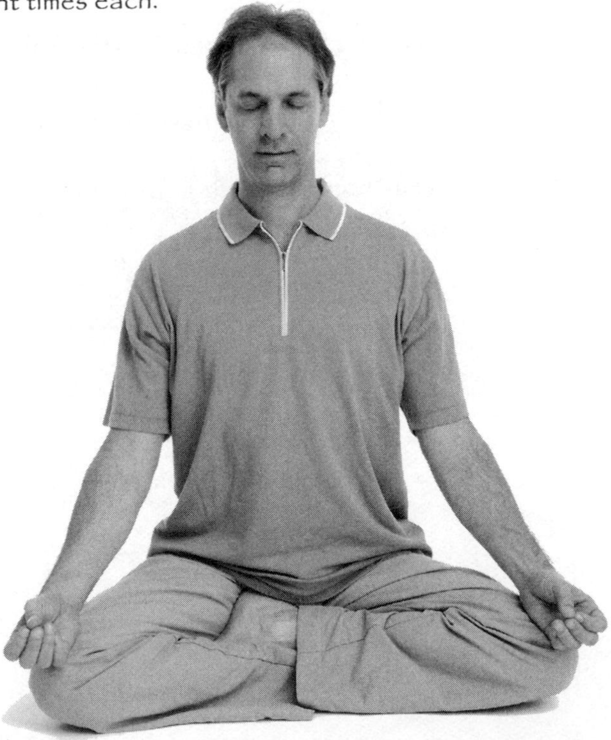

DETAILS:

On inhale: Follow the downward flow of inhalation, expanding progressively from chest to belly.

On exhale: Follow the upward flow of exhalation, contracting progressively from pubic bone to navel.

B:

EMPHASIS: Reflect on the old Chinese proverb

Nothing that enters through the front gate
can be a family treasure.

TECHNIQUE: Consider this proverb for some time.

2.

POSTURE: *Tāḍāsana*

EMPHASIS: To extend the spine and reach the arms upward. To introduce retention of the breath after inhalation. To chant on exhalation as hands are brought to heart. To strengthen calves and feet.

TECHNIQUE: Stand with arms at side, feet parallel.

On inhale: Raise up on toes while simultaneously raising arms up over head, palms together.

Retain the breath after inhale for five seconds.

On exhale: Lower heels halfway to the floor, while bringing hands to heart, while chanting ***"Ātma Hṛdaye."***

On inhale: Raise up on toes while simultaneously raising arms up over head.

Retain the breath after inhale for five seconds.

On exhale: Return to starting point.

Number: Eight times.

DETAILS: *On inhale:* As you raise your hands toward the heavens, feel as if you are invoking the awakening of your heart.

On exhale: Feel as if you are touching the truth that unending joy comes from within.

INHALE
CHANT
EXHALE
INHALE

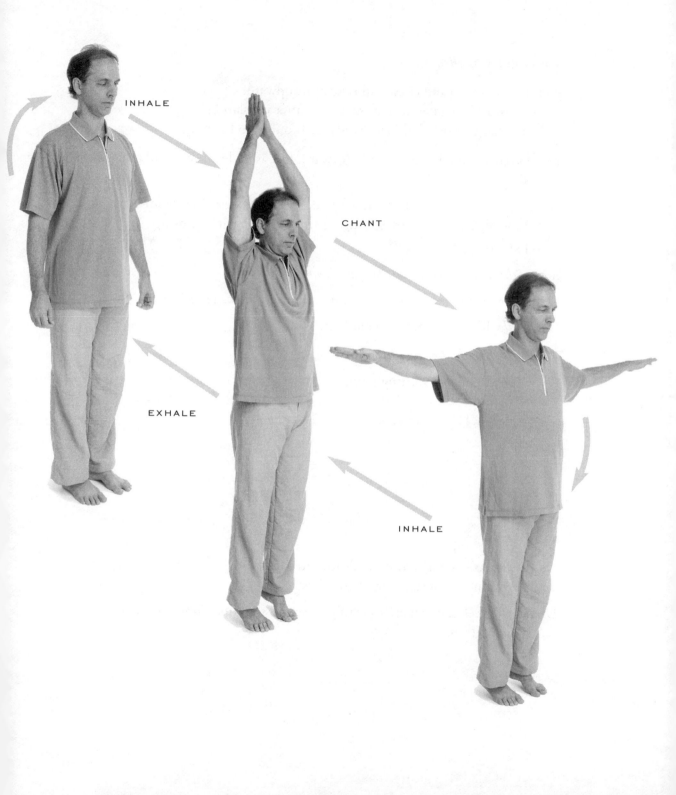

3.

POSTURE: *Vīrabhadrāsana*

EMPHASIS: To expand chest and raise arms upward.
To introduce retention of the breath after inhalation.
To chant on exhalation as hands are brought to heart.

TECHNIQUE: Stand with left foot forward, feet as wide as hips, and arms at sides.

On inhale: Simultaneously bend left knee, displace chest slightly forward and hips slightly backward, and bring arms up and out. Palms up. Arch upper back.

Retain the breath after inhale for five seconds.

On exhale: Bring hands to heart, while chanting ***"Hṛdayam Mayi."***

On inhale: Raise arms upward and out.

Retain the breath after inhale for five seconds.

On exhale: Return to starting point.

Number: Eight times each side.

DETAILS:

On inhale: As you raise your hands toward the heavens, feel as if you are invoking the awakening of your heart.

On exhale: Feel as if you are touching the truth that unending joy comes from within.

INHALE
CHANT
EXHALE
INHALE

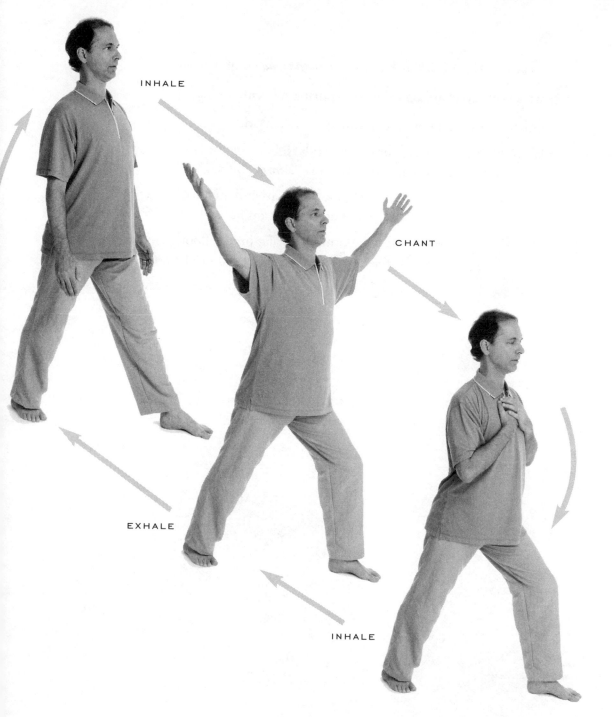

4.

POSTURE: *Vajrāsana/Ūrdhva Mukha Śvānāsana* combination

EMPHASIS: To chant on exhalation during movements.

TECHNIQUE: Stand on knees with arms over head.

On exhale: Bend forward, bringing hands to floor by the side of knees, forehead to the floor, while chanting ***"Aham Amṛte."***

On inhale: Stretch body forward and arch back, keeping only hands and from knees to feet on floor.

On exhale: Lie completely flat on the floor, palms by the shoulders, elbows up, and forehead on the floor.

On inhale: Pushing up with arms, arch to previous position.

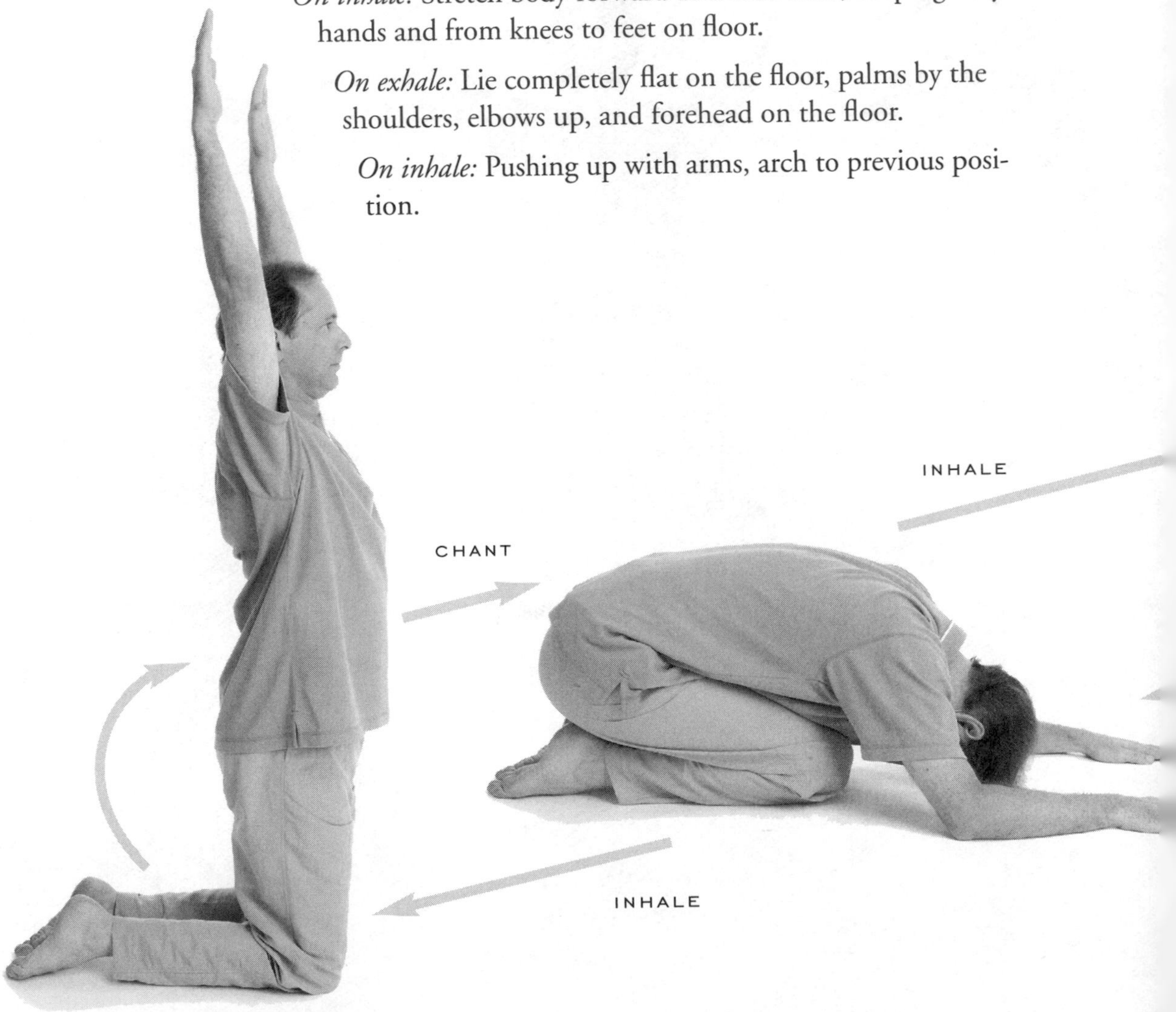

On exhale: Return to the forward bend position, hands on the floor by knees and forehead on the floor, while chanting ***"Amṛtam Ānandam."***

On inhale: Return to starting point.

Number: Eight times. Then rest seated for a few moments.

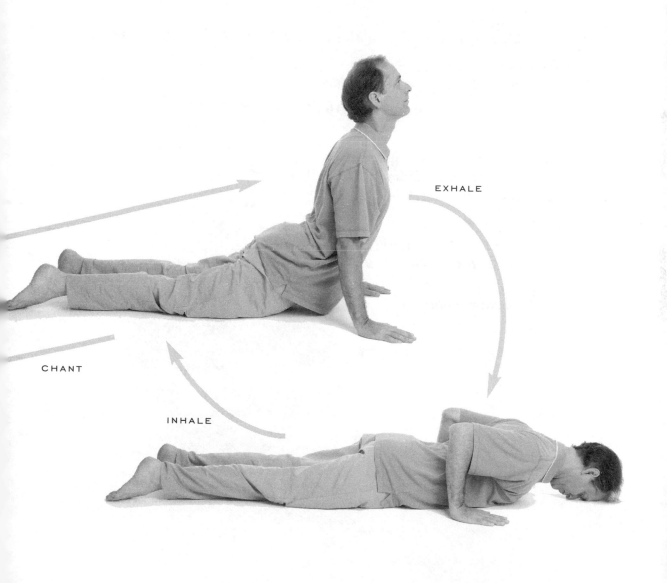

5.

POSTURE: *Siddhāsana*

A: EMPHASIS: To chant entire verse. To chant in ascending pitches.

TECHNIQUE: Chant all four lines of chant, four times in ascending pitches. Do all four lines in one pitch, and raise the pitch with each new round.

Round 1:

Chant in a lower pitch:
Ātmā Hṛdaye, Hṛdayam Mayi, Aham Amṛte, Amṛtam Ānandam

Round 2:

Chant in a slightly higher pitch:
Ātmā Hṛdaye, Hṛdayam Mayi, Aham Amṛte, Amṛtam Ānandam

Round 3:

Chant in a slightly higher pitch:
Ātmā Hṛdaye, Hṛdayam Mayi, Aham Amṛte, Amṛtam Ānandam

Round 4:

Chant in a higher pitch:
Ātmā Hṛdaye, Hṛdayam Mayi, Aham Amṛte, Amṛtam Ānandam

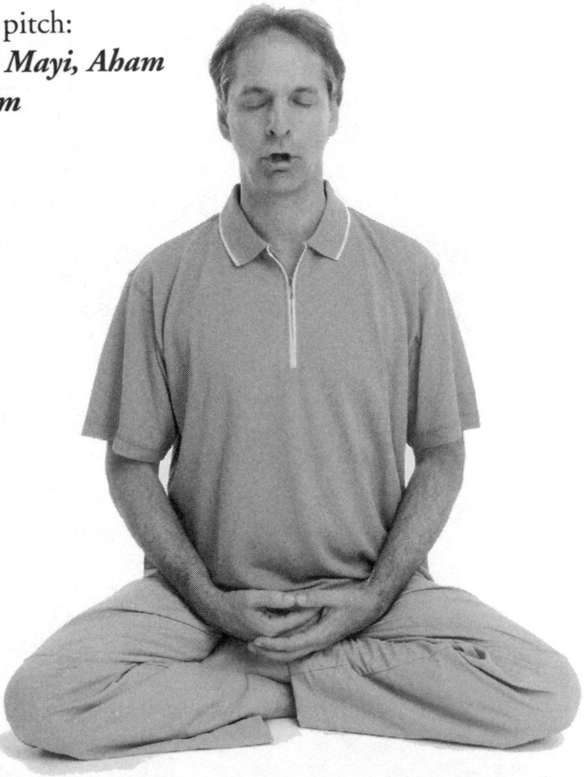

B: EMPHASIS: *Ujjāyī Prāṇāyāma.* To time breath by mental recitation of verse.

Ratio: 1-1-1-1

TECHNIQUE:

Round 1:

Mentally recite, *on inhale:* ***Ātmā Hṛdaye***

Mentally recite, *on retention after inhale:* ***Ātmā Hṛdaye***

Mentally recite, *on exhale:* ***Ātmā Hṛdaye***

Mentally recite, *on suspension after exhale:* ***Ātmā Hṛdaye***

Round 2:

Mentally recite, *on inhale:* ***Ātmā Hṛdaye, Hṛdayam Mayi***

Mentally recite, *on retention after inhale:* ***Ātmā Hṛdaye, Hṛdayam Mayi***

Mentally recite, *on suspension after exhale:* ***Ātmā Hṛdaye, Hṛdayam Mayi***

Round 3:

Mentally recite, *on exhale:* ***Ātmā Hṛdaye, Hṛdayam Mayi, Aham Amṛte***

Mentally recite, *on inhale:* ***Ātmā Hṛdaye, Hṛdayam Mayi, Aham Amṛte***

Mentally recite, *on retention after inhale:* ***Ātmā Hṛdaye, Hṛdayam Mayi, Aham Amṛte***

Mentally recite, *on suspension after exhale:* ***Ātmā Hṛdaye, Hṛdayam Mayi, Aham Amṛte***

Round 4:

Mentally recite, *on inhale:* ***Ātmā Hṛdaye,Hṛdayam Mayi, Aham Amṛte, Amṛtam Ānandam***

Mentally recite, *on retention after inhale:* ***Ātmā Hṛdaye, Hṛdayam Mayi, Aham Amṛte, Amṛtam Ānandam***

Mentally recite, *on exhale:* ***Ātmā Hṛdaye, Hṛdayam Mayi, Aham Amṛte, Amṛtam Ānandam***

Mentally recite, *on suspension after exhale:* ***Ātmā Hṛdaye, Hṛdayam Mayi, Aham Amṛte, Amṛtam Ānandam***

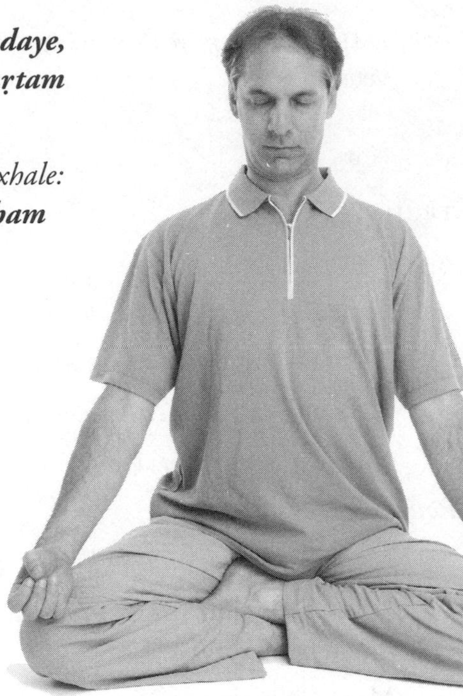

C: EMPHASIS: Silent communion.

TECHNIQUE: Rest awareness in the heart for some time.

D: EMPHASIS: Proclamation (*saṅkalpa*).

TECHNIQUE: Return to the reflection on the Chinese proverb "Nothing that enters through the front gate can be a family treasure." Then affirm your commitment to uncover that source of bliss that "constantly calls from within," to awaken to truth that resides in your heart.

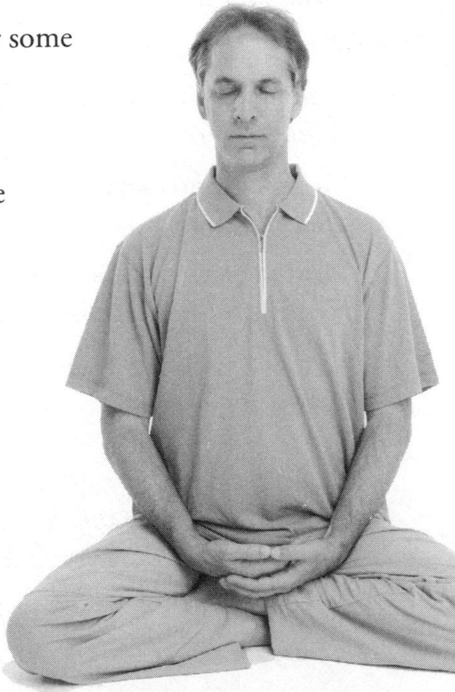

6.

POSTURE: *Siddhāsana*

EMPHASIS: To gesture to the heart while reciting:

aham ānandam—The source of unending bliss resides within my heart.

TECHNIQUE: Sit with arms extended out and upward.

On exhale: Lower palms to heart while chanting.

Add one line with each successive exhalation until you are chanting the entire verse.

On inhale: Extend arms out and up.

DETAILS: *On inhale:* As you raise your hands toward the heavens, feel as if you are invoking the awakening of your heart.

On exhale: Feel as if you are touching the truth that unending joy comes from within.

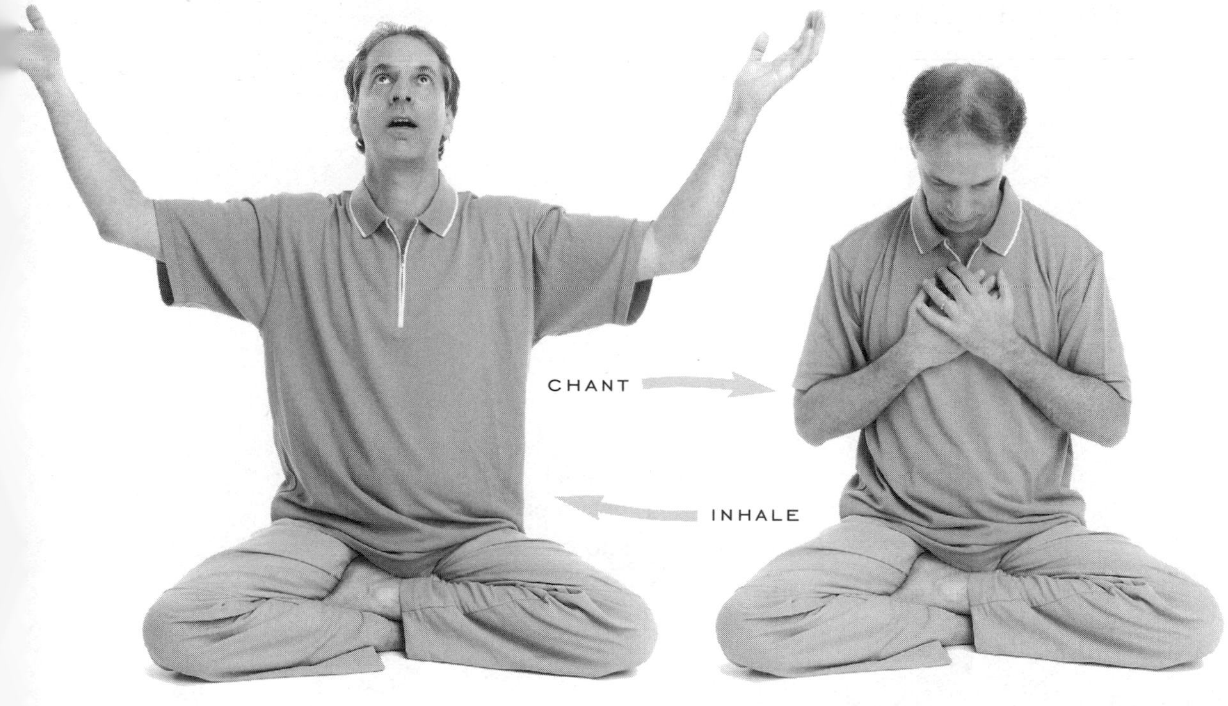

7.

POSTURE: *Samasthiti*

EMPHASIS: Dedication (*maṅgala*).

TECHNIQUE: Stand with your hands folded on your heart facing north.

As you extend your arms and palms outward, chant:

ānandam bhavatu bhavatu—Let this unending bliss be established everywhere.

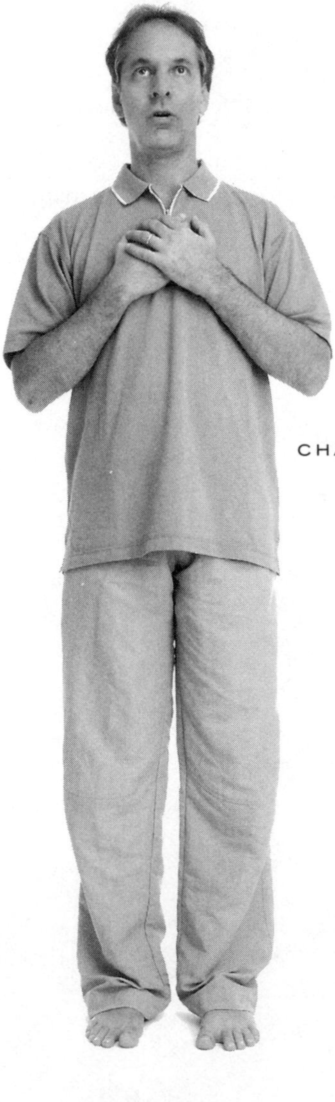

CHANT

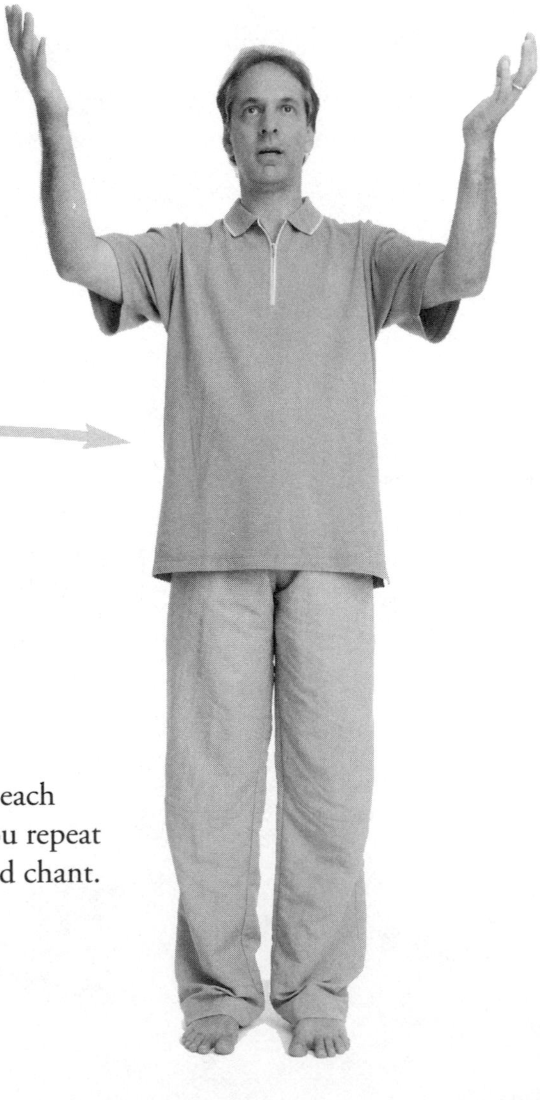

DETAILS:

Turn and face each direction as you repeat this gesture and chant.

Control the breath

Focus your mind

And direct it into the heart

That is the meaning of Spirituality

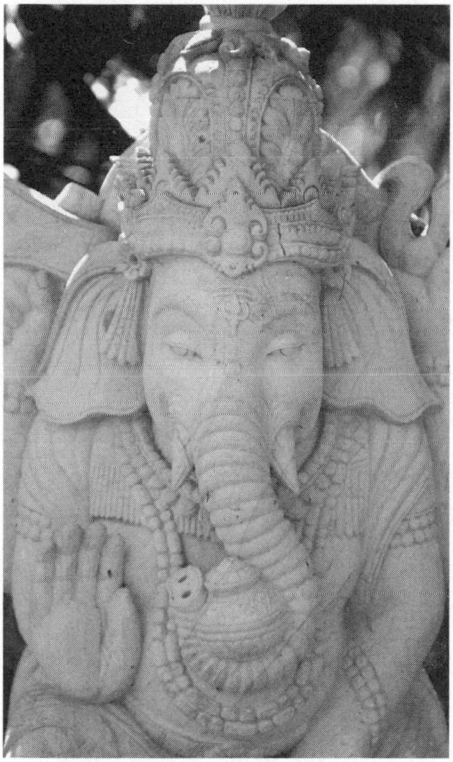

Adapted from the writings of
T. Krishnamacharya

Pronunciation Guide

I. -(Hyphen) denotes a pause during recitation.

II. There are three accents (*svaras*) or levels of pitch that fall on the vowels. They are called:

1. *Svarita* indicated by the absence of any markings. This is the prime or reference note.
2. *Udātta* indicated by a vertical line over the syllable. This has a pitch that is above the reference note.
3. *Anudātta* indicated by a horizontal underline. This has a pitch that is below the reference note.

III. Pronunciation guide for the transliteration

Guttural (pronounced from throat)

vowels	a	as in but
	ā	as in father
plain	k	as in kin
	g	as in good
aspirate	kh	as in sinkhole
	gh	as in leghorn
	h	as in hand
nasal	ṅ	as in encore

Palatal (pronounced from palate)

vowels	i	as in tin
	ī	as in teeth
plain	c	as in church
	j	as in judge
aspirate	ch	as in coachhorse
	jh	as in hedgehog
semivowel	y	as in you
sibilant	ś	as in sure

Retroflex (pronounced with tip of tongue curled up)

vowels	ṛ	as in sabre
	ṝ	as in chagrin
plain	ṭ	as in cart
	ḍ	as in ardent
aspirate	ṭh	as in carthorse
	ḍh	as in Fordham
nasal	ṇ	as in friend
semivowel	r	as in rib
sibilant	ṣ	as in hush

Dental (pronounced with tip of tongue against upper teeth)

vowels	ḷ	as in able
	ḹ	(is rare)
plain	t	as in theater
	d	as in they
aspirate	th	as in withheld
	dh	Buddha
nasal	n	as in boon
semivowel	l	as in lip
sibilant	s	as in sun

Labial (pronounced from lips)

vowels	u	as in bull
	ū	as in rule
plain	p	as in pat
	b	as in bee
aspirate	ph	as in uphill
	bh	as in abhor
nasal	m	as in man

Gutteral and Palatal

vowels	e	as in prey
	ai	as in aisle

Gutteral and Labial

vowels	o	as in go
	au	as in cow

Dental and Labial

semivowel	v	as in van

Nasal

Gutteral and Palatal

ṁ or ṅ makes preceeding vowel nasal

Aspirate

ḥ makes preceeding vowel aspirate

Āsana and Prāṇāyāma Glossary

Apānāsana (apāna=vital air of lower abdomen): apāna posture
Baddha Koṇāsana (baddha=bind; koṇā=angle): bound angle posture
Bakāsana (baka=crane): crane posture
Bandha: lock
  Jālandhara Bandha: chin lock
  Mūla Bandha: root lock
  Uddīyāna Bandha: abdominal lock
Bhāradvājāsana (Bhāradvāja=name of a Vedic *sage)*
Bhastrikā: bellows breathing
Bhujaṅgāsana (bhūjaṅga=cobra): cobra posture
Bhujāsana (Bhuja=shoulder)
  Dvihasta Bhujāsana (dvihasta=two arms, or hands): two arms *(over)* shoulder posture
Cakravākāsana (cakravaka=ruddy goose): ruddy goose posture
Candrabhedana (candra=moon): left nostril breathing
Daṇḍāsana (danda=stick): stick posture
Dhanurāsana (dhanura=bow): bow posture
Dvipāda Pīṭham (dvipāda=two feet; pītham=pose): two-footed posture
Ekapāda Śirṣāsana (ekapada=one foot; śirṣa=head): one foot *(behind)* head posture
Gorakṣāsana (Gorakṣa=name of a great yogī*)*
Hanumānāsana (Hanumān=chief of monkeys from Rāmāyaṇa*)*
Jānu Śirṣāsana (jānu=knee; śirṣa=head): head *(to)* knee posture
Jaṭhara Parivṛtti (jaṭhara=abdomen; parivṛtti=twist): abdominal twist
Kapālabhāti: (Kapālabhāti=skull shining): rapid forceful exhalation
Lolāsana (lola=swing): swing posture
Mahāmudrā (mahāmudrā=great seal): great seal posture
Matsyendrāsana (Matsyendra=name of a yogī*)*
  Ardha Matsyendrāsana (ardha=half)
Mayūrāsana (mayura=peacock): peacock posture
Nāḍī Śodhana: purification of the channels
Naṭarājāsana (Naṭarāja=name of a god)
Navāsana (nava=boat): boat posture

Pādahastāsana: (pāda=feet; hasta=hands): feet *(holding)* hands posture
Pādāṅguṣṭhāsana (pādāṅguṣṭha=big toe): hold toe posture
    Supta Pādāṅguṣṭhāsana (supta=supine)
Padmāsana (padma=lotus): lotus posture
Pārśvottānāsana (pārśva=side; uttāna=upright, stretched out): side stretch posture
    Ardha Pārśvottānāsana (ardha=half)
Paścimatānāsana (paścimatāna=stretching the west - back)
Śalabhāsana (salabha=locust): locust posture
    Ardha Śalabhāsana (ardha=half)
Samasthiti (sama=equal; sthiti=stable): equal stability posture
Sarvāṅgāsana (sarvāṅga=all parts), commonly: shoulderstand
Śavāsana (śava=corpse): corpse posture
Siddhāsana (siddha=accomplishment)
Śirṣāsana (śirṣa=head): headstand
Śītalī: (śītalī=cooling): curled tongue inhalation breathing
Sītkārī: alternate tongue inhalation technique
Sukhāsana (sukha=at ease): easy *(seated)* posture
Sūryabhedana (sūrya=sun): right nostril breathing
Śvānāsana—
    Adho Mukha Śvānāsana (adho mukha=face down; śvāna=dog): downward facing dog posture
    Ūrdhva Mukha Śvānāsana (ūrdhva mukha=face up; śvāna=dog): upward dog posture
Tāḍāsana (tāḍa=straight tree): straight tree posture
Trikoṇāsana (trikoṇa=triangle): triangle posture
    Utthita Trikoṇāsana (utthita=standing): standing triangle posture
    Utthita Trikoṇāsana Parivṛtti (parivṛtti=with twist): twisting standing triangle posture
Ujjāyī (ujjāyī=uplifting): breathing with partial glottal constriction
Upaviṣṭhha Koṇāsana (upaviṣṭha=to sit): seated triangle posture
Ūrdhva Prasṛta Pādāsana (ūrdhva=upward; prasṛta=spread; pāda=foot)
Utkaṭāsana (utkaṭa=squat): squat posture
    Ardha Utkaṭāsana (ardha=half)
Uttānāsana (uttāna=upright, stretched out): upright stretch posture
    Ardha Uttānāsana (ardha=half)
Vajrāsana (vajra=diamond, kneel, spine): kneeling posture
Vimanāsana (vimana=chariot of the gods): airplane posture
Vīrabhadrāsana (vīrabhadra=a hero): warrior posture

INDEX

Adho Mukha Śvānāsana, 76
adhyātmika (self-realization), 42
age model, 32–35
  midday, 34
  sunrise, 33
  sunset, 35
agni, 159
aims of life, four basic, 11–13
air element, *cakra* corresponding to, 160
ājña cakra, 161, 181–82
ākāśa, 5
am, 161, 182
anāhata cakra, 160, 177–78
ānanda, 9, 10, 13
ānandamaya level, 215–44
  being rooted in the heart, 218
  common elements of communal worship, 219–23
  developing *ānanda* through relationship, 216
  natural progression toward deeper meaning, 219
  personal ritual and, *see* personal ritual
  practice, 230–44
    intention of, 230
    using the *Vedic* Sanskrit chant, 230–31
ancient foundation, 1–42
annamaya level, 45–88
  alignment of the spine, noticing the, 54
  becoming aware of our bodies, 45–58
  exploring *āsana* in personal practice, 59–68
  joints, noticing condition of our, 55–56
  muscular structure, awareness of, 57
  neuromuscular patterning, awareness of, 58
  practice, 69–88
  skeletal structure, awareness of, 46
    exercises, 47–53
  symbolism of *āsana,* 68–69
anuloma (with the grain) *ujjāyī,* 121
apāna, 5, 90
Apānāsana, 83, 144, 170
Ardha Matsyendrāsana, 86, 108, 209
  adaptation, 39
Ardha Śalabhāsana, 137
Ardha Uttānāsana, 58
artha, 12, 13
āsana practice, xiii, xvii, 4–5, 45–46, 133, 157
  adapting postures to suit practitioner's needs, 64–65
  breathing in postures, 66
    see also prāṇāyāma
  categories of, 59–62
  chanting introduced to, 162–83
  combining postures, 66–68
    direction of movement with respect to the spine, 67
    using various positions in sequencing, 67–68
  deciding which *āsana-s* to pick, 59–62
  deeper symbolism of, 68–69
  glossary, 249–50
  holding postures, 63–64
  as integral part of holistic practice, 5
  as preparation for meditative self-reflection, 190
  as preparation for *prāṇāyāma,* 133
  questions asked when exploring personal practice, 59–68
  repetition of postures, 63–64
  ways to do postures, 63–64
  Western perception of Yoga and, xi
ascetic practices, 20
asthma, 114
atha, 220
attention:
  basic steps in meditation and, 188–90
  goals of meditation, 187
  normal patterns of, 186–87
authenticity, 218
avidyā, 17
awareness of our bodies, *see annamaya* level
Ayurveda, xi

Bakāsana, 62
bandha-s, 126–30, 146–48
  jālandhara bandha, 128, 147–48
  mūla bandha, 130, 148
  practicing only with qualified teacher, 133

bandha-s (*cont.*)
symbolism of, 127
techniques, 128–30
uddīyāna bandha, 128–29, 148
Bhāradvājāsana, 34, 61, 64, 173
bhastrikā, 124
bhāvana (establishing intention), 224–26
bhogī, 13, 14
Bhujaṅgāsana, 81, 193
bīja mantra, 157
for *ājña cakra,* 161
for *anāhata cakra,* 160
for *maṇipūraka cakra,* 159
for *mūlādhāra cakra,* 158
for *sahasrāra cakra,* 162
for *svādhiṣṭhana cakra,* 158
for *viśuddhi cakra,* 160
brahman, 9
breath, controlling, *see prāṇāyāma*
bṛhmana practices, 131
Buddha, 20, 22
Buddhism, "taking refuge" in, 220

cakra-s, 68–69, 156–63
ājña, 161, 181–82
anāhata, 160, 177–78
maṇipūraka, 159, 174–76
manomaya practice and, 162–83
mūlādhāra, 158, 164–68
sahasrāra, 162, 183
seven major, 157–62
svādhiṣṭhana, 158–59, 171–75
symbolism of wheels and lotuses, 156–57
viśuddhi, 160–61, 179–80
Cakravākāsana, 194
candrabhedana, 122
chanting, xvii
in *ānandamaya* practice, 230-44
energetics of sound, 154–55
learning to listen, 154
in *manomaya* practice, 163–83
symbolism of sound, 155–56
for training and developing the mind, 6–7, 26, 154, 156
transmission of scriptures and teachings through, 6, 153, 155
in *Vedic* Sanskrit, 230–44
chronic diseases, 151–52
commitment, expression of, 222
communal worship, common elements of, 219–23
adapting, 223
first step: turning within to the source, 219
second step: confessing our faith or taking refuge, 220–21
third step: joyous expression of praise, 221
fourth step: petitionary prayer, 221
fifth step: communion, 222
sixth step: return to ordinary life and thanksgiving, 222
seventh step: expressions of commitment, 222
eighth step: dedication of merit, 222
communication, *cakra* associated with, 160–61, 179–80
communion, 28, 222
Communion, ritual of:
Roman Catholic, 28
compassion, 160
concentration:
developmental goal of improving, 37
conditioning, 187
personality and, 8–9
confession, 24
of faith, 220
consciousness, *cakra* corresponding to, 162, 187
creation *cakra,* 158–59, 171–75

darśana, 25
dedication (*maṅgala*), 228–29
dedication of merit, formal, 222
developmental approach to practice, 36–37
Dhanurāsana, 60, 82
dhāraṇā (first step in meditation process), 188
dharma, 11–12, 13
personal, 11
ultimate, 11–12
dhyānam (second step in meditation process), 188
diet:
poor eating habits, 151
restriction of, 20
digestion, 159
dimensions of the human system, *see* five dimensions of the human system
dirty vessel, 15
Divine, *cakra* corresponding to the, 162, 183
Dvihasta Bhujāsana, 36
Dvipāda Pīṭham, 77, 104–105, 142–43, 169, 206

earth element, *cakra* corresponding to, 158
education, 39
continued, 39, 151
transmission of knowledge by chant, 6, 153

Ekapāda Śirṣāna, 56
emotions:
cakra associated with, 160
ānandamaya level, *see ānandamaya* level
energy level:
developmental goal of building our, 37
prāṇāyāma and, *see prāṇāyāma*
establishing intention (*bhāvana*), 224–26
evaluation, *cakra* corresponding to, 161, 181–82
exercise, 151
exhalation, *see prāṇāyāma*

faith, 190
confession of, 220
crisis, in contemporary society, 230
fatigue, xvii
fire element, *cakra* corresponding to, 159
five dimensions of the human system, 4–10
first dimension: the physical body, 4–5
second dimension: the vital body, 5–6
third dimension: the intellectual mind, 6–7
fourth dimension: the personality, 7–9
final dimension: the heart, 9–10
see also individual levels of personal practice, e.g. annamaya level; *vijñānamaya* level
flexibility, 55
foundation *cakra,* 158
manomaya practice, 164–68
Francis of Assisi, Saint, 20, 22, 29

gesture (*nyāsa*), 227–28
glossary, *āsana* and *prāṇāyāma,* 249–50

ham, 160, 180
Hanumānāsana, 37
hearing, sense of, 160
heart as final dimension of human system, 9–10
five aspects of, 9–10
see also ānandamaya level
Hinduism, 28
human system, five dimensions of, *see* five dimensions of the human system

iḍā 125, 156
imperfect vessels, 14–15
inhalation, *see prāṇāyāma*
inspiration, strengthening our connection to the source of our, 216
intellectual mind, 6–7
chanting and, *see* chanting
role of, 151–52
see also manomaya level
intelligence, *cakra* corresponding to, 161
intuition, 161
Īśvara praṇidhāna (recognition and dedication to our source), 27–30
Islam:
self-reflection in, 24
Shahada of, 220
Iyotisha, xi

jālandhara bandha, 128, 147–48
Jānu Śirṣāsana and *Mahāmudrā* combination, 140–41
Jaṭhara Parivṛtti, 38, 107, 139, 171, 208
joints:
awareness of condition of, 55–56
joyous expression of praise, 221
Judaism:
self-reflection in, 24
Shema, 220

kāma, 12, 13
kapālabhāti, 124, 211
knowledge, natural progression toward deeper meaning and, 219
Kraftsow, Gary, xiii–xiv
Yoga for Wellness, xviii, 40, 60
Krishna, xi
Kriyā Yoga, 16–30
Īśvara praṇidhāna (recognition and dedication to our source), 27–30
purpose of, 18
svādhyāya (self-reflection), 22–27
tapas (purification), 19–22
as threefold approach to practice, 19–30

lam, 158, 164–68
langhana practices, 131
Lao-Tzu, 185
leaky vessel, 15
learning, *see* education; *manomaya* level
ligaments, noticing the condition of our, 55–56
listening, 6–7, 154
Lolāsana, 33

Mahāmudrā, 34
and *Jānu Śirṣāsana* combination, 140–41
mahat, 7, 8
maṅgala (dedication), 228–29
maṇipūraka cakra, 159–60, 174–76
manomaya level, 150–83
breakdown of traditional cultures, 152–53
cakra model, *see cakra-s*
chant, training the mind through, *see* chanting
role of the intellect, 151–52
mantra-s, 24, 115
to direct our attention, 226–27
meditation, xvii, 42, 157, 185–90
āsana as preparation for, 190
basic steps in process of, 188–90
faith and motivation to practice, 190
first step: *dhāraṇā,* 188
function of, 185–86
initial goals of, 187
meditative absorption, 226
one-pointed, 186
prāṇāyāma as preparation for, 150, 190
second step: *dhyānam,* 188
self-reflective, 186
third step: *samādhi,* 189
memory, developmental goal of improving, 37
moda, 9–10
mokṣa, 12
mūla bandha, 130, 148
mūlādhāra cakra, 158, 164–68
multidimensional self, 3–10
muscular structure, awareness of, 57

nāḍī-s, 68–69, 156, 161
nāḍī śodhana, 122, 132, 181
Naṭarājāsana, 56
nature as source of inspiration, 216
neuromuscular patterning, awareness of, 58
Nicene Creed, 220
nutrition:
poor eating habits, 151
restriction of diet, 20
nyāsa (gesture), 227–28

om, 162, 183
orientation model, 36
Orthodox Church:
Communion ritual, 222
Nicene Creed of, 220

pace of chanting, 155
Padmāsana, 191, 195–96, 204–205, 211–13
paścimatāna, 60
Paścimatānāsana, 58, 60, 84–85, 109, 174–75, 210
Panikkar, Raimundo, 28n
parivṛtti, 61
parśva, 61
Parśvottanāsana, 61, 71
Patañjali, xi, xiii, 18, 27, 186, 187, 220
patterning, unconscious, 18
perception, 161, 187, 230
meditation and development of, 185, 186
personality, 7–9
conditioning and, 8–9
five aspects of the, 7
see also vijñānamaya level
personal practice:
Viniyoga, see Viniyoga
see also specific dimensions of personal practice, e.g. manomaya level; *prāṇāyāma*
personal ritual, 216–18
common elements of communal worship as model for, 219
ingredients of, 218
science of, practical tools of, 223–31
dedication (maṅgala), 228–29
establishing intention (*bhāvana*), 224–26
gesture (*nyāsa*), 227–28
meditative absorption, 226
petition, 226–27
preparation (*pūrvaṅga*), 223–24
proclamation (*saṅkalpa*), 227
personal transformation, xi, 4, 218
petition, 226–27
petitionary prayer, 221
phonetics of chanting, 154
physical body:
five aspects of, 4–5
working through the, *see annayama* level
pilgrimages, 219
piṅgalā, 125–26, 156
pitch of chanting, 154–55
pramoda, 9, 10
prāṇā, 5, 90
flow of, to the *cakra-s,* 157
prāṇāyāma, xvii, 5, 157
bandha-s, see bandha-s
classical theory of practice, 130–33
application, 132–33
basic paradigm, 131
relationship between ratio and technique, 132

classic techniques, 119–24
exhalation, 66, 94–96
ratio and, *see* ratio, science of breathing
exploring the breath, 90–96
exploring your inhale and exhale, 91–92
how to inhale and exhale, 92–96
glossary, 249–50
inhalation, 66, 92–94
caution, 114
ratio and, *see* ratio, science of breathing
as method of *tapas,* 21
personal practice and, 89–90
practice, 97–112, 133–49
as preparation for meditation and prayer, 150, 190
ratio, science of, *see* ratio, science of breathing
symbolism of, 125–26
pratiloma ujjāyī, 121
prayer, xvii, 42
common elements of communal worship, 219–23
prāṇāyāma as preparation for, 150
preparation (*pūrvaṅga*) for personal ritual, 223–24
preventative approach to practice, 38–39
priya, 9
proclamation (*saṅkalpa*), 227
pronunciation guide, 247
pṛthivī, 5
purification, *see tapas* (purification)
pūrvaṅga (preparation for personal ritual), 223–24
pūrvatāna, 60

rakṣana krama, 38–39
ram, 159, 174–75
ratio, science of breathing, 113–19
cautions in ratio development, 119
developing, 115–18
finding our threshold, 118–19
four parts of the flow of the breath, 113
progressive steps in building a ratio during practice, 117–18
relationship between technique and, 132
samavṛtti ratios, 115–16
understanding, 113–14
viṣamavṛtti ratios, 116
refuge, taking, 220–21
relation *cakra,* 160, 177–78
relationships, developing *ānanda* through, 216
ritual, xvii, 28
developing relationship through, 217
fulfillment of our highest potential and, 217–18
personal, *see* personal ritual
as way of sanctifying our daily activity, 217
rogī, 13, 14
Roman Catholicism:
Communion, 28, 222
confession as self-reflective practice, 24
ṛta, 7

sādhana, 3
sahasrāra cakra, 162, 183
samādhi (third step in meditation process), 189
samāna, 90
Samasthiti, 244
samavṛtti ratios, 115–16
saṅkalpa (proclamation), 227
śarīra samyama, 36
Sarvāṅgāsana, 80
satya, 7
Śavāsana, 88, 145, 214
variation, 40
self-acceptance, 160
self-esteem, 159
self-importance, misapprehension of our, 18, 29
self-reflection, *see svādhyāyā*
Shahada of Islam, 220
Shema of Judaism, 220
shortness of breath, xvii
Siddhāsana, 97, 146–49, 168, 174, 176, 179–83, 232–33, 240–43
Siddhāsana Praṇayama: Anuloma Krama two stage inhale; three stage inhale, 102–103, 111–12
sight, sense of, 159
śiksana krama, 36
Silence of God, The (Panikkar), 28n
Śirṣāsana, 62, 79
Śītalī, 123, 179, 204–205
Śītkārī, 124
skeletal structure, awareness of, 46
exercises, 47–53
smell, sense of, 158
space element, *cakra* corresponding to, 160–61
speech, limiting, 20
spine, awareness of alignment of the, 54
spiritual center, *see ānandamaya* level
śraddhā, 7
substance abuse, 151
suffering:
freedom from, 12–13, 28
natural progression toward deeper meaning and, 219

suffering (*cont.*)
recognition of, 13, 17, 19, 219
roots of, 17–18
Sukhāsana Parivṛtti, 35
Supta Pādāṅguṣṭhāsana adaptation, 138
sūryabhedana, 122
suṣumnā, 126, 156–57
svādhiṣṭhana cakra, 158–59, 171–75
svādhyāya (self-reflection), 22–27, 28, 30
mutual relationship with *tapas,* 22–23, 25–27
Svoboda, Robert E., xi–xii
symbolism:
of *āsana,* 68–69
of *bandha-s,* 127
to direct our attention, 224–26
of *prāṇāyāma,* 125–26
of sound, 155–56
of wheels and lotuses, 156–57

Tāḍāsana, 70, 98, 197, 234–35
Taittirīya Upaniṣad, 3–10, 215
Taittrīya Upaniṣad, 5n
tantric Buddhism, 28
tapas (purification), 19–22, 28, 30
mutual relationship with *svādhyāya,* 22–23, 25–27
taste, sense of, 159
thanksgiving, expressions of, 222
therapeutic approach to practice, 39–40
"third eye," 161
Tibetan Buddhism, self-reflection in, 24
tilted vessel, 15
touch, sense of, 160
transcendental approach to practice, 41–42
transformation *cakra,* 159–60, 174–76
transformation through practice, *see Kriyā Yoga*
Triple Refuge of Buddhism, 220
turning within to the source, 219

udāna, 90
uddīyāna bandha, 128–29, 148
ujjāyī, 120–21, 133, 146, 212
Upaviṣṭha Koṇāsana, 55
upside-down vessel, 14–15
Ūrdhva Prasṛta Pādāsana, 78, 106, 207
Ūrdva mukha Śvānāsana variation, 35
Uttānāsana, 134, 199
Uttānāsana/Ardha Utkaṭāsana combination, 164–65
Uttānāsana/Pādahastāsana, 74–75
Utthita Trikoṇāsana, 72–73
Utthita Trikoṇāsana pavivṛtti, 63

Vajrāsana, 87, 192
with gesture and chant, 177
Vajrāsana/Cakravākāsana/Adho Mukha Śvānāsana/Ūrdhva Mukha Śvānāsana, 166–67, 202–203
Vajrāsana/Ūrdhva Mukha Śvānāsana combination, 100–101, 136, 238–39
values, 219
vam, 158, 171
Veda-s, 3–10, 6
vijñānamaya level, 184–214
meditation at, *see* meditation
nature of personality, 184–85
practice, 191–214
viloma (against the grain) *ujjāyī,* 121
Vimanāsana, 38
viśeṣa, 61
Viniyoga, 15
adaptation of the practice to the individual and, 31
age model, 32–35
midday, 34
sunrise, 33
sunset, 35
developmental approach to practice, 36–37
methodologies of, 31
orientation model, 36
preventative approach to practice, 38–39
therapeutic approach to practice, 39–40
transcendental approach to practice, 41–42
viśuddhi cakra, 160–61, 179–80
viparīta, 62
Vīrabhadrāsana, 33, 99, 135, 198, 236–37
variations, 65, 200–201
viṣamavṛtti ratios, 116
vital body:
energizing the, *see prāṇāmāya*
five aspects of the, 5–6, 90
volume of chanting, 155
vyāna, 5, 90

water element, *cakra* corresponding to, 159
wholeness, 10–11
worship, common elements of communal, *see* communal worship, common elements of

yam, 160, 177
yantra, 157
  for *ājña cakra,* 161
  for *anāhata cakra,* 160
  for *maṇipūraka cakra,* 159
  for *mūlādhāra cakra,* 158
  for *sahasrāra cakra,* 162
  for *svādhiṣṭhana cakra,* 158
  for *viśuddhi cakra,* 160
Yoga:
  definitions of, xi
  as state of mind, 7
  in the West, xi–xii, xiii
Yoga for Wellness: Healing with the Timeless Teachings of Viniyoga (Kraftsow), xviii, 40, 60
Yoga Sūtra, xiii, 27, 186, 220
yogī, 13, 14
yogī-s, 162

CONTACT INFORMATION

For more information on Gary Kraftsow's *Viniyoga* Teacher and Therapist Programs, as well as retreats, workshops, and educational products, please contact:

Gary Kraftsow
American Viniyoga Institute
P.O. Box 88
Makawao, HI 96768

telephone: 808-572-1414
e-mail: *info@viniyoga.com*
Web site: *www.viniyoga.com*

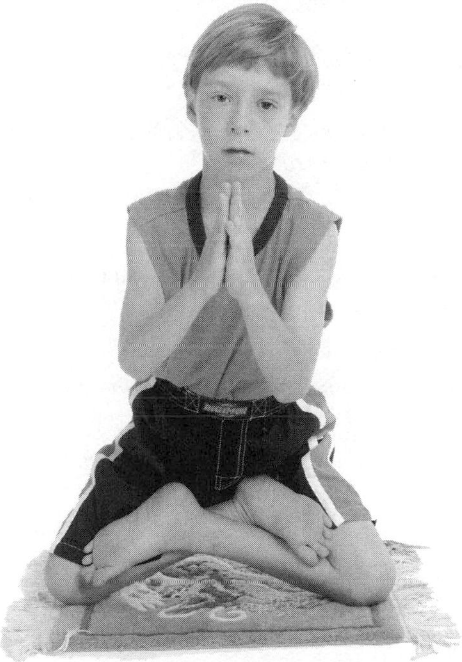